HARVARD SERIES ON POPULATION AND INTERNATIONAL HEALTH

Health and Social Change in International Perspective

Lincoln C. Chen
Arthur Kleinman
Norma C. Ware

Department of Population and International Health
Harvard School of Public Health
Boston, Massachusetts

Distributed by Harvard University Press

Library of Congress Cataloging-in-Publication Data

Health and social change in international perspective / [edited by]
    Lincoln C. Chen, Arthur Kleinman, Norma C. Ware.
        p. cm. -- (Harvard series on population and international health)
    "April 1993"
    Includes bibliographical references.
    ISBN 0-674-38562-4 : $15.00
    1. Health transition. 2. World health. 3. Social medicine.
4. Medical policy. I. Chen, Lincoln C. II. Kleinman, Arthur.
III. Ware, Norma C. IV. Series.
RA441.I143 1993
362.1--dc20   93-1755
                                                             CIP

RA441
.H43
1994

March 1994

© 1994, Harvard School of Public Health, Boston, Massachusetts

Books in the Harvard Series on Population and International Health

Population Policies Reconsidered: Health, Empowerment and Rights
Edited by Gita Sen, Adrienne Germain and Lincoln C. Chen

Power & Decision: The Social Control of Reproduction
Edited by Gita Sen and Rachel Snow

Health & Social Change in International Perspective
Edited by Lincoln C. Chen, Arthur Kleinman and Norma C. Ware

Assessing Child Survival Programs in Developing Countries
By Joseph J. Valadez

Table of Contents

Section III
Rediscovering the Social Nature of Mortality Change

Section IV
Social, Behavioral, and Cultural Mediators

Section V
Health, Policy and Promotion

Acknowledgments

The richness, diversity, and liveliness of these contributions would not have been possible without the intellectual contributions of many participants in the Health Transition Program — contributors, Harvard faculty, and students alike. Especially worthy of acknowledgment are Joe Potter and Jack and Pat Caldwell, who helped shape the structure of the seminar program and the papers for this volume. Many participants from developing countries joined the program, especially from Africa and South Asia. The editorial process was greatly assisted by Colleen Murphy at the Harvard University Center for Population and Development Studies, Hannah Doress of the Library in the Department of Population and International Health at the Harvard School of Public Health, Joan Gillespie of the Medical Anthropology Program in the Harvard Department of Anthropology, and Holly Angell and Toni Tugenberg of the Department of Social Medicine at Harvard Medical School. A debt of gratitude is owed to the Rockefeller Foundation — especially Kenneth Prewitt, Scott Halstead, and Sheldon Segal — for the generous financial support for the program. The book's shortcomings, of course, are the sole responsibility of the editors.

Lincoln C. Chen
Arthur Kleinman
Norma C. Ware

Cambridge, Massachusetts
March 1994

Author Affiliations

David E. Bell is Clarence Gamble Professor of Population and International Health, Emeritus, in the Department of Population and International Health at the Harvard School of Public Health and the Harvard Center for Population and Development Studies.

Nancy Birdsall is Executive Vice-President of the Inter-American Development Bank in Washington, D.C. She was formerly Director of the Policy Research Department of the World Bank.

José-Luis Bobadilla is a public health specialist in Population, Health, and Nutrition at the World Bank in Washington, D.C.

John Caldwell is Director of the Health Transition Centre, Associate Director of the National Centre for Epidemiology and Population Health, and Professor of Demography at the Research School of Social Sciences at the Australian National University.

Pat Caldwell is at the Health Transition Centre and the National Centre for Epidemiology and Population Health of the Australian National University.

Lincoln C. Chen is Taro Takemi Professor of International Health at the Harvard School of Public Health, where he chairs the Department of Population and International Health and also directs the Harvard Center for Population and Development Studies.

Nicholas A. Christakis is a Robert Wood Johnson Foundation Clinical Scholar, Fellow at the Division of General Internal Medicine, and Senior Fellow at the Leonard Davis Institute of Health Economics, at the University of Pennsylvania.

Gretchen Condran is Assistant Professor of Sociology at Temple University.

Clara Sunderland Correa is a psychologist in private practice in Mexico.

Göran Dahlgren is Senior Advisor on Public Health Policies to the Director-General of the Swedish International Development Agency (SIDA). Dr. Dahlgren was formerly Assistant Undersecretary of State at the Swedish Ministry of Health and Social Welfare and has served overseas in Ethiopia and Kenya.

Veena Das is Professor of Sociology at the Delhi School of Economics, University of Delhi, India.

Tomas Frejka is a population expert in the Population Activities Unit of the Economic Commission for Europe.

Julio Frenk is former Director of Mexico's National Institute of Public Health in Cuernavaca. He is currently a visiting professor at the Harvard Center for Population and Development Studies.

Kris Heggenhougen is Associate Professor of Medical Anthropology at the Department of Social Medicine, Harvard Medical School, and Associate Professor of Population and International Health, Harvard School of Public Health.

Arthur Kleinman chairs the Department of Social Medicine at Harvard Medical School, where he is the Maude and Lillian Presley Professor of Medical Anthropology and Professor of Psychiatry. Dr. Kleinman is also Professor of Anthropology at Harvard University.

Stephen J. Kunitz is Professor in the Department of Community and Preventive Medicine at the University of Rochester School of Medicine.

Robert A. LeVine is Roy E. Larsen Professor of Education and Human Development, and Professor of Anthropology at the Harvard Graduate School of Education.

Sarah E. LeVine is Research Associate in Education at the Harvard Graduate School of Education.

Rafael Lozano is Associate Researcher at the National Institute of Public Health, Mexico.

David Mechanic is University Professor and René Dubos Professor of Behavioral Sciences with the Institute of Health, Health Care Policy and Aging Research at Rutgers University.

Christopher J. L. Murray is Assistant Professor of International Health Economics at the Harvard Center for Population and Development Studies.

Joseph E. Potter is Professor of Sociology in the Population Research Center of the University of Texas at Austin.

Samuel H. Preston is Frederick J. Warren Professor of Demography at the Population Studies Center at the University of Pennsylvania.

Michael R. Reich is Professor of International Health in the Department of Population and International Health, at the Harvard School of Public Health.

Amy Richman is Director of the Quality Department at Work-Family Directions, Inc. in Boston, MA.

Amartya Sen is Lamont University Professor and is a Professor in the Departments of Philosophy and Economics at Harvard University.

Claudio Stems is Senior Researcher with El Colegio de Mexico.

Jonathan A. Sugar is Training Director in Child and Adolescent Psychiatry and Director of Pediatric Liaison Psychiatry at the University of Michigan Medical Center.

F. Medardo Tapia Uribe is a researcher and Coordinator of the Program of Studies on Education, Culture, and Survival Strategies from a Regional Perspective at Centro Regional de Investigaciones Multidisciplinarias at the Universidad Nacional Autónoma de México.

Norma C. Ware is Assistant Professor of Medical Anthropology in the Department of Social Medicine at Harvard Medical School.

Overview

Looking back, in future years, the dramatic improvements in health and declines in mortality worldwide may represent one of the most important human achievements of the twentieth century. In the early 1900s, few would have dreamed that one-fifth of the world's people — about 1 billion living in privileged circumstances — would enjoy an average life expectancy approaching 80 years. In these industrialized societies, health improvements have been underway for well over a century and have attained levels far beyond earlier expectations. For most economically poor nations, so-called "developing countries," however, health status was poorer and mortality higher in these early years. Accelerated improvements began during the post-colonial period in the second half of the century. While virtually all developing countries have made some progress, the pace and degree of their health gains vary greatly. Life expectancy in developing countries today ranges from 45 to 70 years.

When considered from another perspective, these health and mortality changes can appear in a very different — less positive, even negative — light. Violence and substance abuse, family breakdown with spouse or child abandonment, teenage pregnancy and sexually transmitted diseases including AIDS, depression and anxiety disorders, and social dislocation due to ethnic conflict and structural breakdown — all speak to another, darker side of global social change. The direction of these social disturbances suggests a changing health picture that is diametrically opposed to the story of declining infectious diseases and increasing life expectancy. If the pessimistic version can be exaggerated, so too can the progressive developmental version be overly optimistic.

Transitions in health, positive and negative, characterize the human condition in our time. The challenge for research is not simply to produce knowledge for health action, but also to advance understanding of the factors — social and biological — that have accompanied these health transitions. Critical questions include: What are the forms and structures of health transitions — in terms of demography, causes of death, morbidity and social and cultural dimensions? Do these changes assume universally regularized patterns, or are health transitions particularistic to space, time, and community? What methodological issues arise in definition and measurement? And how can an understanding of health transitions improve health policy, interventions, and the research agenda?

These questions constitute the themes of this collection. The volume represents the product of an extremely rich research seminar series on the Health Transition that was conducted at the Harvard Center for Population and Development Studies from 1987-1990. The aim of the Health Transition Program was to promote understanding of the social dimensions of health change. Although the scope was global, special emphasis was given to health in developing countries. A major objective of the Program was to foster interdisciplinary dialogue across a range of relevant fields. Scientists in demography, epidemiology, anthropology, economics, sociology, political science, and public health — from North America and many developing countries — all participated in a joint endeavor to advance understanding. Intellectual consensus was not required; rather, the intent was to use various disciplinary perspectives to identify areas of uncertainty and sharpen debate surrounding common themes.

The health transition concept, as it evolved in the Program and as presented in this volume, moves beyond the established theories of the "demographic transition" and the "epidemiologic transition." The "demographic transition" theory is based on patterns observed in now-industrialized countries. From high levels of fertility and mortality in earlier eras, these societies attained low levels of fertility and mortality in contemporary times through a transitional process that involved an earlier and more rapid decline of mortality and a slower decline in fertility. Before and after the transitional phase, the proximity of fertility and mortality levels resulted in slow rates of population growth. During the transitional phase, persistently high fertility and earlier decline in mortality resulted in marked acceleration of population numbers. The "epidemiologic transition" theory focuses on changing patterns in the causes of death in high versus low mortality populations. Whereas infectious, nutritional, and reproductive health problems are the most frequent causes of death in high mortality populations, these problems are displaced by the chronic and degenerative diseases in low mortality populations.

A major argument of this volume is that these demographic and epidemiologic theories are woefully inadequate for understanding health and social change. For us, the concept of the health transition moves beyond demography and epidemiology to explore sociocultural, economic, political, historical, and public health dimensions of health change. The recognition of cultural variation in influences on health change is critical to this conceptualization, as is an acknowledgement of the role of micro- as well as macro-level contextual factors. That is, along with the sociocultural, economic and other dimensions of the health transition, it is essential to examine the impact of interpersonal relations — local social worlds — on changes in individual health status.

Thus, this volume represents a substantial advance over earlier works on demographic and epidemiologic theories. These works have provided the intellectual base for a recent proliferation of research activities. Jamison and Mosley, for example, have just completed a major study for the World Bank on the epidemiologic transition and its implications for health care policy. Caldwell and Findley recently explored the behavioral dimensions of health change. The recently released World Development Report 1993 on "Investing in Health" by the World Bank (1993) further builds upon these earlier works on health policy. The approach adopted in this volume, however, is broader. The breadth is enriching because of its diversity of perspectives, the linkages across disciplines, the theoretical examination of definition and measurement, and a consideration of the social mediators that accompany health change. Our process of exchange and debate, moreover, has highlighted critical areas of intellectual consensus and sharp divergence.

This volume's contributors share a common recognition that while generalized patterns of health change may be postulated, there is no single health transition. As mortality levels decline, for example, the causes of death may shift from infectious diseases, nutritional deficits, and reproductive problems among children to chronic and degenerative diseases in adults and the elderly. Virtually undocumented are the direction and intensity of changes in illness and morbidity that accompany these mortality shifts. For most developing countries today, there is no inexorable progression from high to low mortality and from bad to good health. Indeed, it is even questionable whether such inexorable progression has ever existed in industrialized societies. The deteriorating health circumstances reported in industrialized Eastern European countries illustrate the fragility of health change. Rather, the pattern and composition of mortality and illness display considerable uncertainty in their relative weight and even direction. Indeed, if health may be considered a key measure of development, it is misleading to lump together under the rubric of "developing countries" diverse societies at very different stages of socioeconomic and health change. In health, this grouping may be more a vestige of history than a contemporary reality or a future direction.[1]

The inadequacy of current definitions and measurements of health status is also made clear in this volume. The customary dependence on mortality as the indicator of health status leads to biases. Undermining scientific validity and practical usefulness, it distorts our understanding of health and the consequent prioritization of health action. An overfocus on mortality, for example, may have led to the privileging of the health of high-risk children over that of adults and the elderly, an emphasis on life-threatening diseases rather than chronic and debilitating illness, and the conceptualization of health as episodic medical events instead of the fundamentally social, human process that it is.

Debates also emerged. The definition and measurement of health status itself, not surprisingly, became an area of considerable uncertainty. Moving away from very practical definitions and measurement instruments, we explored the methodological, philosophical, and ethical bases of health assessment. "Objective" approaches by an external observer and "subjective" reporting by the person himself or herself were compared. The dissonance is both disturbing and edifying, with the resolution of such uncertainty certain to rank high on the future research agenda. Controversial also was the nature or character of health problems — ranging from specific diseases to human illness experiences to health defined in moral terms. Especially divisive debates surfaced over the comparative importance of behavioral, mental, and psychological dimensions of health and whether they were receiving sufficient attention from entrenched and powerful professional communities.

As noted above, the question of what constitutes contemporary social change is equally vexing. Economic structures, social institutions, national and local cultures and governance are all inextricably related to health change. Generalizations are difficult; it is not easy to come to terms with global processes that affect radically different societies. While we have no easy resolution, the chapters that follow offer a panoply of views on what health and social change may entail.

The Chapters

Together, the 18 chapters in this volume advance understanding of the social dimensions of health change. The volume represents an integration of information, theories, and empirical analyses from diverse disciplinary fields. A solid conceptual approach backed by particularistic understanding of unique societies, it is postulated, is fundamental to basic understanding and the practical application of knowledge for effective health policies and interventions. So too would the shaping of a future research agenda be made possible by an improved understanding of the health transitions.

The volume is organized into five sections. The first section contains three chapters on the patterns of health and social change, and the second addresses conceptual and methodological issues in the assessment of health. Rediscovering the social nature of mortality change is the theme of the third section, and social, behavioral, and cultural mediators of change are addressed in the fourth. The final section examines the political economy of health, health promotion, health policy and intervention strategies.

The three chapters in *Section I: Patterns of Change* examine the theory and empirical evidence related to health, mortality, and social change. The chapters by Murray and Chen and by Frenk and colleagues focus on changing patterns of mortality and causes of death, while the last chapter by Sugar, Kleinman and Heggenhougen discusses health in sociobehavioral terms. These works, as a whole, directly challenge the primary thrust of current thinking regarding the universality of mortality and cause of death change, as well as the dynamic balance between mortality and illness, the latter inadequately appreciated and assessed.

In Chapter 1, Murray and Chen conclude that while overall declines in mortality may be experienced by many societies, these patterns are not uniform. Rather, great diversity is exhibited — by age, gender, social class, cause of death, and even the rate and direction of mortality change. Frenk and colleagues, in Chapter 2, move beyond these empirical data to propose basic elements in a new theory of the epidemiologic transition, including concept definition and the determinants, attributes, and consequences of health change.

The next chapter moves the terrain beyond disease and mortality into the realm of social, behavioral, and human dimensions of transitions. Sugar, Kleinman, and Heggenhougen, in Chapter 3, underscore the explosive growth of sociobehavioral pathologies that have accompanied "socioeconomic development" in both industrialized and developing societies. Substance abuse, violence, mental illness, drug and alcohol addiction, all arise in and disturb social routines, the daily rhythm of life, and social support systems. The authors argue that traditional studies neglect these significant health problems and misdirect priorities to medicalized responses.

The four chapters in *Section II: Conceptual and Methodological Issues* grapple with the very definition of health itself. Taken as a whole, the section challenges the established wisdom that we understand how to define health and know how it should be measured. These chapters explore the fundamental underlying basis of health constructs and measurements.

Chapter 4, by Murray and Chen, takes a systematic approach to the concept and measurement of morbidity, while Sen, in Chapter 5, moves the basis of assessment into the philosophical and ethical realms through consideration of the "positionality" of observers. In Chapter 6, Kleinman assumes a distinctly anthropological perspective on measurement, arguing that ethnographic approaches possess inherently powerful insights into illness experience. Das, in Chapter 7, moves beyond traditional definitions of health to encompass a more complete definition: "well-being." She views health from the perspective of human experience and moral categories, defining it as a sociomoral construct involving power, justice, and pain. To her, ill-health is human suffering and powerlessness. Two case studies from India — ethnic violence and the Bhopal chemical disaster — illustrate Das's conclusion that "medicalizing" health problems may cloud, indeed pervert, our understanding of the politics and morality of human suffering.The four chapters together offer a rich dialogue on fundamental issues related to definition and measurement that constitute the very basis of our understanding of health and social change.

Section III: Rediscovering the Social Nature of Mortality Change examines the history of health improvements in industrialized society, highlighting the sociobehavioral dimensions of health transitions. Written by demographers, an economist, and a historian, these chapters enrich our customary explanations of mortality change in relation to health transitions.

Condran and Preston, in Chapter 8, review the empirical experience for the mortality decline in the United States over the period 1900-1930. They underscore the importance of changes in personal health care habits, mass education, and hygienic practices as important determinants of the reduction in mortality. Disease prevention resulted more from personal behavioral change than the capabilities of the U.S. medical system. Examining differing patterns of marriage and childbearing, household structure, and cultural contexts in Eastern and Western Europe, Kunitz, in Chapter 9, warns against overly simplistic generalizations and inappropriate extrapolations of diverse experiences across space and time. Generalizations may obscure or mislead, and an appreciation of "particularism" can powerfully advance understanding by demonstrating historical effects in concrete contexts. Chapter 10, by Potter, compares mortality and fertility transitions. Potter observes that customary approaches focus on sociobehavioral factors in explaining fertility decline but mortality change is often attributed to medical forces. Potter argues that, contrary to traditional thinking, fertility and mortality reflect parallel interconnected social processes.

The three chapters in *Section IV* review *Social, Behavioral, and Cultural Mediators* of health transitions. Social constructs of illness, the impact of maternal education, and the nature of patriarchial societies and their consequences for health are explored. Chapter 11, by Christakis, Ware and Kleinman, employs an anthropological perspective to examine illness experience and help-seeking behavior. Chapter 12, by LeVine, LeVine, and colleagues, examines field data from Mexico to propose a model for understanding how maternal behavior operates as a mediator of the well-documented relationship between maternal education and improvement in child health. Chapter 13, by John and Pat Caldwell, presents a cultural approach to health change. The Caldwells argue that patriarchy in Eurasian family structures, which are organized to protect property and inheritance in agrarian societies, leads to the subordination of women, thereby retarding health and fertility modernization.

Health, Policy and Promotion is addressed in *Section V.* The first two chapters examine health policy from the perspective of economic theory and political science. Birdsall's Chapter 14 offers an analytical framework for health care policy that identifies appropriate roles for government in the social sector, the optimization of the power of the marketplace, and balance in the level of decentralization of decision making. Birdsall offers a mixture of liberal objectives (equity and basic needs) and conservative approaches (market competition) for arriving at an optimal policy mix. Reich, in Chapter 15, challenges economic approaches as politically naive. The contrasting schools of government intervention and market forces are described as oversimplifications, and the often employed explanations of "political will" are considered lacking in analytical rigor. Instead, Reich offers a novel "political feasibility" approach to the study of the political economy of health transitions.

Chapter 16, by Dahlgren, moves political economy from theory into real world practice. Dahlgren describes and analyzes the factors that shaped decisions on health care financing strategies in Kenya, 1987-90. Failure to attain optimal policy decisions was not due to the lack of theory, information, or better alternatives. Rather, the policy process required the accommodation of diverse interests serving multiple objectives.

Chapter 17, by Mechanic, brings a sociological and psychological approach to the application of the health transition to health promotion and education. Mechanic argues that health education often fails because human behavior is not atomized and responsive to targeted specific messages. Rather, Mechanic proposes that health behavior is powerfully shaped by group structures and social norms. Change in health behavior comes from the reorganization of everyday activities and life contexts. Basic education operates paradigmatically through its fundamental impact on "psychological modernity" rather than through its specific content. Chapter 18, by Bell and Chen, distills the lessons of the health transition chapters and proposes practical ways of applying the health transition concept to health policy formulation and implementation.

Overall, this volume of 18 chapters recognizes that, like social change, the health transition can be depicted along more positive or more negative trajectories. The picture depends upon the size of the canvas, the breadth of the brush, and the perspective of the artist. That we aspire to a summary view of global change is understandable. Yet, much of what we know draws attention to the complex, multi-sided processes of change in particular societies and even communities. After all, aggregated regional or global change is the net outcome of diverse historical patterns of specific political, economic and cultural processes at work in local worlds of human experience where diversity and pluralism abound. Those mediating social processes may have more to do with the actual health outcomes than health care *per se*. A number of the contributions to this volume support this line of analysis in which the unique historicity of local social worlds shapes the response to larger-scale social forces with varied consequences for health.

As a whole, the contributions to this volume offer fertile ground for future research. One critical challenge is to identify the "mediators" that link social and health change, and to dissect the causal and consequential processes they contain. Another challenge is to achieve greater clarity and precision to the development and use of "indices" of health status. More sophisticated instruments are needed, which include not only mortality but also illness, quality of life, and human suffering as assessments of health change. Gender perspectives, the growing role of the physical environment, and social dislocation among refugees, ethnic conflict, and societal breakdown, are only several of the major thematic areas that deserve greater attention. Finally, these studies should increasingly incorporate the global and universal with the local and particularistic, as health transitions take place across different aggregations of the human experience. These transactions can be captured only through embedding our understanding in the social relations between people in diverse communities, nations, and regions that together make up an ever-shrinking world.

Lincoln C. Chen
Arthur Kleinman
Norma C. Ware
Cambridge, Massachusetts
March 1994

Notes

1   There is no satisfactory term available to refer to the poorer countries of Asia, Africa and Latin America that are the focus of this volume. "Third World" sounds pejorative to some; others find "developing countries" misleading; "non-industrialized" or "industrializing" has other shortcomings. In the absence of universally acceptable terminology, we have not imposed an artificial consensus in the text.

Section I
Patterns of Change

1

Dynamics and Patterns of Mortality Change

Christopher J.L. Murray
Lincoln C. Chen

Initially proposed by John Caldwell, the term "health transition" has been used by many to capture the social dimensions of health improvement and mortality decline, particularly in developing countries. In 1988, a series of international workshops — in Canberra, London, and Cambridge, Massachusetts — explored the concept of the health transition (Caldwell et al. 1990, Cleland and Hill 1991, Chen et al. 1992). Subsequently, Caldwell (1989) proposed that the concept of the health transition be viewed as an extension of "the epidemiologic transition," which focuses on the changing patterns in the causes of death. The shift of nomenclature from "epidemiologic" to "health," according to Caldwell, is intended to emphasize the "social and behavioral changes which parallel the epidemiological transition and may do much to propel it" (p. 1). Indeed, both Caldwell and Findley (1989) emphasize the social and behavioral dimension of health change, relegating to insignificance the role of economic, political, demographic, ethical, and other factors associated with health change.

This chapter deals with the basic question: What is a "health transition"? The term "transition" connotes change from one state of affairs to another. This interpretation does not imply a predetermined change either from or to any particular state. Nor is it restricted to any particular set of socioeconomic determinants or consequences of health change.

When the concept of transition is applied to health, the term becomes even more problematic because a spectrum of definitions of health may be employed. The World Health Organization defines health as a "complete state of physical, mental and social wellbeing, not simply the absence of disease" (WHO 1984). Many variants of this definition have been proposed (e.g., Goldsmith 1972; Culyer 1983; Holland, Ipsen, and Kostrzewski 1979). More restrictive definitions, such as those that focus on the death rate, the absence of disease, or freedom from disability, are often necessary in order to measure and quantify health.

It is important to recognize that defining health is not simply semantics; definitions have theoretical and practical implications. Rifkin and Walt (1986), for example, argue that fundamentally different definitions of health lie at the heart of the debate over "selective" versus "comprehensive" primary health care strategies. The very basis of a health transition depends on the definition adopted. As a consequence, a health transition can mean different things to different people.

The most common measurable parameter employed to define health is mortality. The mortality rate, as an indicator of health, is useful because death is a definitive event, it is relatively easily measured, and it may be quantified and verified. Even so, assuming that mortality can fully reflect the state of health is a mistake since other indicators of health, such as morbidity and disability, should be included to capture a fuller range of health states. Beyond these three indicators — mortality, morbidity, and disability — however, the definition of health becomes more ambiguous. Broadly encompassing definitions such as "well-being" blur boundaries, making health indistinguishable from general welfare.

In this chapter, we examine the concept of and empirical evidence for health transitions around the world, focusing particularly on mortality change in developing societies. We conclude that there is no universally applicable pattern of mortality change. Rather, within overall declines in death rates, enormous diversity in the pattern of mortality dynamics exists among and within developing countries. Such heterogeneity is noteworthy with regard to mortality level, its age-sex-social structure, the causes of death, and even the pace and direction of change. Many unsubstantiated assumptions implicitly accepted in measuring and interpreting mortality change are examined. We find a lack of both solid theory and sufficient empirical evidence regarding the structure and cause of death patterns in mortality change. As a consequence, the chapter deals in depth with varying age-sex-social patterns of mortality change as well as the apparently puzzling simultaneous decline of infectious diseases along with the emergence of chronic diseases in populations experiencing mortality decline. In concluding this chapter, we propose a tentative theory of how and why health improves in diverse populations.

The Demographic and Epidemiologic Transitions

As a field of study, "health transition" echoes several earlier theories of health change. Two of the most prominent are the demographic transition and the epidemiologic transition. Stolnitz (1964) and Teitelbaum (1975), summarizing a good deal of earlier work, noted that demographic transition theory seeks to describe and explain the historical changes of fertility, mortality, and population dynamics in now-industrialized populations over the past century. These societies progressed over time from very high levels of fertility and mortality to very low levels of both. Although exceptions exist, the shift between these two steady states was characterized initially by mortality decline, followed, after variable lag periods, by fertility decline. A new equilibrium was achieved when both mortality and fertility reached low levels. During the transition period, the gap between an earlier declining mortality and a later declining fertility resulted in a major difference between birth and death rates. Thus, while population growth rates were very modest during the pre- and post-transition periods, the rates accelerated during the transition period.

One derivative of demographic transition theory is the hypothesis that many of today's developing societies are in the midst of their own demographic transitions, repeating the experience of now-industrialized countries. In its full form, the theory postulates various social and economic forces that shaped the initial mortality and later fertility decline. Since the theory includes both fertility and mortality change, it contains the implication that fertility and mortality processes are interlinked — through, for example, the possibility that improved child survival can influence reproductive decision making and fertility.

Demographic transition theory deals with changes in both fertility and mortality as well as their social and economic antecedents. To analyze the mortality component of demographic change, Omran (1971) coined the term "epidemiologic transition" to focus on "the complex change in patterns of health and disease *and* on the interactions between these patterns and their demographic, economic and sociologic determinants and consequences" (p. 510; emphasis in original). In shifting from high to low mortality levels, all populations experience a shift in the major causes of illness and disease. Whereas infectious diseases and nutritional and reproductive health problems predominate in high mortality populations, the chronic and degenerative diseases predominate in low mortality populations.

Health Improvement and Mortality Decline

In many ways, demographic and epidemiologic transition theories characterize well the mortality experiences of contemporary societies, industrialized and developing alike. For the world as a whole, the last century and a half has witnessed unprecedented declines of mortality (Stolnitz 1955, 1956; Preston, Keyfitz and Schoen 1972; United Nations 1989). Nearly all populations have shared in these mortality improvements, but by no means have these declines been enjoyed to the same extent by all. For example, in the United States, life expectancy at birth for both sexes increased from about 47 years in 1900 to about 75 years in 1985 (NCHS 1988). Virtually all industrialized populations have experienced a roughly similar pattern of mortality decline.

Many developing countries have also enjoyed widespread mortality improvements. The United Nations estimates that for the developing world as a whole, life expectancy at birth was 41.0 years in 1950–55, increasing to 61.5 years by 1990–95.

Demographic transition theory assumes that mortality declines in a monotonic, linear fashion. Little subtlety is hypothesized regarding potential deceleration, reversals, or other deviant patterns of mortality change. In contrast, fertility decline is presumed to vary markedly among societies. This oversimplification of mortality change has pervaded the demographic and public health literature and has dominated the interpretation of population and health statistics. Two illustrations of this simplification are the assumptions associated with the use of model life tables in estimating trends in mortality, and the inappropriate use of aggregate health indicators as measures of health and social change.

Models of population change are used by academics and international agencies to estimate mortality levels for countries with insufficient data or to make projections of future population trends. These models often assume simple linear decline of mortality levels, virtually regardless of the health circumstances in or the policies pursued by different countries (Murray 1987). There has been little empirical validation of the use of such model tables. Another dubious practice is the reliance on aggregate indicators, usually life expectancy at birth or the infant mortality rate, as single measures to characterize health changes. An underlying assumption is that mortality change across age groups follows a predetermined pattern that can be captured by a single indicator. Various models may be used, but once a model life table is selected, the population is assumed to follow a particular pattern of age-specific mortality decline (Coale and Demeny 1966). Neither the assumption of steady rates of decline nor that of constant age patterns of mortality change is substantiated by available evidence. When such assumptions are used carelessly, a wealth of detail on the dynamics of mortality change in various age groups is bypassed, and the complex determinants and risk factors shaping health are neglected.

Age

In general, while dramatic gains in life expectancy have occurred in most countries, these gains have not been experienced by all age groups uniformly. One example of this is Sri Lanka, renowned for the steepness of its post-World War II mortality decline. From 1950 to 1980, the infant mortality rate of both sexes declined from 82 to 34 per one thousand live births per year. Between 1952 and 1985, life expectancy in Sri Lanka also improved for adults, but not uniformly. Life expectancy at birth increased from 57.6 to 66.1 years for men and from 55.5 to 70.2 years for women (Fernando 1985). Yet adult mortality improved only for women, and virtually stagnated for males (Murray, Yang and Qiao 1992). This should be contrasted with the situation in a number of other countries — Chile, Italy, and Sweden, for example — where declines in male and female adult mortality were nearly simultaneous and comparable in magnitude. Clearly, the forces shaping the health of populations can have a different impact on different age groups of a population.

Other evidence for the heterogeneity of age-specific mortality change is provided by Bucht (1985). She has shown that the pattern of mortality in some countries appears to change from one Coale-Demeny model life table pattern to another as mortality declines. Indeed, data on specific risk factors and causes of death suggest that changes in the mortality age pattern would not be uniform. For example, rising homicides, suicides, and accidents, which tend to be concentrated among young adults, could alter the age structure of mortality. So too could smoking, which would elevate mortality rates among the elderly. The World Bank, for instance, estimates that life expectancy in China, which has been improving, may level off with rapid increases in lung cancer and cardiovascular disease caused by a recent surge in smoking rates (World Bank 1990a). The diversity of age patterns of mortality may also be magnified by the numerous technologic interventions, such as WHO's Expanded Programme on Immunization (EPI), which targets life-saving vaccinations to young children. If the efforts of the last decade directed to children have been at all successful, child mortality should have declined faster relative to adult mortality in many developing countries (UNICEF 1990).

Sex Structure

How do men and women fare in the mortality transition? Studies in South Asia consistently have shown that female age-specific mortality rates are higher than male rates throughout childhood and early adulthood (D'Souza and Chen 1980; Sen 1989; Dyson 1984). In India, the age at which male and female mortality rates cross over has been moving to steadily younger ages; it is now estimated to be in the early 30s. Dyson (1984) concludes that the Indian pattern of excess female mortality at younger ages is a recent phenomenon, dating from about 1921. Before that time, male mortality was higher in all age groups. Preston (1976), analyzing historical life tables for 43 mostly Western populations, showed that the pattern of excess female-to-male mortality is highly variable across countries and time periods. In some countries, males had higher rates than females in all age groups. An increased likelihood of higher female-to-male mortality rates in ages 1 to 39 years was associated with very high overall mortality levels. As the mortality level declined, excess female-to-male mortality became less common and was increasingly confined to the age groups 10 to 39 years. Perhaps the most remarkable aspect of Preston's data was the great variability in sex patterns of mortality between populations.

Heligman (1982) analyzed sex-specific life tables for 36 developing countries. In these populations, the pattern of higher female-than-male mortality was bimodal, peaking in early childhood and the reproductive ages. Summary data in Table 1-1 illustrate the diversity of these patterns. Even at high mortality levels (Column 1), 40 to 60 percent of the life tables have higher male than female mortality in the reproductive years.

Social Structure

Most studies implicitly assume that the mortality transition is shared equally by all members of a community. In virtually all societies, disadvantaged groups, ethnic minorities, or those living in backward regions experience higher mortality levels than the national average. Indigenous groups throughout the world consistently have worse levels

Table 1-1　Percent of Higher Female-than-Male Mortality by Age
Group and Life Expectancy at Birth, in Developing
Country Life Tables

Life expectancy overall at birth (years)

Age group	Under 50	50-59	60-69	70+
		Percent		
0	20	8	–	–
1–4	80	67	67	–
5–14	40	5	7	–
15–24	60	42	7	–
25–44	40	33	13	–
45–64	–	–	–	–
65–84	40	25	–	–
No. of life tables	5	12	15	4

Source: Heligman (1982:18)

of mortality than more privileged counterparts in the same country. In
Paraguay, in 1981, for example, the national infant mortality rate was
below 50 per one thousand live births, but the rate for indigenous
peoples was 177, or more than three times the national average (Murray
1988). Among New Zealand Maoris, adult mortality was approximately
50 percent higher than among white New Zealanders (Pearce et al. 1985).
In the United States, blacks have a mortality pattern resembling that of
developing country populations. While adult white American males
have only a 16 percent chance of dying from age 15 to 60 years, adult
black males have a 31 percent chance of death between these ages
(Murray 1990). Particularly striking are mortality data by social class (Fox,
Goldblati, and Jones 1985; Duleep 1986), which find a consistently
inferior situation for the disadvantaged classes of virtually all societies.

Pace and Direction of Change

One critical aspect of any health transition is the pace and direction
of change. The vast majority of country experiences indicate that
mortality has been improving steadily with only minor fluctuations.
Gwatkin (1980), however, has postulated that the pace of mortality
decline has been steadily decelerating due to the low levels that mortality

has already attained. Acute crises can temporarily increase mortality rates in all age groups, as in cases of famine (Sudan, Ethiopia), war (Cambodia, Mozambique), and disaster (Iran, Philippines). These reversals of mortality decline are usually temporary or confined to population subgroups.

Nevertheless, there are instances of rising age-specific mortality rates or "counter-transitions," as described by Frenk et al., (1989) reporting on the Mexican experience. We can illustrate counter-transitions with four examples. First, Anderson (1955) noted that age-specific mortality rates for males over age 35 years in France increased by 10 to 20 percent from 1850 to 1900. This slow deterioration of mortality over a half century was followed by more than 50 years of improvements in the adult death rates. Second, in Eastern Europe adult male death rates increased over the period 1952 to 1985 (Uemura and Pisa 1988; Eberstadt 1989). From 1970 to 1985, age-standardized male death rates (ages 30-69 years) did not change in a uniform fashion across Eastern Europe. The changes ranged from an improvement of 3 percent in East Germany to a worsening of 33 percent in Hungary. For most other Eastern European countries, adult male mortality from 1952 to 1985 did not change significantly. Uemura and Pisa (1988) have shown that a significant percentage of the increase was due to a substantial rise in cardiovascular deaths. Third, the Pacific Island state of Nauru has experienced rising adult male mortality largely attributable to accidents, cardiovascular disease, and diabetes mellitus (Taylor and Thomas 1985; Schooneveldt et al. 1988). Finally, the AIDS pandemic is projected to significantly increase adult male mortality in several Central African countries (Anderson, May and McLean 1988).

Transitions in Causes of Death

Age structure or incidence effects?

How do changes in mortality levels relate to dynamics in the pattern of causes of death? Fredrikson (1969) was among the earliest to delineate specific patterns of disease characterizing various levels of mortality. He postulated endemic infections, parasitisms, infestations, and nutritional deficiencies in high mortality populations being replaced by bronchopulmonary and cardiovascular diseases, malignant neoplasms, mental illness, accidents, and obesity in low mortality populations. Omran (1971) described the long-term shift from pandemics of infectious diseases to the prevalence of degenerative and manmade diseases as mortality declines in a population. According to Omran, most of these mortality improvements were concentrated in children and young women.

McKeown's classic works (1976, 1979) on the history of mortality change in England and Wales provide a longitudinal examination of changes in causes of death over nearly a century. McKeown computed the proportion of the decline in standardized mortality rates due to specific causes. Seventy-four percent of the decline in mortality was due to the reduction of infectious diseases. The 26 percent attributable to nonfectious causes was mostly in the category of nephritis, diseases of early infancy and old age, and other diseases. Over the same period, age-standardized mortality rates for cardiovascular disease increased 250 percent; for neoplasms, the age-standardized rates increased 380 percent.

McKeown's and Omran's observations have been influential in establishing a two component model of the transition in the causes of death — a decline of infectious diseases and a concomitant rise of chronic diseases. This model has received significant support from epidemiological studies in many countries on the increasing prevalence of risk factors predisposing to cardiovascular diseases, such as smoking, diabetes, and high cholesterol levels. These risk factors appear to be rising in many developing countries as well, due to "Westernization." In economic terms, these patterns are income elastic in that they are responsive to income change (Pearson, Jamison and Trejo-Gutierrez 1993).

The rise of chronic diseases in developing countries can be explained by two phenomena. First, as fertility and mortality decline, the population age structure shifts from a youthful, pyramidal form to a more elderly, rectangular form. In other words, younger people make up a smaller percent and older people make up a greater percent of the population. In absolute terms, there should be greater chronic rather than infectious disease burdens, as the former are maladies of older age. A second explanation for the rise of chronic diseases is the proposition that the incidence of these diseases is actually increasing due to worsening risk factors. Under this hypothesis, the age-specific death rates for chronic diseases would be expected to increase as mortality declines. In the remainder of this chapter, we examine the empirical evidence for this hypothesis on the transition in causes of death.

Changes in the incidence of chronic disease

In 1976, Preston published an extensive analysis of 165 cause-of-death life tables for 43 countries covering the period 1861 to 1964. Ninety-two percent of these tables represented Western populations; only 8 percent were from developing country populations. Thus, the sample largely reflects the cause-of-death transition in European populations; it is the logical extension to many countries of McKeown's single country study for England and Wales. Preston used age-standardized mortality rates to examine overall changes in the cause-of-death structure across age groups. Each cause-specific age-standardized mortality rate was related to the all-cause standardized mortality rate using linear regression to determine the contribution of each cause to overall mortality decline. In Table 1-2, the slopes of the cause-specific regression lines reflect how much of a unit change in the all-cause mortality rate is attributable to any specific cause. Except for neoplasms in both sexes and cardiovascular mortality in males, all the cause-specific regression line slopes are positive, implying declining cause-specific rates as total mortality declines. The major causes accounting for the decline in all-cause mortality are respiratory tuberculosis (11 to 12 percent), other infectious and parasitic diseases (14 to 15 percent), influenza/pneumonia/bronchitis (24 to 28 percent), and diarrheal diseases (10 to 11 percent). Unfortunately, 33 to 35 percent of the decline is due to changes in the cause category "unknown or others."

Preston's analysis supports McKeown's observations on rising neoplasm and cardiovascular disease mortality paralleling overall mortality decline, at least in men. Preston also noted an interesting inverse correlation between the category "other and unknown" and "cardiovascular and neoplasm" mortality. Where one was high relative to a given mortality level, the other was low. "Other and unknown" deaths occurred mostly in older age groups. Preston postulated that these "other and unknown" deaths may have been poorly classified, possibly genuine cardiovascular disease or neoplastic mortality. The decline in "other and unknown" may be attributable to an improvement in cause of death coding at older ages resulting from a proper assignment of deaths into cardiovascular diseases and neoplasms. Preston recomputed the relationship between cardiovascular disease mortality and all-cause mortality, including "other and unknown" as an independent variable. The new slopes for cardiovascular diseases were large and positive: 0.25 for females and 0.24 for males, indicating that cardiovascular mortality probably declines substantially with mortality reductions. Preston (1976) was aware of the counter-intuitive implications: "(the) somewhat unusual suggestion, based on a variety of indirect evidence, is that cardiovascular

Table 1-2 Coefficients of correlation and linear regression relating
standardized death rates from each cause related to
all causes combined

Cause of Death	Coefficient of correlation with death rate, all causes combined		Simple linear regression	
	Females	Males	Females Slope	Males Slope
Respiratory tuberculosis	0.86	0.87	0.11	0.12
Other infectious and parasitic	0.91	0.88	0.14	0.15
Neoplasms	-0.48	-0.66	-0.02	-0.06
Cardiovascular	0.11	-0.15	0.02	-0.03
Influenza/pneumonia/bronchitis	0.93	0.94	0.24	0.28
Diarrheal	0.8	0.78	0.10	0.11
Certain chronic	0.29	0.31	0.02	0.02
Maternal	0.89		0.02	
Certain diseases of infancy	0.77	0.73	0.04	0.04
Violence	0.22	0.4	0	0.02
Other and unknown (residual)	0.89	0.87	0.33	0.35
All causes			0.9998	1.0002

Source: Preston (1976: Table 2.2).

diseases have in general been important contributors to mortality change,
more important than the specific infectious diseases of childhood
exclusive of tuberculosis" (1976: 7).

Preston's study has three major limitations: the all-age grouping in the
analysis, the bias of data from Western populations, and the restricted
number of disease categories. These limitations have been partially
addressed by recent studies on causes of death in adults (Murray and
Feachem 1990; Murray, Yang and Qiao 1992). These studies divide
causes into three categories instead of the traditional two-part division
of infectious and chronic. The three categories are reproductive and
communicable, noncommunicable, and injuries. The rationale is that
respiratory infections, maternal mortality, diseases of early infancy, and
nutritional deficiencies should all be grouped with infectious and
parasitic diseases. The noncommunicable diseases in this framework

include senile and ill-defined causes, following Preston's observations that these causes may be largely miscoded noncommunicable diseases. Injuries, both intentional and unintentional, are placed in a separate category because they possess determinants that are independent of the other two groupings.

The two studies by Murray and colleagues used cause-of-death data from 60 developing and industrialized countries for a single year in the 1980s and longitudinal data covering up to three and a half decades in five countries — Sri Lanka, Costa Rica, Singapore, Cuba, and Chile. Age-standardized mortality rates were not used; rather, the probability of death from 15 to 60 years (45Q15) was estimated for each of the three groups of causes. The analysis showed that the reproductive and communicable category falls at a faster rate at higher mortality levels than the noncommunicable category, which falls at a faster rate at lower mortality levels. The third group, injuries, has an ambiguous pattern of change. Injury rates are higher in males and there is no consistent trend among females.

Murray and colleagues also measured the association of changes in one cause of death with changes in all other causes of mortality. They found striking positive relationships for tuberculosis, respiratory infections, maternal mortality, digestive diseases, and, in females, cardiovascular mortality. No cause-specific mortality rates increase as total mortality declines. Cardiovascular disease mortality in males does not have a close relationship with total mortality. The category "senile and ill-defined" is gratifyingly less important in these adult years.

By examining recent cross-sectional cause-of-death data for industrialized and developing countries in the 1980s, Murray and colleagues (1991) studied the relationship between detailed causes and overall mortality. The major drawback of this more limited data set is the absence of very-high-mortality populations. In the group neoplasms, the only statistically significant relationship is for lymphatic and hematopoietic neoplasms, which rise as total mortality declines. Among the endocrine diseases, the decline is largely attributable to diabetes mellitus. While overall cardiovascular disease rates decline with total mortality, this appears to be largely attributable to declines in hypertensive heart disease and cerebrovascular accidents. Ischemic heart disease mortality has no statistically significant relationship with total mortality. Both major components of digestive disease mortality — chronic liver disease and ulcers — decline. Finally, among specific causes of injuries, water transport accidents rise and drownings decline with overall declines in adult male mortality.

Similar results for females illustrate strong relationships for two cancers: breast cancers increase and cervical cancers decline with reductions in total female adult mortality. All cardiovascular causes and diabetes mellitus fall as well. Fires, drownings, and homicides in women all have statistically significant slopes indicating declines with total mortality decline.

The correlation coefficient in this study and that in Preston's work concur on an important finding. Many causes of death exhibit no statistically significant relationship with overall mortality. In other words, variations in these causes of death are virtually independent of the overall level of mortality. This finding challenges the assumption underlying studies of most cause-of-death transition — that the cause-of-death structure is largely a function of the overall mortality level. Other variables, such as the presence of risk factors, may be critical for predicting the cause-of-death transition. For example, rising cardiovascular risk factors may not be as closely associated with mortality decline as assumed, but rather could vary independently of mortality levels. In Japan, for example, adult mortality is very low, and cardiovascular risk factors have not yet increased to the level characteristic of Europe and North America. On the other hand, levels of cerebrovascular diseases are higher than in the West.

Trends in Cardiovascular Diseases

The counter-intuitive decline of cardiovascular disease mortality in women and stagnation in men deserves further analysis. The experience of industrialized countries since 1950 illustrates the complexities of analysis and interpretation. Uemura and Pisa (1988) studied mortality change in the age groups 30 to 69 years from 1950 to 1980 in 35 industrialized countries. They found that ischemic heart disease mortality rates increased in the majority of countries from 1952 to 1967 but decreased in the period 1970 to 85. Changes in ischemic heart disease (or any specific cause of heart disease) are difficult to interpret because of changes in coding practices over time and differences in practices between countries. Total cardiovascular mortality rates are a more robust category; these rates in the majority of countries stagnated from 1952 to 1967 but decreased from 1970 to 1985. The discrepancy between total cardiovascular disease and ischemic heart disease is explained by cerebrovascular mortality, which declined in most countries throughout the period 1952 to 1980. An exception to this pattern, mentioned earlier, is Eastern Europe, where cardiovascular disease mortality has been increasing over the past 30 years. All of these trends must be interpreted with caution, as the potentially miscoded "senile and ill-defined causes" also declined over the same time period.

There is consensus that the major risk factors for cardiovascular diseases are smoking, high serum cholesterol levels, and hypertension. Unfortunately, comparable population data on the prevalence of these risk factors are not available. The Monitoring of Cardiovascular Diseases project (MONICA) of the World Health Organization, which will ultimately fill this gap in knowledge, estimated baseline risk-factor prevalence for 27 countries (WHO, MONICA 1988). In this study, the proportion of smokers ranged from 34 to 62 percent in men and 3 to 52 percent in women; rates of hypertension ranged from 8 to 44 percent in men and 12 to 40 percent in women. The prevalence of abnormally high cholesterol levels ranged from 4 to 6 percent. This study shows great heterogeneity in the prevalence of risk factors between populations.

Data on these risk factors from developing countries are scanty. Surveys using comparable methods are simply not available. There is, thus, insufficient evidence supporting the hypothesis of rising cardiovascular mortality in developing countries. For example, Nissinen et al., (1988) reviewed 16 developing countries with sequences of cause-of-death data. They found declining hypertension associated with declining mortality in almost all countries. There are, however, well-known examples of specific populations in the developing world with rapidly rising risk factors and mortality from diabetes mellitus and cardiovascular mortality. Nauru is a powerful example of the potential effects of dietary and behavioral change. Rising per capita incomes on the island have been associated with dramatic increases in caloric intake, smoking, alcohol consumption, and adoption of hazardous behaviors such as motorcycle driving. Although the historical record is poor, the net effect may be to increase adult mortality to some of the highest levels known. In Nauru, 42 percent of deaths are due to injuries, and the next leading cause of death is cardiovascular disease (Taylor and Thomas 1985; Schooneveldt et al. 1988).

The lack of an increase of cardiovascular disease mortality in many countries may be assessed in terms of changes in the underlying risk factors. Not all countries experience rising levels of smoking, hypertension, and cholesterol as overall mortality declines. But how might significant declines in cardiovascular disease be explained? Explanations may lie in the declines of rheumatic fever and related mortality from bacterial endocarditis. There are also other parasitic causes of cardiac mortality. For example, Maguire et al. (1987) found that adult males suffering from Chagas disease (a form of trypanosomiasis widely distributed in South and Central America) with electrocardiographic abnormalities had a sevenfold relative risk of death. And interactions may exist between infectious and parasitic diseases and cardiovascular mortality that are poorly understood — e.g., the cardiomyopathy common in Western and Southern Africa (Hutt and Burkitt 1986).

Our review of the rise of chronic disease mortality in populations with rapidly declining overall mortality leads to two tentative conclusions. First, chronic diseases as a group decline as total mortality declines. The only diseases for which rates may rise are ischemic heart disease in men, breast cancer in women, and lung cancer in both sexes. The evidence for a rise in lung cancer is based on knowledge of rising cigarette consumption in many developing countries, not on clear evidence from cause-of-death data. Second, whether cardiovascular disease rates rise or fall appears to depend on the balance of change in risk factors. The lack of a correlation between changes in cardiovascular mortality and total mortality across countries suggests that change in risk factors may occur independently of mortality decline, making generalizations about rises in specific chronic disease mortality rates untenable.

Conclusion

We have reached several basic conclusions in this chapter. First, while mortality declines have been enjoyed by virtually all populations, industrialized and developing, the dynamics of change have not been uniform across all age, sex, and social groupings among and within countries. Nor has the pace of decline been similar. Indeed, there are instances of a "counter-transition," in which some population subgroups have experienced rising mortality. Thus, we may point to no single pattern of "health transition." Rather, many "health transitions" exist. The future of world health, therefore, is less predetermined than it is predicated upon the changing nature of the determinants of health — physical environment, human behavior, and health care action.

Disaggregated analyses are critical to an understanding of the age, sex, and social structure of mortality change. When analyzing mortality transition, one should distinguish, as a minimum, changes in mortality under age 5 years from deaths in older age groups. Indeed, the balance of under-5 versus over-5 mortality is one of the major factors distinguishing families of Coale-Demeny model life tables (United Nations 1983). Further distinctions are also desirable. We propose examining age-sex-specific mortality in children (0 to 4 years), adolescents (5 to 14 years), young adults (15 to 39 years), older adults (40 to 59 years), and the elderly (60+ years) separately. Each of these groups has characteristically dominant causes of death at different mortality levels that reflect different determinants of life experiences and health hazards. Not only do health risks vary between these age and sex groups, but the consequences of illness and premature death in these groups would be expected to have a distinct impact on families, communities, and the country at large.

The transition in the cause-of-death structure may not follow a universal pattern either. Contrary to general notions, our review suggests that the determinants of specific causes of death may operate independently of the overall level of mortality. Predictive and explanatory power may be found only when causes are disaggregated and assigned to more meaningful groupings.

Given the variability in patterns and causes of mortality change, how and why does health improve in populations? The customary explanation is that mortality levels reflect changing determinants of health, including the use of medical technologies and services. We argue that changes in mortality levels possess enormous intergenerational momentum. For example, mortality rates after acute crises (famines, war, disasters) return briskly to predisaster levels (e.g., Chen 1980; Sen 1989; and Dyson 1989). A simple explanation for this would be that the social, economic, and health care determinants of mortality remain resilient. However, many health-related factors such as income, food supplies, and health services are subject to adverse trends, an observation that poses a major challenge to this explanation. The 1980s world economic recession exemplifies the reversal in many such factors (World Bank 1990 B).

An alternative explanation for improvements in health is that the key determinants of mortality may be insensitive to short- or medium-term reversals. Murray (1988) and Murray and Chen (1993) explain this phenomenon by proposing a distinction between stocks and flows in the determinants of the health of populations. While flows are determinants that are transient, stocks refer to basic aspects of a society's human resources, physical infrastructure, and social systems. Some of our current paradigms for health focus on flows — for example, income or recurrent expenditure on health. Stocks, in contrast, are built up through investment over decades in knowledge, education, social organization, and infrastructure for water supplies and health services. Such stocks do not change quickly, even in times of hardship. The resistance of mortality to temporary reversals could be explained by the importance of these stocks as critical determinants of health.

The stocks approach is a relative argument. Some flows clearly matter; with no income, everyone will soon die. Among stocks, some are reversible after prolonged depreciation, such as water supply systems, health care systems, or educational institutions. Others, such as community or individual knowledge, are practically irreversible. Several observations, nevertheless, lend support to the importance of stocks and the consequent resistance of mortality to reversal. In Guyana, economic decline over the last 15 years, with concomitant decreases in food availability, health service expenditure, and standards of living, was not associated with increases in mortality (Murray 1988). Likewise, UNICEF set out to study the impact of the world recession on children; the summary report by Cornia (1984) concluded that infant mortality rate and other child welfare indicators continue to show signs of improvement even under a moderate economic recession (Cornia 1984: 216). The World Bank, in its 1990 review of the world economic recession, observed that during the same period in which many countries in the developing world suffered economic setbacks, mortality rates continued to decline (World Bank 1990b).

If stocks of knowledge, infrastructure and social institutions are key determinants of health change, our time frame for analyzing health change must become broader. A focus on short-term changes in health flows or health outcomes would be misguided. Even attempts to assess the impact of health programs over short periods would need to be reconsidered. Further work to clarify the importance of health stocks and flows is needed.

References

Anderson, O.W. 1955. "Age-specific mortality in selected western European countries with particular emphasis on the nineteenth century: Observations and implications." *Bulletin of the History of Medicine,* 29(3): 239–254.

Anderson, R.M., R.M. May, and A.R. Mclean. 1988. "Possible demographic consequences of AIDS in developing countries." *Nature,* 332: 228–234.

Bucht, B. 1985. "Child mortality change in developing countries and its relationship with Coale and Demeney model life tables." Paper presented to International Union for the Scientific Study of Population Conference, Florence, Italy.

Caldwell, J. 1989. "Introductory thoughts on the health transition. Paper for the health transition workshop: Cultural, social and behavioral determinants of the health transition: What is the evidence?" Canberra: National Center for Epidemiology and Population, Australian National University, May 15–19.

Caldwell, J.C., S. Findley, P. Caldwell, G. Santow, W. Cosford, J. Braid, and D. Broers-Freeman. 1990. *What We Know About the Health Transition: The Cultural, Social and Behavioural Determinants of Health, Health Transition Series,* No. 2, Volumes 1 and 2. Canberra: Health Transition Centre, Australian National University.

Cleland, J., and A.G. Hill. 1991. "The health transition: Methods and measures." The proceedings of an international workshop, London, June 1989. *Health Transition Series,* No. 3.

Coale, A.J., and P. Demeney. 1966. *Regional Model Life Tables and Stable Populations.* Princeton, NJ: Princeton University Press.

Cornia, G.A. 1984. "A summary and interpretation of the evidence." In R. Jolly and G.A. Cornia, eds. *The Impact of the World Recession on Children.* Oxford: Pergammon Press.

Culyer, A.J., ed. 1983. *Health Indicators.* London: Martin Robertson.

D'Souza, S., and L.C. Chen. 1980. "Sex differentials in mortality in rural Bangladesh." *Population and Development Review,* 6(2): 257–270.

Duleep, H.O. 1986. "Measuring the effort or income on adult mortality using longitudinal administrative record data." *Journal of Human Resources,* 21: 238–426.

Dyson, T. 1984. "Excess male mortality in India." *Economic and Political Weekly,* 19(10): 422–426.

Dyson, T. 1989. "Demography of famines in South Asia." Paper presented to Health Transition Seminar, Harvard Center for Population and Development Studies. December 13.

Eberstadt, N. 1989. "Health and mortality in Eastern Europe 1965 to 1985." In *Pressures for Reform in the East European Economies,* Vol. 1. Study papers submitted to the Joint Economic Committee, Congress of the United States. Washington, DC: US GPO.

Fernando, D.F.S. 1985. "Health statistics on Sri Lanka, 1921–1980." In S.B. Halstead, J.A. Walsh, and K.S. Warren, eds. *Good Health at Low Cost.* New York: Rockefeller Foundation.

Findley, S.E. 1989. "Social reflections of changing morbidity during health transitions." Revised paper for health transition workshop: Cultural, social and behavioral determinants of the health transition: What is the evidence? Canberra: National Center for Epidemiology and Population, ANU. May 15–19.

Fox, A.J., P.O. Goldblati, and D.R. Jones. 1985. "Social class mortality differentials: Artifact, selection or life circumstances?" *Journal of Epidemiology in Community Health,* 39: 1–8.

Frederiksen, H. 1969. "Feedback in economic and demographic transition." *Science,* 166: 837–847.

Frenk, J., J.L. Bobadilla, J. Sepúlveda, and M. López-Cervantes. 1989. "Health transition in middle-income countries: New challenges for health care." *Health Policy and Planning,* 4(1): 29–39.

Goldsmith, B. 1972. "The status of health indicators." *Health Service Reports,* 88(10): 937–941.

Gwatkin, D.R. 1980. "Indications of change in developing country mortality trends: The end of an era?" *Population and Development Review,* 6(4): 615–644.

Heligman, L. 1982. "Patterns of sex differentials in mortality in less developed countries." In L.T. Ruzicka, and A.D. Lopez, eds. *Sex Differentials in Mortality Trends, Determinants and Consequences.* Canberra: Australian National University.

Holland, W.W., J. Ipsen, and J. Kostrzewski. 1979. *Measurement of Levels of Health.* Copenhagen: World Health Organization, Regional Office for Europe.

Hutt, M.S.R., and D.P. Burkit. 1986. *The Topography of Non-Infectious Disease.* Oxford: Oxford University Press.

Maguire, J.H., R. Hoff, I. Sherlock, A.C. Guimaraes, A.C. Sleigh, N.B Ramos, K.E. Mott, and T.H. Weller. 1987. Cardiac morbidity and mortality due to Chagas' disease: Prospective electrocardiographic study of a Brazilian community. *Circulation*, 75(6): 1140–1145.

McKeown, T. 1976. *The Modern Rise of Population.* London: Edward Arnold.

McKeown, T. 1979. *The Role of Medicine: Dream, Mirage or Nemesis?* Oxford: Basil Blackwell.

Murray, C.J.L. 1987. "A critical review of international mortality data." *Society of Scientific Medicine,* 23(7): 773–781.

Murray, C.J.L. 1988. "Determinants of health improvement in developing countries: Case-studies of St. Lucia, Guyana, Paraguay, Kiribati, Swaziland and Bolivia." [D. Phil Thesis]: Oxford University.

Murray, C.J.L. 1990. "Mortality among black men." *New England Journal of Medicine*, 322(3): 205–206.

Murray, C.J.L. and R.G. Feachem. 1990. "Adult mortality in developing countries." *Transactions of the Royal Society of Tropical Medicine and Hygiene*, 84(1): 1–2.

Murray, C.J.L., G. Yang, and X. Qiao. 1991. "Adult mortality in developing countries: Levels, patterns and causes." In R.G. Feachem, T. Kjellstrom, C.J.L. Murray, M. Over, and M. Phillips, eds. *The Health of Adults in the Developing World*. Washington, DC: World Bank.

Murray, C.J.L., and L.C. Chen. 1993. "In search of a contemporary theory for understanding mortality change." *Social Science and Medicine*, 36(2):143–55.

National Center for Health Statistics. 1988. *Vital Statistics of the United States 1985*. Volume II — Mortality Part *A*. Hyattsville, Maryland: National Center for Health Statistics.

Nissinen, A., S. Bothig, H. Granroth, and A.D. Lopez. 1988. "Hypertension in developing countries." *World Health Statistics Quarterly*, 41(3&4): 141–154.

Omran, A.R. 1971. "The epidemiologic transition: A theory of the epidemiology of population change." *Milbank Memorial Fund Quarterly*, 49: 509–538.

Pearce, N.E., P.B. Davis, A.H. Smith, and F.H. Foster. 1985. "Social class, ethnic group, and male mortality in New Zealand, 1974–8." *Journal of Epidemiology and Community Health*, 39: 9–14.

Pearson, T.A., D.T. Jamison, and J. Trejo-Gutierrez. 1993. "Cardiovascular disease." In D.T. Jamison, W.H. Mosley, A.R. Measham, and J. Bobadilla, eds. *Disease Control Priorities in Developing Countries*. New York: Oxford University Press.

Preston, S.H. 1976. *Mortality Patterns in National Populations with Special Reference to Recorded Causes of Death*. New York: Academic Press.

Preston, S., N. Keyfitz, and N. Schoen. 1972. *Causes of Death: Life Tables for National Populations*. New York: Seminar Press.

Rifkin, S., and G. Walt. 1986. "Why health improves: Defining the issues concerning 'comprehensive primary health care' and 'selective primary health care.'" *Social Science and Medicine*, 23: 559–566.

Schooneveldt, M., T. Songer, P. Zimmet, and K. Thomas. 1988. "Changing mortality patterns in Nauruans : An example of epidemiological transition." *Journal of Epidemiology and Community Health*, 42: 89–95.

Sen, A. 1989. "Women's survival as a development problem." Paper presented at the American Academy of Arts and Sciences, Cambridge, MA, March 8.

Stolnitz, G.J. 1955. "A century of international mortality trends." *Population Studies*, 9(1): 24–55.

Stolnitz, G.J. 1956. "A century of international mortality trends: II." *Population Studies*, 10(1): 17–42.

Stolnitz, G.J. 1964. In R. Freedman, ed. *Population: The Vital Revolution.* New York: Double-Day-Anchor.

Taylor, R., and K. Thomas. 1985. "Mortality patterns in the modernized Pacific island nation of Nauru." *American Journal of Public Health*, 75(2): 149–155.

Teitelbaum, M. 1975. "Relevance of demographic transition theory for developing countries." *Science*, 188: 420–425.

United Nations. 1989. *World Population Prospects: 1988 Assessment.* New York: United Nations.

Uemura, K., and Z. Pisa. 1988. "Trends in cardiovascular disease mortality in industrialized countries since 1950." *World Health Statistics Quarterly*, 41: 155–178.

UNICEF. 1990. *State of the World's Children 1990.* Oxford: Oxford University Press.

World Bank. 1990a. *China: Long-Term Issues in Options for the Health Sector.* Washington, DC: World Bank.

World Bank. 1990b. *World Development Report.* Oxford: Oxford University Press.

World Health Organization. 1984. *Basic Documents: Thirty-Fourth Edition.* Geneva: World Health Organization.

World Health Organization Monitoring of Cardiovascular Diseases Project. 1988. "Geographical variation in the major risk factors of coronary heart disease in men and women aged 35–64 years." *World Health Statistics Quarterly*, 41: 115–140.

2

Elements for a Theory of the Health Transition

Julio Frenk
José-Luis Bobadilla
Claudio Stern
Tomas Frejka
and Rafael Lozano

Introduction

Over the past years, the world has witnessed the decline of many old certainties. The health field has not been an exception to the process of fast and vast transformation. Times when priorities were obvious and the direction of progress was clear-cut have been left behind. The only certainty today is an increasing complexity. Nations are experiencing a health transition; its characteristics must be fully understood if we are to anticipate changes and not only react to them once they have occurred.

Transformations take place in all nations, but they are particularly complex in middle income countries, where the model of economic development has been marked by deep social inequality, thus creating a mosaic of living conditions (Frenk, Bobadilla et al. 1989). In these countries, the health transition is expressed by an epidemiological pattern where the sharp decline in the level of mortality has been accompanied by a differentiation in its causes. General mortality levels are lower, but the composition by causes of death is much more complex. Thus, infectious diseases lose their previous predominance, but still maintain a major position in the epidemiologic profile. At the same time, the absolute and relative importance of noncommunicable diseases and injury increases. Apart from social inequality in the quantitative levels of mortality, there is now a qualitative inequality in the distribution of causes of death by geographic region and social class.

Increasing complexity also characterizes the organization and functioning of health systems. Generally speaking, these are systems that have not solved old problems, such as insufficient population coverage, urban concentration of resources, technological lag, and low productivity. At the same time, they face the new challenges posed by institution building and expansion, greater diversity of human resources, growing costs, scientific and technological dependence, and inadequate quality of care.

In order to understand the dynamics of health change, it is necessary first to define a conceptual and theoretical base that allows us to arrange and give coherence to the growing body of empirical evidence. This article outlines the general elements needed to delve into the theory of the health transition. In this endeavor, there have been important advances since the publication of the seminal paper by Omran (1971). Nevertheless, the original formulation of the theory and many of its revisions are still insufficient to give full account of the complexity of several transition patterns observed within and between different countries. Our purpose in this article is therefore to systematize the main components of the theory and thus contribute to reducing the conceptual confusion usually experienced by academic developments at their initial stage. We do not intend to offer a finished theory, but rather some elements that will make progress possible towards building a research paradigm.

Building a theory

Every theory must include at least the following components:

1. *Concepts:* What is the definition of the object of analysis that the theory intends to account for?
2. *Determinants:* What are its causes?
3. *Mechanisms:* Which factors explain changes in the object?
4. *Attributes:* How is the object characterized?
5. *Consequences:* What effects does it have on other processes?

This article attempts a preliminary answer to each of these questions as they relate to the health transition. While we appreciate the specificity of each national reality at each historical moment, the purpose is to derive propositions that can be generalized, so as to provide a comprehensive theoretical basis for comparative studies of health dynamics.

Concepts

After the classical writings of authors like Virchow, Malthus, Marx, and Engels, an early attempt to analyze the health implications of demographic and economic transitions was published by Frederiksen (1969) more than two decades ago. In 1971, Omran coined the term epidemiologic transition and thus made possible a major breakthrough in our understanding of the dynamics of causes of death in populations. Almost simultaneously, and apparently independently, Lerner (1973) presented a paper postulating a "health transition", a broader concept than the one used by Omran, since it included elements of the social conceptions and behaviors regarding health determinants.

Not many conceptualization and research activities were carried out during the decade that followed those pioneering works, even though some of their particular aspects, such as the analysis of mortality causes, produced both theoretical advances and empirical results. In contrast, recent years have witnessed a rediscovery of the epidemiologic transition, with many groups of researchers, national institutions, and international agencies becoming interested in this concept as a useful explanation of the intense changes that have occurred in the health of populations (see, for example, Caldwell et al. 1990).

Largely owing to this renewed interest, the concept of epidemiologic transition has been given various meanings that need to be clarified in order to achieve any theoretical progress. In particular, it is common to refer to the transition as a period rather than as a process of change. From this viewpoint, the epidemiologic transition is regarded as a time interval, with a beginning, when infectious diseases were predominant, and an end, when non-communicable diseases have finally dominated the causes of death. Instead of this rather static perspective, it is necessary to conceive the transition as a dynamic process, whereby the health and disease patterns of a society evolve in diverse ways as a response to broader demographic, socioeconomic, technological, political, cultural, and biological changes. The theory of the epidemiologic transition should then aim to understand the characteristics, determinants, and consequences of such a process (Omran 1982). If we accept that health conditions are continuously being transformed, as different diseases disappear, appear or re-emerge, it can be stated that the transition is an ongoing process, rather than a relatively simple and unidirectional period of time. Obviously, a transition is not just any change; it is change that follows an identifiable pattern and that occurs over a relatively long time.

Another source of conceptual confusion arises from interchanging the terms "epidemiologic transition" and "health transition". In a previous paper (Frenk, Frejka et al. 1989), we proposed to define the latter as the broader concept, of which the former is a component. Let us consider that, in an abstract sense, the study of health in populations comprises two major objects: on the one hand, the health conditions of the population; on the other, the response to those conditions. According to this simplifying dichotomy, the health transition may be divided into two main components. The first is the epidemiologic transition strictly speaking, which is defined as the long-term process of change in the health conditions of a society, including changes in the patterns of disease, disability, and death. The second component, which may be called the healthcare transition, refers to the change in the patterns of the organized social response to health conditions. Our definition is consistent with the formulations of other authors, such as Lerner (1973) and Caldwell (1990), who also conceive of the epidemiologic transition as part of a broader health transition.

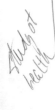

Finally, one more cause of confusion often comes from including in the definition of epidemiologic transition, processes that really constitute mechanisms through which the transition occurs. This confusion may be observed particularly with regard to fertility changes. Since the original work by Omran (1971), there has been a tendency to include fertility decline as a defining element of the different epidemiologic transition models. This tendency is even more explicit in a later revision by Omran himself (1983). Fertility decline is one of the main mechanisms through which prevailing morbidity and mortality patterns change, but is not in itself part of the definition of the epidemiologic transition.

If the typology and definitions proposed above are accepted, then it is possible to address the next component of the theory, which consists of postulating the main relationships of determination regarding the defined phenomena. The remainder of this article focuses mostly on the epidemiologic transition, but the last section attempts to draw out some of its main implications for the health care transition.

Determinants of health

Since the epidemiologic transition refers to changes in the patterns of health and disease in a society, it is clear that any complete theory in this field must include a formulation about the determinants of health status. Indeed, in order to understand the dynamics that drive health change, it is necessary to account for the factors that determine health at a given point in time. The conceptual scheme that follows attempts to identify those factors, while specifying their interrelationships in a framework of hierarchical multicausality where factors operate at different levels of determination. The final link in this chain is the individual, in whom disease processes must express themselves. Higher levels of determination impose structural limits to variation in lower levels.

There is a growing consensus that health and disease are determined in a multicausal way (Dubos 1959; MacMahon and Pugh 1970; Rothman 1986), and that they need to be approached from a comprehensive and interdisciplinary perspective. In order to do so, it is necessary to integrate the multiple determinant factors into a coherent analytical framework. Several attempts have been made to identify and elucidate such factors (see, for example, Mosley and Chen 1984; San Martin 1985; Breilh 1986; Cornia 1987; Almeida 1989). The framework we propose next tries to organize conceptually the complex multicausality of health conditions and systems. This framework is summarized in Figure 2-1, where the main relationships between health and its determinants are outlined. We do not attempt to examine thoroughly each of those relationships, nor do we review the available empirical evidence pertaining to them; instead, we concentrate on the basic analytical aspects.

The starting point in Figure 2-1 is the relationship between the population and its physical environment. From the standpoint of health determination, the most important population attributes are size, growth rate, age structure, and geographic distribution. The environment, altitude, climate, natural resources, and types of parasites and vectors continue to exert important influences for specific disease processes. However, the fundamental attribute shaping the nature of the human habitat is the extent and quality of urbanization.

Population and environment are linked through two major bridges. The first one is social organization, through which human beings develop the necessary structures and processes to transform nature. The second one is represented by the genome, which transforms the deepest constitution of human populations in response to changes in the environment. These four elements set the broadest limits for the analysis of health determination. Indeed, all health phenomena occur in a population whose members have a certain genetic constitution and

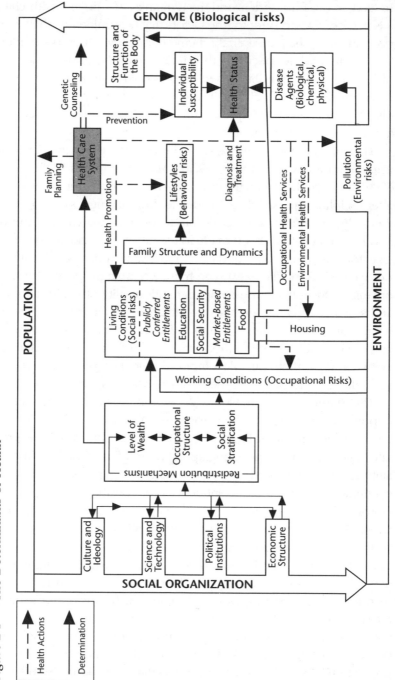

Figure 2-1   The Determinants of Health

Figure 2-2   Types of Determinants and Levels of Analysis in Health

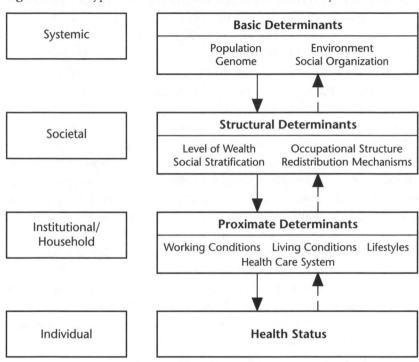

organize themselves socially to transform the environment. Specific relationships of determination take place within this basic frame. It should be pointed out that our conceptual formulation does not assume a diffuse multicausality, where everything influences everything. Instead, it arranges determinants according to a hierarchy; this principle is schematized in the right-hand side of Figure 2-2, which summarizes the main relationships proposed in Figure 2-1.

In order to analyze these relationships in greater detail, it is convenient to start from the left of Figure 2-1, which focuses on the social determinants. As can be seen, there are four major dimensions of social organization: economic structure, political institutions, science and technology, and culture and ideology. Together, these dimensions determine the total level of wealth of a society and the rules for stratifying different groups. Two major factors mediate the differential access of those groups to the total wealth pool: on the one hand, the occupational structure; on the other, the redistribution mechanisms used by the state, notably taxes and subsidies. It is beyond the scope of this paper to elaborate on the complex relationship among these various categories, which is the subject of many of the most lasting and profound debates in the social sciences. For our purposes, suffice it to say that these elements constitute the structural determinants of the health and disease process. Together, they constrain the variation of a set of proximate determinants, namely, working conditions, living conditions, lifestyles, and the health care system (see Figure 2-2).

The separation between working and living conditions is, of course, arbitrary. The purpose is to highlight the critical importance of work both as a direct determinant of the worker's health status and as an indirect contributor to the health of the rest of the family. In recognition of its direct effect, working conditions are portrayed in Figure 2-1 as part of the immediate environment of the worker. Such an effect is due to the occupational risks that derive from working conditions.

At this point, it is necessary to highlight the central position given to the category of risk in our analysis. Risk is defined by Last (1983) as "a probability that an event will occur, e.g., that an individual will become ill or die within a stated period of time or age". For the purposes of this article, health determinants can be conceived of as risk factors, that is to say, processes, attributes or exposures that determine the probability of occurrence of disease or other health outcomes.

As shown in Figure 2-1, living conditions occupy a central position among the proximate determinants of health. In turn, living conditions depend mainly on what Sen calls the "exchange entitlement" of an individual or family; i.e., the alternative bundles of goods and services that a person can acquire in exchange for the resources that he or she owns or commands (Sen 1981: 3-6). For our present purpose, it is very important to distinguish two types of entitlements, according to whether they are publicly conferred or market-based. This distinction is based on the rules governing access to goods and services. Simply stated, market-based entitlements are goods and services that can be obtained through trade or production exchanges that are governed by the logic of the market. In contrast, publicly conferred entitlements are goods and services that, through the intervention of some collective actor, generally the state, are removed from market distribution and made available either as a supplement to market exchanges or as a social right; they are considered a requisite for equality of opportunity, which provides the ethical foundation for market competition (see Briggs 1961). Evidently, it is not enough for the state to declare certain goods or services to be a social right, e.g., through a constitutional amendment; it is necessary to analyze the extent to which such a declaration is put into practice (see Fuenzalida-Puelma and Scholle-Connor 1989). The distinction between market-based and publicly conferred entitlements varies across time and among societies. Furthermore, access to the same goods (e.g., certain foodstuffs) may be governed by the market for some social groups but by the state for others (e.g., those earning less than a specified minimum). Despite these complexities, it is possible, in almost all circumstances, to make the proposed distinction.

Within the sphere of market-based entitlements, food and housing are of special interest because of their effects on health (McKeown 1976). Among other processes, food intake involves nutrition, which conditions biological development and thus affects the structure and function of the body, including its resistance to infection. In turn, housing is represented in Figure 2-1 as a bridge between living conditions and environment, since it constitutes the immediate habitat of human beings. Moreover, while a house in good condition may be a protection against environmental risks, poor housing conditions add to deleterious environmental factors because they, too, are sources of pollution (Hardoy and Satterthwaite 1987). Among the principal elements that link housing with the environment are water supply and sanitation, which have been proposed as important determinants of health (Shuval et al. 1981; Feachem 1985).

Health effects, education and social security systems stand out among the most important publicly conferred entitlements. In particular, female education has been shown to be a critical factor in child health, although the precise mechanism through which this effect is exerted remains a matter of debate (Caldwell 1979; Ware 1984; Caldwell and Caldwell 1985; United Nations 1985; Cleland and van Ginneken 1988; Grosse and Auffrey 1989; LeVine et al. in this volume). With respect to formal social security systems, it is convenient, for the purposes of this article, to distinguish them from health care services, even though in many countries a single institution may be responsible for both. Strictly speaking, social security services refer to benefits that assure minimum levels of economic and social well-being. They include social insurance services, considered as economic and social fringe benefits for workers who pay premiums, as well as social assistance services for vulnerable persons who are not required to pay.

Apart from being a means for redistributing access to certain goods and services, publicly conferred entitlements also have economic, political, and ideological value. In an economic sense, they represent a means for the survival of large sectors of the population. They also have political value in a double sense: on the one hand, they are the object of demands by social groups; on the other, they are means to exercise political control. In this last sense, the ideological value of entitlements must also be understood as a way of legitimizing a social system. These multiple values explain, at least in part, the unequal character of publicly conferred entitlements in many countries, which often contradicts the declared universality of access to them. Hence these entitlements — notably social security — have been mainly directed towards groups involved in the formal sector of the economy, where the aforementioned values can be more effectively realized.

As indicated earlier, the summation of market-based and publicly conferred entitlements defines the total set of goods and services to which a person has access, thus determining living conditions. Through the mediation of family structure and dynamics, living conditions in turn affect the next proximate determinant of health status: lifestyles. Lifestyles are also directly affected by culture and ideology, as well as laws, regulations, taxes, subsidies, and the pressures of commercial enterprises (though these relationships are not portrayed in Figure 2-1 for reasons of simplification). As Coreil et al. (1985) have argued, the notion of lifestyle has gained wide currency in the health field without an adequate conceptual analysis. The most common usage reduces its meaning to specific individual behaviors that are interpreted as risk factors. This usage does not take proper account of the sociocultural context of behavior, which was central to the original sociological meaning of lifestyle. Coreil et al. (1985) propose that this concept be applied to behaviors that are shared by a social group in a specific context. In this sense, it represents a conceptual bridge between cultural and behavioral patterns.

In accordance with this broader perspective, Figure 2-1 makes a fundamental distinction between living conditions and lifestyles. The former refer to the objective material situation in which the different social groups exist; the latter represent the manner in which those social groups translate their objective situation into patterns of behavior. Therefore, living conditions generate what could be called "social risks", while lifestyles produce "behavioral risks". Considered as a whole, both define the quality of life. Undoubtedly, an exhaustive conceptual development will require an operationalization of the categories of living conditions and lifestyles. However, for the time being, it suffices to establish their position in the determination of health status.

Up to this point, our analytical scheme has defined different kinds of risks that are generated throughout the determination chain. As we pointed out previously, the concept of risk has a central role in our frame of reference. Indeed, a dynamic conception cannot be restricted to visualizing an ideal state of health and a state of disease as the two extremes of a continuum (Terris 1975); instead, it must incorporate the various gradations within the continuum, that is, the risk levels. It can be postulated that the complex interaction among basic, structural, and proximate determinants (Figure 2-2) defines a whole spectrum of risk levels.

Since the concept of risk indicates a certain probability of suffering a loss of health, it necessarily refers to population groups, which offer the denominators for estimating probabilities. At a given moment, a high-risk situation may experience a change of state and bring about a health loss. It is in this step between risk and loss that the individual dimension of health is realized. Indeed, the population attribute of risk is translated, at the individual level, into a corresponding attribute that might be called "susceptibility" to disease agents. As Figure 2-1 shows, susceptibility is a phenomenon where working conditions, living conditions, and lifestyles, determined by social processes, converge with body structure and function, determined by biological processes. Susceptibility is also a product of the interaction between the internal and the external milieux, the balance of which determines health, according to Dubos (1959) and other advocates of the ecological conception. Thus, the transformation of the environment by human beings generates pollution, understood in a broad sense as the presence of biological, chemical, and physical agents that may act upon susceptible individuals and potentially produce disease. It should be noted that this broad definition of pollution includes not only the active introduction of disease agents into the environment as a result of human activity, but also the failure to remove agents that occur naturally.

In summary, health status is the final result of the balance between exposure to disease agents and individual susceptibility resulting from a complex network of risks; this, in turn, is the product of an articulated set of social and biological determinants. The rich topic of health status measurement is beyond the scope of this article; for three successive reviews, see Donabedian 1973:136-192; Bergner & Rothman 1987; Schlaepfer and Infante 1990. A related topic refers to the social and individual perceptions about the set of human experiences included in the domain of health, as well as the thresholds that mark the limits of normality (Riley 1990; Murray and Chen in this volume). Despite the importance of these issues for a thorough understanding of health status, they are not discussed here; it is sufficient to mention that health status, like risks, manifests itself in various degrees that range from positive health, a concept including bio-psychic development and well-being, to death. In between are various states that include uncomplicated disease and temporary or permanent disability.

We also do not enter into the debate on the relative importance of the previously described factors and the health care system as determinants of health levels (Caldwell 1986; Frenk-Mora 1988). In any event, every society has various means to intervene at different points of the determination process; that is, the transformation of determinants, risk modification, reduction of individual susceptibility, and repair of a health loss. The relative importance, effectiveness, and efficiency of the interventions targeted at each of these points depend on various economic, political, scientific, cultural, and ideological conditions. Indeed, Figure 2-1 shows that the health care system is mainly a product of the interaction among the spheres that we have termed structural determinants (Frenk and Donabedian 1987). Clearly, a complete picture of the health care system cannot be limited to this aggregate level of determination, but must also analyse the organizational arrangements and the set of behaviors, both of people and of providers, that define the physical and cultural accessibility of the system. In addition, a thorough account should include informal and traditional forms of practice. Such a detailed analysis of the health care system falls, however, outside the limits of our present purpose, which concentrates on determinants.

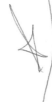

In a feedback loop of determination, the health care system may, in its turn, influence: (1) the basic and structural determinants, by family planning, environmental health services, and, still incipiently, genetic counselling; (2) the proximate determinants, by means of occupational health services and health promotion; (3) individual susceptibility, through preventive actions in a restricted sense, such as vaccinations, and (4) health status, once it has been determined, through diagnostic and therapeutic services.

The complete set of processes included in our theoretical framework can be summarized as portrayed in Figure 2-2. A fundamental element of the framework is that, as shown on the left side of this figure, five analytical levels can be distinguished: systemic, societal, institutional, household, and individual. The systemic and societal levels correspond to the basic and structural determinants respectively. In turn, the proximate determinants can be analyzed at two levels: the social institutions that give them an organizational expression and the family processes that articulate their expression in the household (DaVanzo & Gertler 1989). Finally, health status is defined, as mentioned earlier, at the individual level. From top to bottom, each analytical level "explains", or sets the limits of variability of the factors operating at the level below; from bottom to top, "explanations" of elements at each level (or the limits of actual existing alternatives) have to be sought through the characteristics and operation of factors from the levels above.

This figure should be seen simply as a schematic device to portray the notion of hierarchical multicausality that underlies our theoretical framework. The figure does not suggest that the higher analytical levels are intrinsically more important or complex than the lower ones. On the contrary, many of the breakthroughs in explaining and improving health status will come from a better understanding of the subtle interactions operating at the institutional, household, and individual levels. Furthermore, our formulation does not imply a unidirectional flow of determination. While the solid arrows in Figure 2-2 do postulate a dominant direction of determination, the dotted arrows illustrate the existence of important feedbacks.

The frame of reference that has been developed here still requires much further elaboration. Nevertheless, it allows us to appreciate the complex determination of health processes and to identify areas for future research. This framework also provides the basis to understand the mechanisms for change, which constitute the next element in articulating a theory of the epidemiologic transition.

Mechanisms

As indicated earlier, health status is expressed at the individual level, its aggregation defines the epidemiological profile of a population, and the long-term change in such a profile constitutes the epidemiologic transition. Having specified the determinants of individual health status, a theory of the transition must also account for the mechanisms that drive change at the aggregate level.

Three major mechanisms are involved in the epidemiologic transition (Mosley et al. 1990). Each of them also refers to long-term transformations. They are: fertility decline, which alters the age structure; changes in risk factors, which affect the incidence of diseases, and improvements in health care technology and organization, which modify case-fatality rates.

Fertility decline. This process, which is part of the demographic transition, involves a shift from a situation in which fertility is dominated by natural and biological factors, to another in which fertility is controlled to a large extent by the decisions of couples.

As a result of reductions in fertility, societies fundamentally change their age structures. From a distribution biased towards young ages, they move to one in which adults predominate. Earlier in the demographic transition, the absolute number of adults increases as a result of population growth caused by a decrease in mortality combined with high fertility. Subsequently, when the latter declines, the adult population continues growing because of the aging of persons born under the past conditions of high fertility. At the same time, the relative preponderance of adults becomes evident, since the decline of fertility causes the number of new persons in the youngest ages to be smaller than would be the case with higher fertility.

In epidemiological terms, the result of this process is an increase in the absolute number and the proportion of persons exposed to non-communicable diseases, such as cardiovascular problems and cancer. Thus, even with constant age-specific incidence rates, the absolute volume of patients and deaths resulting from this type of disease increases substantially. Moreover, the total number of deaths also rises as a result of the new age structure. (For empirical support for this phenomenon with data from Mexico and other countries, see Bobadilla, Frenk et al. 1990 and Mosley et al. 1990.)

Changes in risk factors. Unlike the previous, this mechanism acts primarily on the probabilities of becoming ill, that is, on the incidence of diseases. According to our analytical framework, the underlying force in the modification of such probabilities is the change in the various types of risks: biological, environmental, occupational, social, and behavioral (Figure 2-1).

Many of those changes are associated with the process of modernization. A detailed analysis of its social, economic and cultural dimensions
is beyond the scope of this article, but mention should be made of the
manifestations of modernization that most significantly influence health
risks. Overall, they include the shift from a society dominated by
agricultural production to one in which industrial production predomi-
nates, which also implies a notable increase in productivity. Closely
related is the change in population distribution, from rural to predominantly urban settlements. These socioeconomic changes have occurred
parallel with two cultural transformations: the expansion of education,
which provides access to a minimum level of schooling common to most
members of society; and the increased participation of women in the
labor force, which is related to profound modifications in the dynamics
of families and communities. An important condition accompanying
these changes is the average improvement in nutrition, housing, water
supply, and sanitation, which significantly decreases health risks (McKeown
1976; Evans et al. 1981).

From the point of view of the epidemiologic transition, most
economic, social, and cultural changes usually associated with modernization have a double face: some help to reduce the incidence of
infectious diseases and of problems related to reproduction, others
generate an increase of non-communicable diseases and injury. For
example, the introduction of basic urban infrastructure and the adoption
of hygienic measures considerably reduce the incidence of infections.
Also, the acceptance of effective contraceptive methods, which is
associated with the increased participation of women in the labor force,
not only decreases fertility levels, but also alters reproduction patterns,
for example, by extending birth intervals. There is evidence that these
modified patterns influence maternal and neonatal survival by reducing
exposure to high risk pregnancies (Fortney 1987; Bobadilla, Schlaepfer
and Alagon 1990).

But not all aspects of modernization have a positive effect on health.
The working and living conditions of many urban dwellers produce a
high incidence of injuries. Similarly, the adoption of certain patterns of
consumption and behavior increase the overall risk of becoming ill and
dying. For instance, Berkman and Breslow (1983) have demonstrated
that individuals who smoke cigarettes, drink alcohol excessively, are
overweight, do not get enough exercise, and get little sleep, have
increased probabilities of dying prematurely. The practical importance

of these findings is that, far from considering the rise of non-communicable diseases a sign of "progress", less developed countries should now start adopting preventive strategies that obviate the repetition of the negative experiences observed in industrialized nations (Soberon, Frenk and Sepúlveda 1986).

Improvement in case-fatality rates. Several changes have occurred in the quantity, distribution, organization, and quality of health services that have contributed to the epidemiologic transition. Mainly during the past century, medical research and technological development have resulted in major advances for the effective management of many diseases, both infectious and non-communicable. An important part of improved survival is due to the decrease in case-fatality rates achieved by the application of effective diagnostic and therapeutic technologies.

Therapeutic interventions, such as the treatment of pulmonary tuberculosis with specific drugs, acute respiratory infections with antibiotics or acute diarrhea with oral rehydration salts, do not modify the probability of becoming ill, except insofar as early treatment reduces the risk of spreading the disease to others in the population. The main effect of therapeutic interventions is to diminish the probability of death among those who are already ill. In the case of chronic diseases, this type of intervention actually produces the paradoxical effect of increasing the absolute morbidity level by extending the average duration of the disease (Donabedian 1973:154-155; Gruenberg 1977; Riley 1990). In contrast, primary preventive interventions, such as immunization, do act on the probability of becoming ill. In any event, the main effect of both types of intervention in underdeveloped countries has been a reduced proportion of deaths caused by infectious and parasitic diseases, thus contributing to the initial stages of the epidemiologic transition. In more advanced stages of the transition, technological innovations may produce a decrease in the case-fatality rates or even, although less commonly, in the incidence of some non-communicable diseases. Together with other factors, this may result in an epidemiological pattern that Olshansky and Ault (1986) characterize as the postponement of deaths caused by degenerative diseases.

The diversity of modalities that each of the three mechanisms may assume in different historical contexts explains why the epidemiologic transition is not a uniform process in every nation or region. Indeed, the characteristics of each mechanism, as well as their interrelationships, establish important differences in the epidemiological dynamics of a country. This poses the need for careful study of the specific attributes of such dynamics.

Attributes

Among the main attributes that characterize different epidemiologic transition experiences are the patterns of change, the pace and direction of changes, the sequence of stages, the starting moment, and the distribution of health profiles among different groups.

Basic patterns of change. Beyond its various manifestations, the epidemiologic transition always includes three fundamental change processes in the configuration of a population health profile: patterns of mortality, morbidity, and disability. Such changes refer to the composition of cause-specific mortality, the age structure of mortality, and the relative weight of morbidity versus mortality in the epidemiological situation.

First, the mortality decline that accompanies the start of the transition is selectively concentrated on infectious diseases, which thereby tend to be displaced by noncommunicable diseases, injuries, and recognized mental illnesses. Second, the burden of death and diseases shifts from the younger to the older groups. As mentioned above, this process is due primarily to two mechanisms: a decline in the incidence and case-fatality rates of infectious diseases, which benefits mainly the young population, since infections are more frequent and severe among them; and a change in the age structure of the population resulting from the demographic transition, which generates a higher proportion of adults. The third direction is the change from a health picture dominated by mortality to one where morbidity is the predominant force. Indeed, the epidemiologic transition implies a profound transformation in the social meaning of disease. Instead of being something acute, from which one either recovers or dies, disease becomes a chronic, frequently stigmatizing condition, with increasing psychological, social, and economic burdens. Assuming that these three patterns are in fact the basic processes in the epidemiologic transition, it is important to ask when they start, how fast they progress, and whether or not their progression varies among different social strata.

Stages or eras of the epidemiologic transition. The original theoretical formulations of the epidemiologic transition envisaged a progression of ages or stages. According to Frederiksen (1969) the predominant patterns of morbidity, mortality, and fertility, as well as the organization of health care, correspond to four "stages" of society: "traditional", "early transitional", "late transitional", and "modern". Omran (1971) identifies three sequential ages: "pestilence and famine", "receding pandemics", and "degenerative and man-made diseases". Similarly, Lerner (1973) presents three stages, which he calls "low vitality", "increasing control over mortality, and "broadened conception of health". Later authors (e.g., Olshansky and Ault 1986, Rogers and Hackenberg 1987) have proposed additional stages.

The usefulness of these classifications is limited, since they tend to create a linear and unidirectional view of the transition. In a previous work (Frenk, Bobadilla et al. 1989), we have suggested that, at least in the case of middle-income countries, this view should be modified regarding the next four attributes.

Direction of change. The fundamental attributes of the epidemiologic transition are limited to the three change patterns already described. Beyond that, it seems incorrect to assume that change must always occur smoothly and in one direction. In fact, a reversal of trends may occur. The most outstanding example is the emergence of AIDS, a viral disease. Also, there may be relapses of infections that had been previously controlled, such as malaria and dengue fever. In other words, small or large "counter-transitions" may take place.

Sequence of stages. The sequence of stages described by earlier authors could suggest that each era is clearly separated from the one preceding it. In reality, several periods or stages may overlap. For instance, the decline of infectious diseases may be slow or even stagnant among important population strata, while non-communicable diseases may be increasing rapidly in another segment of the same population, thus causing an "overlap of stages."

Starting point and pace. In his seminal article, Omran (1971) recognizes that there may be different transition models. He specifically proposes three: the "classical or Western model", characteristic of Europe and North America; the "accelerated model", illustrated by Japan; and the "contemporary or delayed model", typical of some developing societies such as Sri Lanka and Chile. The criteria used in this classification are the historical time at which the transition starts and the pace at which each country goes through the stages. What Omran has done is to select the starting point and the velocity of the epidemiologic transition in Western

Europe as the standard for comparison. The experiences of other countries are then labelled according to their differences from the European standard. Such an approach is justified for the purposes of defining the starting point and the pace of the transition. These two attributes are necessary but not sufficient to characterize the nature of the epidemiologic transition in a country. In addition, other attributes of the transition should be analyzed, including the direction of change, the sequence of stages, and the distribution of health conditions among population groups.

Distribution of epidemiological profiles. What has happened, and is still happening in many societies, is that the three basic change patterns described above proceed at different rates among the different social strata and regions of a country (Possas 1989). For example, if changes are slower among the poor than the rich, then the former will necessarily have a higher incidence of infectious diseases affecting their larger proportion of the young population. An "epidemiological polarization" is thus produced, which, as pointed out at the beginning of this article, worsens health inequalities.

The summation of all the analyzed attributes suggests that, together with the models described by Omran, a "protracted and polarized" transition model seems to be appearing in recent years, in which the overlap of stages persists during a long period of time and the social distribution of changes is very heterogeneous among social groups (Frenk, Frejka et al. 1989). In any event, it is clear that the dynamics of epidemiological change vary substantially among and within countries. For this reason, Murray and Chen (in this volume) suggest the need to use the plural in referring to the varied health transitions.

Consequences

The growing complexity of the health field is highlighted by the intricate effects that the epidemiologic transition has on its own determinants. Thus, the demographic processes that contribute to the epidemiologic transition are themselves accentuated by further changes in age structure and population growth rates caused by that transition. There are also important economic consequences derived from shifting health conditions, such as the effects on labor force productivity, retirement allowance plans, and medical care costs. The protracted and polarized transition model has social effects as well, since it aggravates the inequality from which it originated. In addition, the dependency burden shifts from children to the old and from the family to the corporation and the state.

Of course, the epidemiologic transition has (or should have) a profound effect on the health care system. The emergence of non-communicable diseases usually aggravates the pressure on more complex services, such as hospitals. The growing demand for more specialized human resources and more elaborate technologies, which are not necessarily more effective, tends to increase costs. The epidemiological polarization is then more likely to produce a competition for the definition of priorities among types of pathology and for the corresponding allocation of resources (Evans et al. 1981). In order to manage the conflicts that may result, it is necessary to develop innovative service models that use the epidemiologic transition as a guide to achieve a corresponding health care transition (Bobadilla, Frenk et al. 1993).

Conclusion

This article has attempted to develop some of the building blocks for a theory of the health transition. These blocks find their foundation in the original formulations of the theory, but attempt to take them one step further by specifying the concepts, determinants, mechanisms, attributes, and consequences of the transition.

Three major tasks seem to lie ahead for further theoretical advances. The first one is to elaborate with greater detail each of the building blocks that we have presented here. In particular, there is need to give more analytical attention to the consequences of the epidemiologic transition, including the precise feedback mechanisms through which it affects its own determinants and the manner in which it interacts with the health care transition. The second task is probably the most difficult, since it involves connecting the building blocks among themselves in order to develop a real theory from which to derive propositions that may be subject to empirical verification. Even in the absence of such connections, it is necessary to move forward along the third task: increasing our empirical knowledge about actual transition experiences. This endeavor requires an important amount of new research, which should adopt a comparative perspective, both in the diachronic dimension of analyzing each country through time, and in the cross-national dimension of contrasting a number of countries with different social, economic, political, and cultural conditions. In defining a research agenda, particular attention should be given to the subnational level, so that social and regional inequalities in health may be better documented. In addition, the quest for valid findings makes it mandatory to address the issues of the varying cultural definitions about health and of the quality of historical and contemporary information.

Simultaneous progress in these three tasks would help to build a more solid theory, which could provide conceptual guidance to the renewed interest in the health transition. We are still far from having the level of theoretical development demanded by the complexity of our object of analysis. Nevertheless, there is no doubt that we are in a field with the potential of transforming our ways of thinking about and acting upon health.

Acknowledgments

This article originally appeared in *Health Transition Review,* 1991, 1 (1): 21–38. Earlier versions were presented at the following meetings: Health Priorities Review, organized by the World Bank, Puebla, Mexico, 20 January 1990; IV National Meeting on Demographic Research, organized by the Mexican Society for Demography, Mexico City, 25 April 1990; International Symposium 'Evolution and Revolution in Health', organized by El Colegio Nacional and the National Institute of Public Health, Mexico City, 9 July 1990. We are grateful to Avedis Donabedian, Fernando Cortés, Catalina Denman, W. Henry Mosley, Brian Abel-Smith, Lincoln Chen, David Bell, Dean Jamison, and Carlos Cruz for their valuable comments on the manuscript. The responsibility for the content remains solely with the authors.

References

Almeida, N. 1989. *Epidemiología sem Numeros. Una Introducción Crítica a Ciencia Epidemiológica.* Rio de Janeiro: Campus.

Bergner, M., and M.L. Rothman. 1987. "Health status measures: An overview and guide for selection." *Annual Review of Public Health,* 8: 191–210.

Berkman, L.F., and L. Breslow. 1983. *Health and Ways of Living: The Alameda County Study.* New York: Oxford University Press.

Bobadilla, J.L., J. Frenk, T. Frejka, R. Lozano, and C. Stem. 1993. "The epidemiologic transition and health priorities." In D.T. Jamison, W.H. Mosley, A.R. Measham, and J. Bobadilla, eds. *Disease Control Priorities in Developing Countries.* New York: Oxford University Press..

Bobadilla, J.L., L. Schlaepfer, and J. Alagón. 1990. *Family Formation Patterns and Child Mortality in Mexico*. Population Council and Institute for Resources Development. New York: Macro Systems.

Breilh, J. 1986. *Epidemiología, Economía, Medicina y Política*. Mexico: Fontamara.

Briggs, A. 1961. "The welfare state in historical perspective." *European Journal of Sociology,* 2: 221–258.

Caldwell, J.C. 1979. "Education as a factor in mortality decline: An examination of Nigerian data." *Population Studies,* 33: 395–413.

Caldwell, J.C. 1986. "Routes to low mortality in poor countries." *Population and Development Review,* 12: 171–220.

Caldwell, J.C. 1990. "Introductory thoughts on health transition." In Caldwell, J.C., S. Findley, P. Caldwell, G. Santow, W. Cosford, J. Braid, and D. Broers-Freeman. 1990. *What We Know About the Health Transition: The Cultural, Social and Behavioural Determinants of Health, Health Transition Series,* No. 2, Vol. 1. Canberra: Health Transition Centre, Australian National University.

Caldwell, J.C., and P. Caldwell. 1985. "Education and literacy as factors in health." In S.B. Halstead, J.A. Walsh, K.S. Warren, eds. 1985. *Good Health at Low Cost.* New York: Rockefeller Foundation.

Caldwell, J.C., S. Findley, P. Caldwell, G. Santow, W. Cosford, J. Braid, and D. Broers-Freeman. 1990. *What We Know About the Health Transition: The Cultural, Social and Behavioural Determinants of Health, Health Transition Series,* No. 2, Volumes 1 and 2. Canberra: Health Transition Centre, Australian National University.

Cleland, J.G., and J. van Ginneken. 1988. "Maternal education and child survival in developing countries: The search for pathways of influence." *Social Science and Medicine,* 27: 1357–1368.

Coreil, J., J.S. Levin, and G. Jaco. 1985. "Life style – an emergent concept in the sociomedical sciences." *Culture, Medicine and Psychiatry,* 9: 423–437.

Cornia, G.A. 1987. "Economic decline and human welfare in the first half of the 1980s." In G.A. Cornia, R. Jolly, and F. Stewart, eds. *Adjustment with a Human Face. Vol.1: Protecting the Vulnerable and Promoting Growth.* Oxford: Clarendon Press.

DaVanzo, J., and P. Gertler. 1989. "Household production of health: A microeconomic perspective of health transitions." Paper presented at the Health Transition Workshop on Measurement of Health Transition Concepts. London.

Donabedian, A. 1973. *Aspects of Medical Care Administration: Specifying Requirements for Health* Care. Cambridge, MA: Harvard University Press.

Dubos, R. 1959. *Mirage of Health: Utopias, Progress and Biological Change.* New York: Harper and Row.

Evans, J.R., K.L. Hall, and J. Warford. 1981. "Shattuck lecture—Health care in the developing world: Problems of scarcity and choice." *New England Journal of Medicine*, 305: 1117–1127.

Feachem, R.G. 1985. "The role of water supply and sanitation in reducing mortality in China, Costa Rica, Kerala State (India) and Sri Lanka." In S.B. Halstead, J.A. Walsh, and K.S. Warren, eds. *Good Health at Low Cost*. New York: Rockefeller Foundation.

Fortney, J.A. 1987. "The importance of family planning in reducing maternal mortality." *Studies in Family Planning*, 5: 109–115.

Frederiksen, H. 1969. "Feedbacks in economic and demographic transition." *Science*, 166: 837–847.

Frenk, J., J.L. Bobadilla, J. Sepúlveda, and M. López-Cervantes. 1989. "Health transition in middle income countries: New challenges for health care." *Health Policy and Planning*, 4: 29–39.

Frenk, J., and A. Donabedian. 1987. "State intervention in medical care: Types, trends and variables." *Health Policy and Planning*, 2: 17–31.

Frenk, J., T. Frejka, J.L. Bobadilla, C. Stern, J. Sepúlveda, and M.V. José. 1989. "The epidemiologic transition in Latin America." In *International Population Conference, New Delhi*, Vol.1, Liege:International Union for the Scientific Study of Population.

Frenk-Mora, J. 1988. "Morbimortalidad, sistema de salud y Estado." In M. Bronfman and J. Gómez-de León, eds. *La Mortalidad en México: Niveles, Tendencias y Determinantes*. México: El Colegio de México.

Fuenzalida-Puelma, H.L., and S. Scholle-Connor, eds. 1989. *El Derecho a la Salud en las Americas: Estudio Constitucional Comparado*. Washington, DC: Pan American Health Organization.

Grosse, R.N., and C. Auffrey. 1989. "Literacy and health status in developing countries." *Annual Review of Public Health*, 10: 281–297.

Gruenberg, E.M. 1977. "The failures of success." *Milbank Memorial Fund Quarterly*, 55: 3–24.

Halstead, S.B., J.A. Walsh, and K.S. Warren, eds. 1985. *Good Health at Low Cost*. New York: Rockefeller Foundation.

Hardoy, J.E., and D. Satterthwaite. 1987. "Housing and health." *Cities*, August: 221–235.

Last, J. 1983. *Dictionary of Epidemiology*. New York: Oxford Medical Publications.

Lerner, M. 1973. "Modernization and health: A model of the health transition." Paper presented at the annual meeting of the American Public Health Association, San Francisco, November.

MacMahon, B., and T. Pugh. 1970. *Epidemiology, Principles and Methods.* Boston: Little Brown.

McKeown, T. 1976. *The Modern Rise of Population.* London: Edward Arnold.

Mosley, W.H., and L.C. Chen. 1984. "An analytical framework for the study of child survival in developing countries." In W.H. Mosley and L.C. Chen, eds. *Child Survival: Strategies for Research.* A supplement to Volume 10 of *Population and Development Review.*

Mosley, W.H., D.T. Jamison, and D.A. Henderson. 1990. "The health sector in developing countries: Prospects for the 1990s and beyond." *Annual Review of Public Health,* 11: 335–358.

Olshansky, S.J., and A.B. Ault. 1986. "The fourth stage of the epidemiologic transition: The age of delayed degenerative diseases." *Milbank Memorial Fund Quarterly,* 64: 355–391.

Omran, A.R. 1971. "The epidemiologic transition: A theory of the epidemiology of population change." *Milbank Memorial Fund Quarterly,* 49: 509–538.

Omran, A.R. 1982. "Epidemiologic transition. l. Theory." In J. Ross, ed. *International Encyclopedia of Population.* New York: Free Press.

Omran, A.R. 1983. "The epidemiologic transition theory. A preliminary update." *Journal of Tropical Pediatrics,* 29: 305–316.

Possas, C. 1989. *Epidemiologia e Sociedade: Heterogeneidade Estrutural e Saude no Brasil.* Sao Paulo: Hucitec.

Riley, J.C. 1990. Long-term morbidity and mortality trends: Inverse health transitions." In J.C. Caldwell, S. Findley, P. Caldwell, G. Santow, W. Cosford, J. Braid, and D. Broers-Freeman. 1990. *What We Know About the Health Transition: The Cultural, Social and Behavioural Determinants of Health, Health Transition Series,* No. 2, Vol. 1. Canberra: Health Transition Centre, Australian National University.

Rogers, R.C., and R. Hackenberg. 1987. "Extending epidemiologic transition theory: A new stage." *Social Biology,* 34: 234–243.

Rothman, K. 1986. *Modern Epidemiology.* Boston: Little Brown.

San Martin, H. 1985. *Crisis Mundial de la Salud.* Barcelona: Ciencia.

Schlaepfer, L., and C. Infante. 1990. "La medición de salud." *Salud Pública de México,* 32: 141–152.

Sen, A. 1981. *Poverty and Famines: An Essay on Entitlement and Deprivation.* Oxford: Clarendon Press.

Shuval, H.I., R.L. Tilden, B.H. Perry, and R.N. Grosse. 1981. "Effects of investments in water supply and sanitation on health status: A threshold-saturation theory." *Bulletin of the World Health Organization,* 59: 243–248.

Soberón, G., J. Frenk, and J. Sepúlveda. 1986. "The health care reform in Mexico: Before and after the 1985 earthquakes." *American Journal of Public Health,* 76: 673–680.

Terris, M. 1975. "Approaches to an epidemiology of health." *American Journal of Public Health,* 65: 1037–1045.

United Nations, Department of International Social and Economic Affairs. 1985. *Socio-Economic Differentials in Child Mortality in Developing Countries.* New York: United Nations.

Ware, H. 1984. "Effects of maternal education, women's roles, and child care on child mortality." In W. H. Mosley and L.C. Chen, eds. *Child Survival: Strategies for Research.* A supplement to Volume 10 of *Population and Development Review.*

WHO/UNICEF. 1978. *Primary Health Care: Report of the International Conference on Primary Health Care,* Alma Ata, USSR, 6–12 September. World Health Organization, Geneva.

3

Social and Behavioral Pathologies

Jonathan A. Sugar
Arthur Kleinman
Kris Heggenhougen

The dominant forces in international health have traditionally been the public health administrators and physicians with expertise in infectious disease, epidemiology, and organizational development. Impressive gains have been made with respect to diarrhea, malaria, hepatitis, schistosomiasis, tuberculosis, leprosy, and other ailments, although in some regions of the world (sub-Saharan Africa and India, for example), the burden of communicable disease remains high. We would like to add the voices of anthropologists and psychiatrists to those of the experts named above. The anthropologic perspective encourages us to question what the experiential human problems are in the health domain of international development, and permits a focus on forms of suffering that have been traditionally left out of discussions in public health and economic development. Our position is also that mental health concerns of psychiatrists and psychologists are central to health and social change, but such concerns have not been addressed adequately in the past. Our aim is to provide an overview of this area, address the epidemiology of psychiatric and behavioral conditions in developing countries, relate these problems to an anthropological perspective on social and economic development, and then briefly explore policy implications. We see our chapter as pointing towards an emergent international mental health policy agenda that we believe will become, in the 1990s, a major component of global health policy.

"Social and Behavioral Pathologies" is loose terminology that refers to behaviors with general health status implications (such as nicotine addiction, alcohol abuse, and illicit drug use), major mental illnesses (schizophrenia, affective illness, and a spectrum of anxiety disorders), behavioral manifestations of other illnesses (such as epilepsy and HIV related mental status changes) and problems in the life cycle with behavioral presentations (such as mental retardation, attention deficit disorder, and dementia). Other "disorders" that accompany social change, urbanization, and economic development will also be discussed, such as hypertension, cardiovascular disease, and overall vulnerability and resistance to disease (Berkman and Syme 1979; Marmot and Syme 1976). Included also is the seemingly associated increase in suicide rates (Rubinstein 1987). The resurgence of racism and ethnic conflict as behavioral problems with significant negative health status implications must also be noted (Heggenhougen and Shore 1986).

Economic development, rapid urbanization, and attendant social and political transformations bring with them changes in the epidemiology and ecology of health and disease. There is a predictable shift in morbidity towards "noncommunicable diseases" as countries undergo modernization (Litvak et al. 1987). Alcoholism, drug abuse, and violence become major health and social problems as traditionally oriented populations modernize (Kleinman 1988a), and there are clear and direct health status consequences from such changes. Inter-ethnic violence, social upheaval, forced uprooting and urban migration accompany modernization in many contexts, and have serious mental health consequences (Caplan 1989; House et al. 1988; Kinzie et al. 1984; Kleinman 1986; Mollica et al. 1990; Nguyen 1982a; Nguyen 1982b).

The direct impact of behavior on health status has been shown in several studies: childhood mortality is highly associated with changes in maternal behavior, educational level, and the social autonomy of women (Caldwell 1979; Caldwell 1986). Eisenberg (1986) has shown how recreational, dietary and water use patterns affect the spread of schistosomiasis; and Rosenfeld (1988) and Sawyer (1986) describe how settlers in Brazil have chosen to risk malaria and not use prophylactic measures, in order to better their economic lot. AIDS is, of course, the most dramatic current example of the health consequence of certain behaviors. Care must be taken, however, in how the term "behavioral pathology" is applied.

House et al. (1988) conclude from meta-analysis of major epidemiological studies that weak attachment networks are associated with increased risk of disease and death. Such "webs" of attachment are also crucial in mediating the social and personal effects of disaster and loss. While urbanization, industrialization, and other aspects of social transformation carry increased risks of such upheaval, the population shifts created by such changes often attenuate these attachment networks.

There is a dearth of international mental health policy to guide development endeavors, reflecting little knowledge among international health experts of the extent of psychiatric and behavioral conditions, and the implications for medical care systems, in industrializing countries. Economic development may bring with it significant changes in the incidence and presentation of mental illness, its consequences, and the demands made on the medical care systems of the developing world. "Economic development" may not be synonymous with "social development," in terms of improved quality of life and social welfare, as is often assumed. There is a great need for increased scrutiny of economic development projects, often legitimized as improving social conditions, to determine if they will indeed socially benefit a significant portion of a population rather than simply benefit an elite minority (Agbonifo 1983; Morris and Liser 1978). Any development, of course, implies change, which if too drastic, has negative effects. Care must be taken in the examination of where so-called "development" is headed, the social and behavioral consequences that might ensue from a given project, and, in turn, the health consequences that may result. Indeed, counter to the conclusions drawn by most international health experts, from the anthropological and mental health perspectives there is sufficient evidence of the untoward effects of development on human conditions to warrant concern about the routinely negative personal and group mental health outcomes associated with the current pace and direction of social change worldwide.

Behavioral Conditions Affecting Health Status

As noted above, Litvak and others have shown that there is a predictable progression in overall morbidity to the many diseases of behavior and aging as one looks at countries at different stages in the process of development. Thus, the significant health problems of North America and Western Europe are noncommunicable conditions such as cardiovascular disease, cancer, and fatal injury. Indeed, violent death might profitably be considered an "infectious" disease of developing and certain developed societies alike. Homicide ranks high as the cause of death in developing countries such as Mozambique and El Salvador, and violence is endemic in many countries in Central and South America. The social conditions that invite such "infectious violence" demand elucidation, however, and must be considered in development schemes.

Table 3-1 Cigarette Use

Increases in per capita production and consumption:
1979 – 1983 (Nath 1986)

Kenya	20%
Algeria	25%
Egypt	45%
Indonesia	32%
China	>45%

While the current morbidity experience of Latin American countries is quite different from that of North America, the longitudinal view suggests that these countries are going to face a similar demographic and epidemiologic picture in the future (Litvak et al. 1987). East and Southeast Asian societies, and a number of African countries as well, are headed in the same direction of rising rates of heart disease, diabetes, and cancer. Smoking (with attendant nicotine addiction), alcohol abuse, and illicit drug use are all on the rise in countries undergoing modernization. Indeed, these problems can now be regarded as shared across rich and poor societies, although in the United States, smoking appears to be on the wane.

Cigarette Smoking

Cigarette smoking has an established causal link with heart disease, respiratory illnesses, cancer, and complications of pregnancy; unfortunately, the prevalence of smoking in developing countries is high. The World Health Organization (WHO) notes that the U.S. tobacco industry alone spent over US$2500 million on the global promotion of tobacco products (World Health Organization 1987). The effort has been successful: data show that the per capita production and consumption of cigarettes has increased dramatically from 1979 to 1983 in Kenya (20 percent), Algeria (25 percent), Egypt (45 percent), Indonesia (32 percent), and China (>45 percent) (Nath 1986).

In China, there is a 10 percent increase in the number of cigarettes manufactured annually; over 60 percent of the men 20 years of age and older are smokers. Cardiovascular disease deaths rose by more than 250 percent from 1957 to 1984, and similar increases were seen in the death

Table 3-2 Alcoholism in Developing Countries

Site (source)	% Alcoholic or excessive drinker	Comment
Sri Lanka (Samarasinghe, 1989)	2.9%	men > 25 yrs 90% > 35 yrs
Latin America (Coombs, 1986)	(reviews rates found in studies)	adults
Brazil (urban)	10.3%	
Santiago, Chile	12.9%	
Colombia (village)	13.0%	
Costa Rica	10.2%	
Guatemala	15.0%	
Mexico City	13.5%	

rates for malignancy and stroke (Weng 1988). While successful prevention efforts have occurred in the developed world, they have not generally been undertaken in developing countries.

Alcohol Abuse

Alcohol is thought to contribute to at least 10 percent of the deaths in industrialized nations, and the increase in alcohol consumption and abuse in some less industrialized countries has been described. In addition to direct morbidity, such as alcoholic liver disease, combined system deficiency diseases, dementia, and peripheral neuropathies, the abuse of alcohol contributes to suicide, deaths by violence, and traffic fatalities.

Reviewing available data on Latin America, Coombs and Globetti (1986) state that 15 percent to 20 percent of the adults in Latin America are "excessive drinkers" or "alcoholics." Argondoña (1988) reported that over 20 percent of the men in both the rural and urban areas of one Bolivian region were intoxicated at least once a week, and that about 7 percent of the men in the urban areas were addicted to alcohol. He found that 4 percent of the women over age 31 were addicted to alcohol, posing a serious pregnancy risk to this cohort.

Marshall (1988) found that beer consumption in Papua New Guinea had doubled at least four times from 1962 to 1980. He notes that alcohol was banned for natives during colonial rule (Australia granted limited home rule in 1951; the first representative house of government was formed in 1964.) and the "right" to use alcohol was considered among the issues of freedom and independence. The consumption of alcohol was legalized in 1962. Between 1967 and 1979, there was a greater than 400 percent increase in road traffic fatalities, with alcohol being directly implicated in at least 20 percent of the accidents. A similar picture is found in the injury and death rates from the consumption of methanol, and from blunt injury trauma, and penetrating injuries, including gunshot wounds.

Rubinstein (1987) found that alcohol was implicated in almost half of the suicides recorded in Micronesia from 1960 to 1987. He notes that the period from World War II to the present has been one of extraordinary social change in Micronesia, and that alcohol plays an important role as a culturally recognized "time out" from rules of behavior, including the control of anger and quiet demeanor. Thus he posits that the use of alcohol, especially among adolescents, "permits" the angry emotional displays that frequently precede a suicide.

Alaskan native populations, which might be regarded as a developing sector in an industrialized society quite comparable to populations of non-industrialized societies, have the world's highest rate of alcohol abuse and related violence (Kraus and Buffler 1979). There are Alaskan native villages in which more than 50 percent of adults abuse alcohol. Even Chinese societies, which formerly enjoyed among the world's lowest rates of alcohol problems, are experiencing increasing rates (Lin and Lin 1982).

Illicit Drug Use

There has been an especially dramatic increase in the worldwide use of illegal drugs during the past two decades. While detailed and extensive epidemiologic data on drug use in the Third World is lacking, several studies are available (Acuda 1982; Aslam 1989; Carlini-Cotrim and Carlini 1988; Johnston 1980; Keltzer 1989; National Institute on Drug Abuse 1985; World Health Organization 1987), and the technology for even more accurate studies is at hand (Johnston 1988). Along with the increased demand for opiates in the West, the producing countries of Southeast Asia and the Mideast have developed substantial populations of heroin addicts, and have become active secondary markets. Pakistan, a particularly tragic example, has 700,000 to 1.5 million heroin addicts currently, whereas there were very small numbers in the early 1970s (Aslam 1989; Gossop 1989). The same can be said for Malaysia and Thailand.

Substantial social problems involving the recreational use of illicit drugs are being encountered in the Andean cocaine producing countries, especially among dispossessed children in urban areas (Argondoña 1988). This is distinctively different behaviorally and contextually from the traditional practice of coca chewing of Andean Indian peasants. Argondoña reports that 80 percent of the homeless children in one Bolivian city were deserted by alcoholic parents (Argondoña 1988). Solvent abuse among nine- to eighteen-year-olds in a poor area of Sao Paulo, Brazil was studied by Carlini-Cotrim and Carlini (1988), who found that nearly 24 percent of the respondents reported lifetime use of solvents and that 4 percent had used them within the past 30 days. Children's use of solvents was associated with poor academic performance, the child's being employed outside of home and school, and heavy alcohol consumption among close relatives.

The studies cited above highlight the complex interactions between "modernization" and substance use disorders. Tobacco and alcohol use may represent Western influence on behavioral patterns (note, for example, the increase of women smokers in many developing societies), increasing personal autonomy and freedom of choice, or a "break" from stress (Rubinstein 1987). Population shifts, increases in personal income, and quests for "modern lifestyles" yield new, exploitable markets for established manufacturers of alcohol, cigarettes, and illegal drugs. Such substances may also function as available palliatives for the anomie and distress accompanying the often wrenching social changes in life ways and traditions that constitute "modernization." Elsewhere, alcoholism has been linked with poverty, where drinking provides a periodic numbing effect that shuts out the harsh realities of "no hope" situations and a violent release for resentment and desperation. Alcoholism and drug addiction provide different degrees of escape, and are, in certain respects, coping mechanisms, making destructive social change tolerable. These behaviors have significantly negative outcomes — of which family violence and breakup are among the most brutal — and may thus be considered behavioral pathologies. The root of these behaviors may be more societal than individual, psychiatry's and psychology's claims notwithstanding, and it may be quite accurate to talk of the pathogenic nature of certain social changes involved in economic development. "Social pathology" is a term worth rehabilitating to describe the negative effects of modernization.

Substantial criminal organization mediates the flow of drugs from producing to consuming countries, and such organizations will also figure in the increased incomes and materially improved lives of the peasant growers. Significant government revenues derived from alcohol and tobacco taxes may interfere with aggressive anti-drinking or anti-smoking campaigns by governments (Nath 1986; Rubinstein 1987). Thus, constitutional, cultural, economic, and ultimately political influences shape modernity so as to encourage addictive behaviors while creating obstacles to its prevention.

Problems of Increased Survival

Improved survival leads to growing cohorts of children and the elderly who require more health services, including mental health services. Changes in birthing practices that lead to concomitant decreases in early childhood mortality may also lead to increased malnutrition among older children and increases in numbers of children at risk for developmental and psychiatric disorders. This is especially the case where economic and agricultural production (and distribution) do not keep up with demographic changes, including population increases. Using a two-stage procedure involving door-to-door interviews and clinical examination of children, Stein, Durkin, and Belmont estimated rates of serious mental retardation (IQ<55, with serious functional impairment) in eight developing countries (Stein et al. 1986). Among 3 to 9 year-olds they found the rate of serious mental retardation to range from 5 per 1000 in the Philippines to over 16 per 1000 in Bangladesh. Various "developed" countries under study have shown a fairly uniform rate of about 3.5 per 1000. These authors note their impression that prenatal factors are

Table 3-3 Serious Mental Retardation (IQ < 55)

(Estimated Prevalence from all causes, per 1000 pop.)
(Stein et al. 1986)

Malaysia:	11.2
Karachi, Pakistan:	15.1
(Uppsala, Sweden:	2.8)

responsible for a larger portion of serious retardation in developed countries than in the developing countries studied. This may be due to higher perinatal mortality in the developing countries, with the attendant loss of more children with congenital birth defects. It may also represent the losses due to poorer nutrition and environmental assault on children of poorer societies. The causes of such disability may be different even among developing countries due to regional differences in nutritional status, age-specific fertility rates, environmental factors such as tainted water or lead paint, habits such as smoking and drug use, the social status of women, and other factors.

Urbanization, *per se*, appears to increase the risk for behavioral disorder among children in industrializing societies (Rahim and Cederblad 1984). Childhood psychiatric and behavioral disorders affect at least 10 percent of all children, and the urban rate of childhood disorder is more than twice that of rural children (Earls 1988). Rahim and Cederblad found increased rates of childhood behavior problems, as reported by mothers in Khartoum, Sudan, in 1980 compared to 1965. The authors thought this was associated with rapid urbanization, changing urban demographics, and increasing educational pressure on children (Rahim and Cederblad 1984). Argondoña (1988) found that 80 percent of the street children in Cochabamba, Bolivia had alcoholic parents who deserted them. These children, cut off from the supportive and socializing webs of the family and community, are at high risk of exploitation and child prostitution, and often exhibit anti-social behavior. Having lost their families, they are, at least theoretically, at high risk for later depression and other psychopathology (Bowlby 1988).

Scheper-Hughes (1987) writes compellingly of the attitudes toward child survival held among recent rural migrant women of childbearing years living in an urban Brazilian shanty-town. These women spoke often of life being a struggle between the strong and weak, a constant struggle for resources and survival. The pervasiveness of this struggle affects child tending, Scheper-Hughes claims, such that selective child neglect is part of a parent's pursuit of family survival; that is, the strong children may receive selective parental attention. Nations and Rehbun (1988), studying similar subjects, challenge the idea of neglect, but demonstrate that tragically hard decisions must be made about where meager resources can be applied on behalf of sick children.

It becomes clear that the "pathological" effects of urbanization and industrialization, and the associated family structural changes, are somewhat determined by the age and developmental stage of different members of the family. The adults may increase their alcohol use and change their patterns of use, marital violence may increase, maternal depression may become more common as survival becomes more difficult, and childhood developmental and behavioral disorders may increase.

Childhood, adolescent, and young adult suicide has become a problem shared by all societies (Ganasveram et al. 1984; Rubinstein 1987; Shaffer et al. 1988). The suicide rate among white males aged 15 to 24 in the U.S. has tripled in the past 25 years, peaking at close to 30 per 100,000 at age 23 (Shaffer et al. 1988). Rubinstein's findings in Micronesia (Table 3-4) have been referred to above: looking at the same age range, the rate of suicide among men has increased since 1967 to its present overall rate of 75.4 per 100,000 for 15- to 19-year-olds and 110.6 per 100,000 for 20- to 24-year-olds (Rubinstein 1987).

As we note above, the elderly cohort is growing in developing countries, and increasing numbers of people are living long enough to be at risk for dementing illness. According to WHO, 72 percent of the world's elderly will be living in developing countries by the year 2020 (Litvak 1988). Dementing illnesses afflict between five percent and eight percent of persons over 65; the lifetime cumulative risk of dementia is 15 percent to 20 percent for those aged 80 years and older (World Health Organization 1986). Concomitantly, changes in population structure, combined with urbanization and changes in occupational and gender roles, are compromising traditional patterns of care. This aging population, moreover, has higher rates of chronic disorders and increased disability.

WHO notes that the disabled make up as much as 20 percent of the population in some developing countries (World Health Organization

---

Table 3-4 Suicide Among Young Men (per 100,000)

Site	Rate	Source
United States (age 15-25)	30	(Shaffer et al. 1988)
Micronesia (age 15-19)	75.4	(Rubinstein 1987)
Micronesia (age 20-24)	110.6	(Rubinstein 1987)

1987). Consistent with this, China reports more than 50 million seriously disabled persons, with almost one in five families affected ("First time picture of the nation's handicapped", *China Daily*, December 7, 1987, p.1). As populations are subject to industrializing economic development, industrial accidents (such as occur on poorly maintained building or road sites) may represent a growing cause, along with increased automobile accidents and nonfatal but disabling injuries (Marshall 1988). For example, in Africa and South Asia, lorry drivers with perishable produce and other goods on board may drive whole days without sleep on poorly repaired roads. The aggregate disability from their nonfatal automobile accidents stems from a congruence of factors associated with rapid social change.

These increasing cohorts, the extremes of the age spectrum and the disabled, represent a tremendous reservoir of need for social welfare and medical care services in industrializing countries. Few developing societies have the resources or institutional infrastructures to respond to this burden.

Increased survival translates into more individuals living through personally destructive social changes, and suffering the mental health consequences of the prolonged experience and witnessing of misery. As alluded to above, severe economic deprivation, ethnic conflict, forced uprooting, and forceful repression are all powerful harbingers of endemic suffering. For example, a 65-year-old man in China has lived through the Warlord Period, the Anti-Japanese War (with 20 million civilian deaths and 180 million persons displaced), the anti-counter-revolutionary campaigns of the 1950s (with one million killed), the Anti-Rightist Campaign of the late 1950s, the famine of 1960-62 (with 30 million dead), the Cultural Revolution, and the massacre at Tiananmen Square. That man has witnessed social pressures beyond the experience of most Westerners, and such pressures have been shown to have serious psychological and psychiatric consequences (Kleinman 1986). Such personal histories are likely commonplace in many parts of the developing world, such as Afghanistan, El Salvador, Vietnam, and Cambodia.

Adult Mental Disorders

The overall point prevalence of adult psychiatric disorder is about 2 percent worldwide (Carstairs 1983; Sethi 1985; World Health Organization 1987), and the lifetime prevalence is thought to be about 10 percent (World Health Organization 1987). Colin Turnbull, in 1962, illustrated the anguish among adults in a changing East African society in *The Lonely African* (Turnbull 1987). In 1963, Leighton et al. (World Health Organization 1987), found in Western Nigeria that 21 percent of respondents in villages and 31 percent in cities reported major symptoms of psychiatric morbidity. Sixteen years later, Orley and Wing (1979) found in two villages in Uganda that 24 percent of the men, and 27 percent of the women reported significant psychiatric morbidity and distress on the Present State Examination. (In suburban London, using the same instrument, they found that only 11 percent of women respondents reported symptoms of the same severity.) Hollifeld, using the Diagnostic Interview Schedule in a neighborhood survey in Lesotho, one of the poorest nations, reported that 9.8 percent of the sample met the criteria for a diagnosis of depression, 4.9 percent had generalized anxiety disorder, and 3.2 percent met diagnostic criteria for panic disorder (Hollifeld 1990). Contrary to established myths, mental illnesses are more, not less, prevalent and burdensome in settings of deep poverty.

Schizophrenia affects 2 to 10 per 1000 people in developing and developed countries (Goodwin and Guze 1989; Sartorious and Jablensky 1976) with an annual incidence of 0.7 to 1.4 in various cultures

---

Table 3-5 Adult Psychiatric Morbidity Point Prevalence

Site	Year	% Morbidity	Comment
W. Nigeria (Leighton et al. 1963)	1963	21% villagers 31% city dwellers	"with major psychiatric symptoms" (sic)
Uganda (Orley and Wing 1979)	1979	24% men 27% women	"significant" morbidity on Present State Examination
Lesotho (Hollifeld 1990)	1990	9.8% depression 4.9% generalized anxiety 3.2 % panic disorder	meeting DSM III-R criteria for diagnosis

internationally (Sartorius 1986). The point prevalence of schizophrenia in urban Chinese regions is 6.06 per 1000; in rural China it is 3.42 per 1000. With a population of 1.1 billion and an urban:rural population split of 25:75, there are about 4.5 million schizophrenic persons in China. Less than 2 percent of these persons are hospitalized, and about 90 percent live with their families, compared to about 40 percent of U. S. schizophrenics living with their families (State Statistical Bureau 1989). Based on a conservative prevalence estimate of 5 per 1000, there are about 550,000 schizophrenics in Pakistan, with its population of 110 million.[1]

The prevalence of epilepsy in the developing world ranges from 15 to 50 per 1000, in contrast to 3 to 5 per 1000 in industrialized societies (World Health Organization 1987). In addition, seizure disorders carry significant secondary morbidity from serious accidents in transitional and rural societies (Ben-Tovim 1987).

Acquired Immune Deficiency Syndrome

Acquired Immune Deficiency Syndrome (AIDS) is affecting countries in the West and Third World differently, but it is clearly of universal significance. It is now well-known that nervous system involvement and cognitive impairment occur commonly in the course of AIDS. The increasing numbers of people infected and symptomatic will include a significant proportion of individuals with neuropsychiatric and behavioral presentations, including delirium, seizures, depression, memory impairment, dementia, and psychosis.

As of July 1989, Uganda, Kenya, Tanzania, Malawi, Burundi, Zambia, Rwanda, and the Congo led the African nations in the number of reported cases, but virtually none of the African states were untouched by the disease; the United States, Brazil, Canada, Mexico, and Haiti led the American countries; Sudan, Tunisia, Morocco, Qatar, and Lebanon had the most cases in the eastern Mediterranean region; and the Southeast Asian and Western Pacific states (except Australia) reported the fewest cases overall (World Health Organization 1989). There has, however, been a recent upsurge in reported cases in this region; for example, in Thailand, there were only 8 reported cases of AIDS in 1986, compared with almost 15,000 reported in early 1989 (Smith 1990).

In many cases, mental and behavioral changes are the first signs of the disease, and caregivers in developing and developed countries alike must be prepared to recognize and respond appropriately. This clearly represents an increased demand on health care delivery systems of epidemic proportions. HIV infection demonstrates that behavior is not only a critical element in the causal web of disease, but also an important element in its course and outcome.

Help Seeking for Mental Health and Psychosocial Concerns in Developing Countries

As for other medical conditions, factors impinging on the family and individual seeking care for psychiatric conditions include belief systems and stigma attached to particular symptoms, previous experiences in seeking care in the household and from others, expectations about seriousness and outcome, accessibility of different care providers, and educational and economic levels.

The notion of the "health care system," as elaborated by Kleinman (1980), can be conceptualized as the entirety of "socially organized responses to disease," and includes: the "popular sector" of locally held beliefs, home remedies and family care systems; the "folk sector" of healers such as shamans, herbalists, or bone setters who are neither

Table 3-6 Psychiatrists/Mental Health Professionals to Population Ratio

Country	Est. Population	Est. # Mental Health Professionals	Ratio
Pakistan (Aslam 1988; Aslam 1989)	100,000,000	100 psychiatrists	1:1,000,000
Taiwan (Wen 1990)	20,000,000	200 psychiatrists	1:100,000
China (Kleinman 1988)	1,100,000,000	500 psychiatrists + 2,500 mental health workers= 3,000	1:366,600*
United States (Eiler and Pasko 1988; Kleinman 1988)	248,000,000	34,500	1:7,200

*"Mental Health Worker" includes general physicians, nurses, and technicians working in psychiatric hospitals. In 1993, the total number is closer to 6,000.

professionally organized nor legally sanctioned; and the "professional sector" of designated allopathic and traditional health care professionals with licenses and professional organizations.

The recognition of symptoms and the decision to seek care for them are profoundly molded by cultural and personal beliefs. Such beliefs are involved in seeking help for specific illness episodes; they include notions about the nature of the problem, its cause, clinical course, desired treatment, and expected outcome. For example, if dysphoria, sleepless- ness, inability to concentrate, and weight loss are seen as physical problems caused by an imbalance of bodily fluids, then appropriate treatment will be to restore this balance. (Western psychiatrists often tell patients with these symptoms, diagnosed as major depression, that they are due to a "chemical imbalance.") If the same constellation is seen as moral weakness or as resulting from an interpersonal affront, then a different (likely less somatic) treatment will be sought. Such belief systems profoundly affect the help-seeking process for behavioral and emotional disorders and are culturally and locally specific. Thus, the path to care pursued by a Hindu Brahman will likely be quite different from that taken by an Andean peasant.

The decision to seek care is itself rarely made by an individual; it is rather a social decision involving the patient and significant others surrounding the patient (Janzen 1978). Recognition of this is important in planning for direct services (such as allowing room in infirmaries and hospitals for family members to sleep near the patient) as well as health education efforts aimed not only at patients, but at their families and villages, too.

Kleinman (1980) points out that the aim of help-seeking is ameliora- tion of symptoms and provision of meaning for the experience of illness. Patients and families are quite pragmatic about utilizing providers in different sectors for the same illness, if necessary. Weiss et al. (1986) found, in India, that about half of the patients attending any one of three "allopathic psychiatric service" had first sought care from a traditional source. Li and Phillips (1990) found, similarly, that over 70 percent of rural psychiatric outpatients attending a selected clinic, and a similar percentage of "mentally ill" (sic) persons identified in a rural community in China, reported consulting with folk healers.

Wen (1990) describes an "indigenous" asylum, a temple, for chronic mental patients in Taiwan. In order to be admitted, a patient's family had to present the "master" of the temple with a certificate from a psychiatrist certifying that the patient had a "mental disorder." More than half of the patients had received ambulatory or inpatient psychiatric care within 6 months of the onset of the illness. Wen found that 62 percent of the family respondents had rejected the use of antipsychotic medication for the patients. When queried, the family respondents overwhelmingly stated that they had sought out the asylum because they had exhausted all their other resources, and had no other choice.[2]

In rapidly developing societies, the personal and social standards for distress and behavior may themselves be in flux such that individuals' behavior appropriate to one setting will be considered deviant or ill in another. This may interact, synergistically, with other factors, such as migration and changes in the support network, to change the frequency and characteristics of psychiatric and behavior disorders, as well as to alter patterns of help-seeking for such problems (Carlini et al. 1986; Carlini-Cotrim and Carlini 1988; Garro 1986; Marshall 1988; Rahim and Cederblad 1984; Rubinstein 1987). Such considerations may, in part, explain the findings by Rahim and Cederblad (1984) that more mothers reported more behavioral problems consistent with childhood behavioral disorder, in the same urbanising area of Khartoum, Sudan, in 1980 than in 1965.

Seeking care from a healer trained in Western biomedicine has been repeatedly found to be associated with increasing maternal education (Caldwell 1986; chapters by LeVine et al. and Christakis et al. in this volume) and accessibility. Stock et al. (1983) found, in Nigeria, that the utilization of a government medical clinic declined by 25 percent per kilometer traveled. While such factors have been studied more with respect to physical than psychiatric conditions, it is likely that the cultural and behavioral dimensions of seeking care have greatest impact on the latter, usually stigmatized, problems (Lin and Lin 1982b).

Stigma adds affliction to psychiatric patients in both the developed and developing worlds. Munakata (1986) shows how some Japanese patients with schizophrenia have been confined to poorly maintained mental hospitals because of stigma. Aslam (1989) has described how mentally ill patients in Pakistan are socially rejected and ultimately institutionalized in appallingly inhumane conditions. Two-thirds of the patients in one large psychiatric hospital in Buenos Aires have been abandoned by their families (Christian 1990). Thirty patients in that same hospital died of malnutrition in the first half of 1990; the diet in the hospital reportedly consisted of rice for ten days, then polenta for ten days. Wen (1990) documents how mentally ill family members in Taiwan (a relatively wealthy industrializing society) are often placed in isolated healing asylums or inadequate mental hospitals because of shame. Indeed, Higginbotham condemns biomedical health care facilities for the mentally ill in East and Southeast Asian societies, generally, because of their institutional inadequacies and tendency to provide inhumane care (Higginbotham 1984; Higginbotham and Connor 1989; Wen 1990).

While accessibility has been referred to, the paucity of trained mental health professionals in the industrializing world must be underlined. As shown in Table 3.6, there are about 100 psychiatrists in all of Pakistan to serve 100 million people (Aslam 1989). Consequently children and adults requiring psychiatric hospitalization are treated in the same urban facilities, despite the predominantly rural population and the advantages of specialized treatment for children. As of 1979, there was one psychiatrist serving all of Nepal (Aslam 1989). There is one psychiatrist for each 100,000 people in Taiwan (Wen 1990). There are about 3,000 trained mental health practitioners, including about 500 fully trained psychiatrists for over one billion people in all of China (Kleinman 1988b). Contrast this with the 34,500 psychiatrists (Eiler and Pasko 1988), 60,000 psychologists, and over 90,000 social workers serving the United States population of about 248 million (Kleinman 1988b).

Behavioral Conditions in Primary Care

Area primary care centers are often the most accessible biomedical care providers in regions of the developing world, and several studies have found that significant numbers of primary care patients suffer from psychiatric disorders. Depression, anxiety, and other psychiatric conditions are often present in the form of somatic complaints in non-Western cultures, as in the West (Katon et al. 1982). These diagnoses are often missed or ignored (Kleinman 1986).

Focusing on primary care settings in different regions in China, Kleinman and Mechanic (1979) found that over 20 percent of the patients somatized psychiatric and psychosocial concerns with such symptoms of dizziness, fatigue, headache, and sleep disturbance. Individuals with depression and anxiety disorders were not diagnosed, as such, nor did they receive appropriate treatment. Harding et al. (1983) describes a WHO multicenter, multicultural study in which 10.5 percent to 20 percent of the 1624 patients attending primary care centers in Colombia, the Philippines, India, and Sudan met diagnostic criteria for depressive or

Table 3-7   Behavioral Conditions in Primary Care

Year (source)	Location	Prevalence
1979 (Kleinman and Mechanic 1979)	multiple sites in China	20% of pts. "somatized" psychosocial concerns
1980 (Harding et al. 1983)	multicenter including sites in Colombia, India, Sudan, & Philippines	overall 10.5% - 20% of "psychiatric morbidity" (sic)
1984 (Mari and Williams 1984)	Sao Paulo, Brazil	46% "minor psychiatric morbidity" (sic)
1985 (Jacobsson 1985)	Ethiopia	18% overall, "most with some somatic shading"
1989 (Abiodun 1990)	Nigeria	22.4% overall: 37.5% "anxiety neuroses"; 67.5% "depression neuroses" (sic)

anxiety disorder. Studies in Uganda and Kenya found similar percentages among primary care patients (Dhapdale et al. 1983; German 1972). In Nigeria, it was found that 22.4 percent of the patients presenting to selected primary care centers suffered from anxiety and depressive conditions to the extent that daily functioning was significantly interfered with. Hollifeld, in Lesotho, found that 48 percent of the patients attending a primary care center met DSM III-R criteria for panic disorder and/or depression. Yet only 25 percent of these patients reported that psychiatric symptoms were the main reason for their visit (Hollifeld 1988).

It is important to note that the recognition of psychological symptoms such as anxiety or depression, *per se*, is culturally and linguistically determined. This underscores the import of effective cultural translation of diagnostic instruments, such as questionnaires, as well as queries by physicians.

Many of the conditions described above have prominent somatic components that respond to medication, and several studies have found that simple treatment regimes are effective in these disorders. Essex and Gosling (1983) have developed and successfully applied an algorithm for use by primary caregivers in identifying and treating psychiatric disorders. Several other studies have found that primary care providers can be trained to accurately recognize, triage, and treat selected psychiatric disorders (Ben-Tovim 1987; Harding et al. 1983) and they have found continued positive response at one- to two-year follow-up. Hollifeld (1988) found that a significant majority of the primary care patients identified with depressive and panic disorders in Lesotho showed significant symptomatic and functional improvement with treatment consisting of imipramine, counseling, and relaxation techniques. This improvement was maintained at two- to four-month follow-up. Echoing these findings, one WHO study concluded that over 90 percent of patients with selected psychiatric conditions could be successfully treated with first-line medications from a limited pharmacopeia (Harding et al. 1983).

Refugees

No discussion of economic development and mental health can ignore the growing numbers of refugees worldwide, due to forced uprooting, economic changes, ethnic violence, war, famine, and natural disasters. The refugee experience is, unfortunately, becoming increasingly common, and there are particular health and mental health needs presented by this group.

According to the United States Committee for Refugees, there are about 15 million refugees worldwide, and the number continues to grow (Crisp 1989; U.S. Committee for Refugees 1990). Up to 90 percent of these people may be from, and resettling in, developing countries (Stein 1986). Almost half of the world's refugees are in Africa (Crisp 1990), including 45 thousand Mozambiquan refugees in Zimbabwe (Hiegel and Landrac 1990). Among Southeast Asian refugees, over 220,000 are still in refugee camps: over 56,000 in Hong Kong, 53,000 in Indonesia, 20,000 in the Philippines, and over 100,000 in Thailand (Refugee Reports 1989). In addition, there are over 700,000 Indochinese refugees in the United States (Mollica et al. 1987) and over 50,000 have resettled in Australia.

The refugee experience is distinct from other international migration in that the refugee is *pushed* from home by misfortune, while other migrants are *pulled* to another specific country by opportunity. "Becoming" a refugee involves several phases: the perception of danger, the decision to flee, flight itself, initial asylum (often in a camp), and resettlement or repatriation. Each stage involves particular tasks, decisions, risks, and psychological costs. In addition, it is clear that different types of people will have different experiences in this process. For example, urban professionals may perceive a dangerous political situation on the horizon in their native countries and plan their flight with relative calm; poor members of ethnic minorities do not have the means for such planned flight. In a similar vein, inter-ethnic conflict, such as has occurred in parts of Africa and the Middle East, may displace thousands virtually overnight, leading to almost instant refugee camps.

The nature of the threat, and the flight, too, will in part define the experience, and consequently impact on the vulnerability to psychosocial distress and disorder among the victims. Beiser and Collomb (1981) found that the mental health outcome of major social changes in Senegal, including migration, was largely determined by the social contingencies, i.e., intact social networks and cultural behavioral norms, rather than by change *per se*. Thus, when whole communities flee intact, mental health consequences may be minimal, compared to the effects on disrupted communities and families. Westermeyer (1986b) found little psychiatric illness among the members of Laotian communities that had fled, intact, prior to 1975. In contrast, many authors have found that unaccompanied minors (Harding and Looney 1977; Looney et al. 1975; Szapocznik and Cohen (1986) and widows (Kroll et al. 1989; Mollica et al. 1990; Westermeyer 1986a) are particularly vulnerable. Szapocznik and Cohen (1986) reported that 65 percent of the unaccompanied Cuban teenage refugees in one camp in Florida reported significant levels of sadness or anxiety, 22 percent reported suicidal ideation, and 14 percent stated they had attempted suicide. Another 14 percent of these teenagers reported dysphoric hallucination, and 9 percent were thought to have delusions.

Kinzie et al. (1984, 1990), Mollica et al. (1987, 1990), and others (Beiser et al. 1989; Kroll et al. 1989; Lin 1986; Nguyen 1982a; Shaw and Harris 1989; Stein 1986; Westermeyer 1986a; Westermeyer 1986b) have found that certain groups of Indochinese refugees have experienced multiple serious traumas, such as rape, witnessing the murder of a loved one, and near death; these groups show a very high prevalence of depression and post-traumatic stress disorder that interferes with daily function.

There is a paucity of data about psychiatric illness in refugee camps, the site of first asylum for many refugees (Richard Mollica, personal communication). Case reports and anecdotes suggest that psychiatric morbidity is substantial. Commenting on her experiences as a general physician in the Khao I Dang refugee camp in Thailand, Sughandabhirom, a trained psychiatrist, found that a third of the patients presenting to the clinic for medical care were suffering from a diagnosable "neurotic" (sic) condition or depression (Sughandabhirom 1986). Many authors have remarked on the preponderance of physical symptoms among refugees (Kinzie et al. 1984; Kroll et al. 1989; Lin 1986; Mollica et al. 1990; Nguyen 1982b; Sughandabhirom 1986; Westermeyer 1986a). It has been suggested that one of the factors contributing to the lack of study of psychiatric disorder and distress among refugee camp residents is the need for physicians to distance themselves from the psychological suffering and to focus on physical ailments of the camp residents in order to feel effective (Sughandabhirom 1986; Westermeyer 1986a). This compounds the inherent difficulties of standardized psychiatric diagnosis cross-culturally in refugee camps.

Despite the dearth of epidemiologic studies, the special needs for care of refugees are apparent. Clearly, acute medical needs must be attended to. To the extent possible, however, "health" care provided by host countries in camps should respect the indigenous models of care seeking; at the very least, health care providers among the refugees themselves should be sought out and included in the planning for, and provision of, health care to camp residents (Harding and Looney 1977; Looney et al. 1975).

Generically, the experience of danger and subsequent flight, often with little time to reflect or plan, suggests that a major need for refugees, early on, is a place of true asylum. Concretely, this means a place and opportunity in the refugee camps themselves for the members of the community to discuss the flight and their future plans, and to interact with each other in safety. Concomitantly, as suggested above, "native communities" should be allowed to persist, or develop, among the refugees, in order to ease the impact of major dislocation (Beiser 1988; Beiser and Collomb 1981; Westermeyer 1986a). With respect to unaccompanied minors, this may mean finding foster families among the refugees themselves, rather than the early fostering/adopting of children to families out of the camps and even in other countries (Beiser et al. 1989; Harding and Looney 1977; Lin 1986; Looney et al. 1975; Stein 1986; Westermeyer 1986a).

Particularly "pathogenic" characteristics of camps must be noted: refugees are especially vulnerable to the whims of guards and other "hosting nationals," which may include verbal and physical assault and abuse. The camp experience itself entails a disruption of norms of social interaction and space.

Different age cohorts present different mental health needs, as they have differing developmental tasks and cognitive schemata for mastering change. Thus, Looney and Harding (1977) recommended that play facilities be provided for the young children in the Indochinese refugee camps in the U.S. to allow the children peer experiences and exposure to American playthings, and to allow the parents some free time away from the children. Similarly, occupational and social roles for those in the midst of their productive livelihoods are likely to change dramatically with refugee status, and specific re-education and training in the camps, if possible, may provide some resilience. The particular vulnerability of widows has been alluded to, and presents special problems in terms of providing a support network for these women, often with children requiring care.

While the above measures will hopefully provide some protection against psychiatric morbidity, it is clear that medical care providers must be able to recognize and appropriately treat depressive and anxiety conditions, including post-traumatic stress disorder. This requires awareness of the problems themselves, as well as sensitivity to the often somatic presentation of distress. The clinical predisposition among refugees of different cultures to somatic symptoms has been noted for over 40 years (Mollica et al. 1987; Nguyen 1982a; Sughandabhirom 1986; Westermeyer 1986a). Patience and persistence are required clinically in the elucidation of psychosocial problems and symptoms (Kinzie et al. 1990; Kinzie et al. 1984; Kroll et al. 1989; Mollica et al. 1987; Mollica et al. 1990; Nguyen 1982b). Supportive psychotherapy that attends to direct social concerns and service provision is less threatening and less ethnocentric than attempting to give insight-oriented psychotherapy to non-Occidental refugees (Nguyen 1982b).

Pharmacotherapy, frequently involving antidepressant medications, is often necessary. The prevalence of depressive symptoms may exceed 80 percent in clinic patients; these symptoms are often medication responsive (Nguyen 1982b). Post-traumatic stress disorder has been noted in as many as 70 percent of refugee patients in certain clinics (Kinzie et al. 1990). When considered as a medical problem and treated as such, psychiatric disease may be less stigmatized and access to care improved, with medication "justifying" the visit (Kinzie et al. 1990).

Resettlement ultimately carries with it particular psychological tasks and vulnerabilities. Many authors have found that somatic and psychiatric symptoms of depression, anxiety, and post-traumatic stress disorder persist for many years after resettlement. Beiser (1988) found certain refugees to be at high risk for major depression during the first 10 to 12 months after resettlement (post-camp). These were the people who were without family, lacked access to a similar ethnic community, and who for various reasons remained focused on the past. With these factors in mind, he notes the differing susceptibility to depression among Chinese and non-Chinese Indochinese refugees in British Columbia: the easy accessibility of ethnic Chinese communities in British Columbia may provide some protection for ethnic Chinese immigrants.

Resettlement and potential assimilation presents specific tasks to different family members too. Children and teenagers are often the most exposed to the culture of the host country through schools and peers. They may come to disparage traditional ways and increase family tension. Similarly, primary wage earners may not be able to find work, wives may be forced to work, and depression and marital discord may ensue (Beiser and Collomb 1981; Westermeyer 1986a; Westermeyer 1986b). This may predispose parents to psychological distress, while disrupted family life may predispose the children to behavior disorders (Wolkind and Rutter 1985). Again, the treatment considerations outlined above must be considered in planning for and providing treatment to resettled refugees.

Implications

Several factors emerge from the above review:

1. Social and economic "development" brings with it a change in morbidity and mortality, such that behavioral factors become increasingly important in pathogenesis of disease.

2. There are local differences in the incidence and prevalence of behavioral conditions and psychiatric illness.

3. Adult major mental illnesses, such as affective illnesses and schizophrenia, are a major part of morbidity in developing countries.

4. The expression of "core" syndromes, such as depression or panic disorders, is culturally shaped and thus require culturally appropriate health services.

5. A substantial portion of primary care visits in developing countries is for psychiatric disorders and psychosocial concerns. Many of these conditions are responsive to psychosocial and psychopharmacologic interventions. Local primary care providers can be trained to recognize and appropriately treat these disorders.

6. Typical patterns of program development in the health care systems of developing societies either ignore the mental health sector or foster practices that actually work against the effective recognition and treatment of psychiatric disorders. While preventive programs in mental health are just beginning in industrialized nations, mental health programs are the last to be developed and the first to be cut under economic pressures in developed and developing nations alike.

These factors define specific needs of developing countries in characterizing and responding to behavioral conditions and psychiatric disorder in constructing health care systems. First and foremost, the substantial burden of psychiatric, behavioral, and psychosocial concerns on the health care systems of developing countries must be recognized. This is not "unrecognized" need; it represents need and demand now being made on different parts of the health care system — such as the presentation of somatic complaints for psychosocial concerns in primary care — that can be responded to more appropriately and cost-effectively.

The health care and health status costs of behaviors with direct health consequences must be recognized. Only with this information can the health ministries in developing countries fruitfully enter policy discussions in other domains, such as revenue. For example, the tax revenue obtained from the sales of tobacco and alcohol products must be seen in light of the costs to health status and health systems that cigarette and alcohol use represent.

The epidemiology of behavioral conditions and psychiatric disorders should guide the deployment of specific health care resources. The use of epidemiologic instruments accepted in the West, such as the Present State Examination and the Diagnostic Interview Schedule, will require sensitive modification with respect to local beliefs about illness and patterns of expressing symptoms. The development and transfer of such culturally appropriate "technologies" to the health ministries of developing countries and the dissemination of findings signifying the import of "behavioral conditions" in developing countries are of high priority. Just as important, however, is systematic research on topics that have been politically unacceptable in many poor societies, such as drug and alcohol abuse, child abuse, etc.

Medical anthropologists, who can play a useful role in health policy discussions generally, are especially important for the development of policy and programs for behavioral conditions. Psychiatric illness and psychosocial distress are experienced and labelled in local worlds of experience, and the anthropologist is skilled at eliciting such local knowledge. The ethnographic method employed by anthropologists is most appropriate for studying help-seeking by patients in distress. With this method, the contributions of the household as well as those of traditional healers to the provision of care and the amelioration of distress can be recognized. Indeed, by viewing biomedicine, the household context of care, and traditional healing practices through an "anthropologic eye," it is possible to see how these plural sets of practices can be interrelated in order to most effectively plan and deliver health care to people in resource-poor countries. The recognition of culture-specific psychiatric disorders and psychosocial distress will also be enhanced, as well as the development of triage connections between primary care practitioners, families, and local healers.

Relatively low cost treatments for behavioral conditions are available: it is estimated that about 60 percent of the patients with epilepsy could be effectively treated with phenobarbital at an annual expense of less than US $10 per patient (Norman Sartorious, personal communication 1988; Ben-Tovim 1987). The substantial proportion of psychiatric disorders that are treatable with simple first-line, generic medications has already been noted. The delivery of such care need not occur only in major psychiatric hospitals: Ben-Tovim (1987) has described his experiences in Botswana, working with community primary caregivers to deliver care in widely dispersed local settings. Ben-Tovim used anthropologic data on family and community processes to develop culturally sensitive, socially feasible therapy within a community structure that could support it. Such experiences suggest the value of deploying Western-trained psychiatrists and neuropsychiatrists who are educated and interested in cross-cultural work and prepared to work with anthropologists, local care providers, and local policy makers in devising appropriate treatment strategies in places where there is no mental health service system.

Coda: The Underside of Development

A final implication of our analysis is that many of the behavioral and social pathologies we have charted are the consequences of the current stage of international development. Seen from this perspective, the word "development" is a misnomer. The economic, social and moral transformations that are occurring globally have a mix of effects: improving certain indexes (e.g., GNP and infant mortality rates) and fostering interest in human rights issues and the role of women, while also simultaneously contributing to worsening of a range of social pathologies from violence associated with substance abuse to family breakdown and ethnic conflict. It is important to recognize that economic and political policies have contributed to the latter as much as to the former. It is invalid, and dangerously so, to emphasize the improvements while de-emphasizing the problems. Yet, we would argue, this is precisely what economic planners and health policy experts often do. International health experts, as a result, routinely proceed as if social development meant progressive improvement in health status and health services. This is simply not the case.

As a result, health and development programs frequently fail to address the sources of social pathology and of the global pandemic of mental health problems. Indeed, at times they are part of the problem. An example is when a narrow disease model is fostered for problems like violence, which are so clearly the outcome of broad social disturbances. "Failures of success," as when increasing immunization coverage and other actions designed to reduce infant and child mortality increase widespread malnutrition, are a second illustration. This does not mean that immunization or primary care services should be restricted, but that the way we configure the problems of children contributes to the difficulty in deciding how to respond to problems that fall outside the intervention framework, yet are just as serious as those we prioritize. The priority structure of international health programs is itself a major obstacle to the recognition of and response to mental health problems. Neither traditional mortality nor morbidity statistics adequately project the cost and significance of the mental health pandemic. International health advisers like those working in national ministries are often inadequately prepared to study these problems and to evaluate appropriate interventions. The mental health professions have themselves been remiss. They have failed to produce significant numbers of international mental health experts or to work out the details of an international mental health policy agenda.

There is more than enough blame to go around. What needs to be done is to correct an unacceptable current situation by developing policies and programs that can be applied in industrialized and nonindustrialized societies at the local level where, as we have tried to show, mental health problems have both their roots and their most powerful negative consequences.

It is with this aim in mind that we have reviewed the scope and magnitude of the problem and pointed out the kinds of research required to develop relevant policies and programs. A few such programs are ready to be implemented based on what is currently known. Among these are interventions in primary care settings for the treatment of psychosocial distress and specific psychiatric diseases, and the development of improved specialized treatment and rehabilitation services for the seriously mentally ill and those disabled by mental retardation and other chronic conditions. Such programs need to be complemented by communitywide experiments aimed at controlling substance abuse and violence and their macrosocial sources. Included in this list of policy objectives must be the reformulation of "development" policy itself, to identify and prevent behavioral conditions that are the direct consequences of current political economic policies and social programs. It is toward this end that this chapter seeks to bring the mental health agenda into the discourse of international health and the purview of health policy experts.

Notes

1 Population figure from United Nations data reported in World Almanac and Book of Facts, 1989.

2 Interestingly, Wen found that at 6-month follow-up, the patient group in the asylum showed modest improvement in social functioning, though they suffered much physical morbidity. In contrast, a comparison group of patients in a psychiatric nursing home showed some improvement in psychotic symptoms and in physical health, but slight worsening in social functioning.

References

Abiodun, O.A. 1990. Mental health and primary care in Africa." *International Journal of Mental Health*, 18(4): 48–56.

Acuda, S.W. 1982. "Drug and alcohol problems in Kenya today." *East African Medical Journal*, 59: 642–644.

Agbonifo, P.O. 1983. "The state of health as a reflection of the level of development of a nation." *Social Science and Medicine*, 17(24): 2003–2006.

Argondoa, M. 1988. "Alcohol related problems in developing Latin America." Paper presented to the International Commission on Health Research for Development. Cambridge, MA. November 28.

Aslam, A. 1981. Essential national research in mental health: A case study in Pakistan. International Commission on Health Research for Development, Cambridge, MA.

Aslam, A. 1989. Drug addiction in Pakistan. International Commission on Health Research for Development, Cambridge, MA.

Beiser, M. 1988. "Influences of time, ethnicity, and attachment on depression in Southeast Asian refugees." *American Journal of Psychiatry*, 145(1): 46–51.

Beiser, M., and H. Collomb. 1981. "Mastering change: Epidemiological and case studies in Senegal, West Africa." *American Journal of Psychiatry*, 138(4): 455–459.

Beiser, M., R.J. Turner, and S. Ganesan. 1989. "Catastrophic stress and factors affecting its consequences among Southeast Asian refugees." *Social Science and Medicine*, 28 (1): 183–195.

Ben-Tovim, D.I. 1987. *Development Psychiatry: Mental Health and Primary Care in Botswana.* New York: Tavistock.

Berkman, L., and S.L. Syme. 1979. "Social networks, host resistance, and mortality: A nine-year follow-up study of Alameda County residents." *American Journal of Epidemiology*, 109(2): 186–204.

Bowlby, J. 1988. "Developmental psychiatry comes of age." *American Journal of Psychiatry*, 145(1): 1–10.

Caldwell, J.C. 1979. "Education as a factor in mortality decline: An examination of Nigerian data." *Population Studies*, 33: 395–413.

Caldwell, J.C. 1986. "Routes to low mortality in poor countries." *Population Development Review*, 12: 171–220.

Caplan, G. 1989. "Social Support and Mastery of Stress." In G. Caplan, ed. *Population Oriented Psychiatry.* New York: Human Sciences Press, Inc.

Carlini, B., M. Pires, R. Fernandes, et al. 1986. "Alcohol use among adolescents in Sao Paulo, Brazil." *Drug and Alcohol Dependence*, 18: 235–246.

Carlini-Cotrim, B., and E.A. Carlini. 1988. "The use of solvents and other drugs among children and adolescents from a low socioeconomic background: A study in São Paulo, Brazil." *International Journal of Addiction*, 23(11): 1145–1156.

Carstairs, G. 1983. "Psychiatric problems of developing countries." *British Journal of Psychiatry*, 123: 271–277.

Christian, S. 1990. "Argentine deaths bring focus on health care." *New York Times International*, New York, August 11, p. 5.

Coombs, D.W., and G. Globetti. 1986. "Alcohol use and alcoholism in Latin America: Changing patterns and sociocultural explanations." *International Journal of Addiction*, 21(1): 59–81.

Crisp, J. 1989. "Dossier." *Refugees*, July: 20–23.

Crisp, J. 1990. "Demography and democracy." *Refugees*, March: 11–15.

Dhapdale, M., R. Elison and L. Griffin. 1983. "The frequency of psychiatric disorders among patients attending semi–urban and rural general outpatient clinics in Kenya." *British Journal of Psychiatry*, 142: 379–383.

Earls, F. 1988. "Approaches to the expansion of mental health services for children in developing countries." Paper presented to the International Commission on Health Research for Development, Harvard University. Cambridge, MA. November 28.

Eiler, M.A., and T. Pasko. 1988. *Specialty profiles*. Chicago: American Medical Association.

Eisenberg, L. 1986. "Human ecology and health: Disease prevention and control." Paper presented at the WHO Meeting on Human Ecology and Health. Delphi, Greece. September 30–October 3.

Essex, B., and H. Gosling. 1983. "An algorithmic method for management of mental health problems in developing countries." *British Journal of Psychiatry*, 143: 451–459.

Ganasveram, T., S. Subramaniam, and K. Mahadeven. 1984. "Suicide in a northern town in Sri Lanka." *Acta Psychiatrica Scandanavia*, 69: 420–425.

Garro, L.C. 1986. "Intracultural variation in folk medical knowledge: A comparison between curers and noncurers." *American Anthropologist*, 88: 351–370.

German, G. 1972. "Aspects of clinical psychiatry in Sub-Sahara Africa." *British Journal of Psychiatry*, 121: 461–479.

Goodwin, D.W., and S.B. Guze. 1989. *Psychiatric Diagnosis*. New York: Oxford University Press.

Gossop, M. 1989. "The detoxification of high dose heroin addicts in Pakistan." *Drug and Alcohol Dependence*, 24: 143–150.

Harding, R.K., and J.G. Looney. 1977. "Problems of Southeast Asian children in a refugee camp." *American Journal of Psychiatry*, 134(4): 407–411.

Harding, T., B. d'Arrigo, C. Climent, et al. 1983. The WHO collaborative study on strategies for extending mental health care, III: Evaluative design and illustrative results. *American Journal of Psychiatry*, 140: 1481–1485.

Heggenhougen, H.K., and L. Shore. 1986. "Cultural components of behavioural epidemiology: Implications for primary health care." *Social Science and Medicine*, 22(11): 1235–1245.

Hiegel, J.P., and C. Landrac. 1990. "Voices from the back of the queue." *Refugees*, April: 25–28.

Higginbotham, H.N. 1984. *Third World Challenge to Psychiatry: Culture Accomodation and Mental Health*. Honolulu: University of Hawaii Press.

Higginbotham, N., and L. Connor. 1989. "Professional ideology and the construction of Western psychiatry in Southeast Asia." *International Journal of Health Services*, 19(1): 63–78.

Hollifeld, M. 1988. "Psychiatry in developing countries: Evidence of the burden and intervention efficacy in primary care." Unpublished Manuscript, Department of Psychiatry, University of Washington.

Hollifeld, M. 1990. "Epidemiology of panic, generalized anxiety, and depression in Lesotho." *British Journal of Psychiatry*, 156: 343–350.

House, J.S., K.R. Landis, and D. Umberson. 1988. "Social relationships and health." *Science*, 241: 540–544.

Jacobsson, L. 1985. "Psychiatric morbidity and psychosocial background in an outpatient population of a general hospital in western Ethiopia." *Acta Psychiatrica Scandanavia*, 71: 417–26.

Janzen, J.M. 1978. *The Quest for Therapy. Comparative Studies of Health Systems and Medical Care*. Berkeley: University of California Press.

Johnston, L. 1980. Review of General Population Surveys of Drug Abuse. WHO Monograph #52. Geneva: World Health Organization.

Johnston, L. 1988. "Illicit drug use: Problems and needs at the world level." Paper presented to the International Commission on Health Research for Development. Harvard University, Cambridge, MA. November 28.

Katon, W., A. Kleinman, and G. Rosen. 1982. "Depression and somatization: A review." Part I. *American Journal of Medicine*, 72: 127–135.

Keltzer, K. 1989. "Causative and intervening factors of harmful alcohol consumption and cannabis use in Malawi." *International Journal of Addiction*, 24(2): 79–85.

Kinzie, J.D., J.K. Boehnlein, P.K. Leung, et al. 1990. "The prevalence of posttraumatic stress disorder and its clinical significance among Southeast Asian refugees." *American Journal of Psychiatry*, 147(7): 913–917.

Kinzie, J.D., R.H. Fredrickson, R. Ben, et al. 1984. "Posttraumatic stress disorder among survivors of Cambodian concentration camps." *American Journal of Psychiatry*, 141(5): 645–650.

Kleinman, A. 1980. *Patients and Healers in the Context of Culture*. Berkeley: University of California Press.

Kleinman, A. 1986. *Social Origins of Distress and Disease*. New Haven: Yale University Press.

Kleinman, A. 1988a. *Rethinking Psychiatry*. New York: Free Press.

Kleinman, A. 1988b. "A Window on Mental Health in China." *American Science*, 76: 22–28.

Kleinman, A., and D. Mechanic. 1979. "Some observations of mental illness and its treatment in China." *Journal of Nervous and Mental Disorders*, 167: 267–274.

Kraus, R.F., and P.A. Buffler. 1979. "Sociocultural stress and the American native in Alaska: An analysis of changing patterns of psychiatric illness and alcohol abuse among Alaska natives." *Culture, Medicine and Psychiatry*, 3(2): 111–115.

Kroll, J., M. Habenicht, T. Mackenzie, et al. 1989. "Depression and posttraumatic stress disorder in Southeast Asian refugees." *American Journal of Psychiatry*, 146(12): 1592–1597.

Leighton, A., T.A. Hughes, C.C. Hughes, et al. 1963. *Psychiatric Disorder Among the Yoruba*. Ithaca, NY: Cornell University Press.

Li, S., and M.R. Phillips. 1990. "Witch doctors and mental illness in mainland China: A preliminary study." *American Journal of Psychiatry*, 147(2): 221–224.

Lin, K.M. 1986. "Psychopathology and social disruption in refugees." In C.L. Williams and J. Westermeyer, eds. *Migration and Psychopathology*. Washington, DC: Hemisphere Publishing Corporation.

Lin, T.Y., and D.T.C. Lin. 1982. "Alcoholism among the Chinese." *Culture, Medicine and Psychiatry*, 6: 109–116.

Lin, T.Y., and M.C. Lin. 1982. "Love, denial, and rejection: Responses of Chinese families to mental illness." In A. Kleinman and T.Y. Lin, eds. *Normal and Abnormal Behavior in Chinese Culture*. Boston: Kluwer.

Litvak, J. 1988. "Determinants of healthy aging." Special Program for Research on Aging. Geneva: World Health Organization.

Litvak, J., L. Ruiz, H. Restrepo, et al. 1987. The growing noncommunicable disease burden, a challenge for the countries of the Americas. *Pan American Health Organization*, 21(2): 156–71.

Looney, J., R. Rahe, R. Harding, et al. 1975. "Consulting children in crisis." *Child Psychiatry and Human Development*, 10(1): 5–13.

Marmot, M.G., and S.L. Syme. 1976. "Acculturation and coronary heart disease in Japanese Americans." *American Journal of Epidemiology*, 104: 225–247.

Mari, J.J., and P. Williams. 1984. "Minor psychiatric disorder in primary care in Brazil: A pilot study." *Psychological Medicine*, 14: 223–27.

Marshall, M. 1988. "Alcohol consumption as a public health problem in Papua New Guinea." *International Journal of Addiction*, 23(6): 573–589.

Mollica, R.F., G. Wyshak, and J. Lavelle. 1987. "The psychosocial impact of war trauma and torture on Southeast Asian refugees." *American Journal of Psychiatry*, 144(12): 1567–1572.

Mollica, R.F., G. Wyshak, J. Lavelle, et al. 1990. "Assessing symptom change in Southeast Asian refugee survivors of mass violence and torture." *American Journal of Psychiatry*, 147(1): 83–88.

Morris, M.D., and F.B. Liser. 1978. "The PQLI: Measuring progress in meeting human needs." *Urban Ecology*, 3: 225–240.

Munakata, T. 1986. "Japanese attitudes toward mental illness and mental health care." In A. Alek, T. Lebra and W. Lebra, eds. *Japanese Culture and Behavior*. Honolulu: University of Hawaii Press.

Nath, U.R. 1986. "Smoking in the Third World." *World Health*. pp. 66–67.

National Institute on Drug Abuse. 1985. "Patterns and trends in drug abuse: A national and international perspective." National Institute on Drug Abuse, United States Department of Health and Human Services.

Nations, M.K., and L.A. Rebhun. 1988. "Angels with wet wings won't fly: Maternal sentiment in Brazil and the image of neglect." *Culture, Medicine and Psychiatry*, 12: 141–200.

Nguyen, S.D. 1982a. "Psychiatric and psychosomatic problems among Southeast Asian refugees." *The Psychiatric Journal of the University of Ottawa*, 7(3): 163–172.

Nguyen, S.D. 1982b. "The psychosocial adjustment and mental health needs of Southeast Asian refugees." *Psychiatric Journal of the University of Ottawa*, 7(1): 26–35.

Orley, J., and J. Wing. 1979. "Psychiatric disorders in two African villages." *Archives of General Psychiatry*, 36: 513–520.

Rahim, S., and M. Cederblad. 1984. "Effects of rapid urbanization on child behavior and health in part of Khartoum, Sudan." *Journal of Child Psychology and Psychiatry*, 25: 629–641.

Rosenfeld, P. 1988. "The social determinants of tropical disease." New York: Carnegie Corporation.

Rubinstein, D.H. 1987. "Suicide in Micronesia." Unpublished manuscript.

Samarasinghe D. 1989. "Treating alcohol problems in Sri Lanka." *British Journal of Addiction,* 84: 865–87.

Sartorious, N., and A. Jablensky. 1976. "Transcultural studies of schizophrenia." *WHO Chronicle,* 30: 481–485.

Sartorius, N. 1986. "Early manifestation and first contact incidence of schizophrenia." *Psychological Medicine,* 16: 909–928.

Sawyer, D.R. 1986. "Malaria on the Amazon frontier: Economic and social aspects of transmission and control." *Southeast Asian Journal of Tropical Medicine and Public Health,* 17: 342–345.

Scheper-Hughes, N. 1987. "The cultural politics of child survival." In N. Scheper-Hughes, ed. *Child Survival.* Dordrecht: D. Reidel.

Sethi, B.B. 1985. "Biological psychiatry in developing countries." *Biological Psychiatry,* 20: 357–359.

Shaffer, D., A. Garland, M. Gould, et al. 1988. "Preventing teenage suicide: A critical review." *Journal of the American Academy of Child and Adolescent Psychiatry,* 27(6): 675–687.

Shaw, J., and J.J. Harris. 1989. "A prevention/intervention program for child PTSD." Paper presented at the 142nd Annual Meeting of the American Psychiatric Association, San Francisco, CA.

Smith, D.G. 1990. "Thailand: AIDS crisis looms." *Lancet,* 335: 781–782.

State Statistical Bureau. 1989. *Zhongguo Tonggi Nianjian. (Statistical Yearbook of China).* Beijing, China: Statistical Publishing House. p. 889.

Stein, B.N. 1986. "The experience of being a refugee: Insights from the research literature." In C.L. Williams and J. Westermeyer, eds. *Refugee Mental Health in Resettlement Countries.* Washington, DC: Hemisphere Publishing Corporation.

Stein, Z., M. Durkin, and L. Belmont. 1986. "Serious mental retardation in developing countries: An epidemiologic approach." *Annals of the New York Academy of Sciences,* 42:8–21.

Stock, R. 1983. "Distance and the utilization of health facilities in rural Nigeria." *Social Science and Medicine,* 17: 563–570.

Sughandabhirom, B. 1986. "Experiences in a first asylum country: Thailand." In C.L. Williams and J. Westermeyer, eds. *Refugee Mental Health in Resettlement Countries.* Washington, DC: Hemisphere Publishing Corporation.

Szapocznik, J., and R.E. Cohen. 1986. "Mental health care for rapidly changing environments: Emergency relief to unaccompanied youths of the 1980 Cuban refugee wave." In C.L. Williams and J. Westermeyer, eds. *Refugee Mental Health in Resettlement Countries.* Washington, DC: Hemisphere Publishing Corporation.

Turnbull, C.M. 1987. *The Lonely African.* New York: Simon & Schuster.

United States Committee for Refugees. 1990. 1989 World Refugee Statistics. *World Refugee Survey.* Washington, DC: American Council for Nationalities Service.

Weiss, M., S. Sharma, R. Gaur, et al. 1986. "Traditional concepts of mental disorder among Indian psychiatric patients." *Social Science and Medicine,* 23(4): 379–386.

Wen, J.K. 1990. "The hall of dragon metamorphoses: A unique indigenous asylum for chronic mental patients in Taiwan." *Culture, Medicine and Psychiatry,* 14(1): 1–19.

Weng, X.Z. 1988. Smoking—a serious health problem in China. *Chinese Medical Journal,* 101(5): 371–372.

Westermeyer, J. 1986a. "Indochinese refugees in community and clinic: A report from Asia and the United States." In C.L. Williams and J. Westermeyer, eds. *Refugee Mental Health in Resettlement Countries.* Washington, DC: Hemisphere Publishing Corporation.

Westermeyer, J. 1986b. "Migration and psychopathology." In C.L. Williams and J. Westermeyer, eds. *Refugee Mental Health in Resettlement Countries.* Washington, DC: Hemisphere Publishing Corporation.

Wolkind, S., and M. Rutter. 1985. "Separation, loss and family relationships." In M. Rutter and L. Hersov, eds. *Child and Adolescent Psychiatry: Modern Approaches.* Oxford: Blackwell Scientific Publications.

World Health Organization. 1986. *Dementia in later life—research and action.* Geneva: WHO.

World Health Organization. 1987. Global Review. In *Evaluation of the Strategy for Health for All by the Year 2000.* Seventh Report on the World Health Situation. Geneva: WHO.

World Health Organization. 1989. Statistics from the World Health Organization and the Centers for Disease Control. *AIDS.* 3: 543–553.

———. 1989. Indochinese Refugee Activities. *Refugee Reports,* 10:12:5.

———. 1989. *World Almanac and Book of Facts.* New York: Pharos Books.

Section II

Conceptual and Methodological Issues

4

Understanding Morbidity Change

Christopher J. L. Murray
Lincoln C. Chen

In part because of their singular importance and their relative ease of observation, measures of mortality have been the predominant indicators employed in assessing the health status of populations. Yet, "health" is a far more complex phenomenon. Illness, disability, handicap, and other compromised states of well-being — physical, social, and mental — all constitute critical dimensions of health, however difficult their assessment. For the purposes of this article, these attributes of sickness are termed "morbidity."

For decades, investigators have attempted to ascertain health status by measuring, quantifying, and comparing illness and disease in individuals and populations. These attempts at assessing morbidity have grown in importance as life expectancy increases and mortality declines to very low levels in many populations. But sickness may be equally or even more significant in populations still experiencing very high mortality levels. Both the concept of morbidity and its measurement are plagued by conceptual and methodological difficulties. Different morbidity indicators may capture entirely different aspects of illness and health. Differing definitions of health itself underlie some of the complexities.

In this article, we seek to develop an approach to morbidity definition and measurement. We review specific methods and present a framework for classifying different types of morbidity indicators. We examine various approaches to the interactions between morbidity and mortality change and illustrate them by selected data from India, the United States, and Ghana. Finally, we present an integrated approach to understanding the dynamic transitions of both morbidity and mortality in human populations.

Defining and Measuring Morbidity

Morbidity measures are of two fundamental types: self-perceived and observed. Self-perceived morbidity refers to measures that are perceived and reported by an individual, usually in response to inquiries regarding illness. Observed morbidity, in contrast, is assessed through an independent observer employing specific methods that can be repeated with some degree of consistency. Self-perceived morbidity depends upon an individual's perception of illness, while observed morbidity is influenced by standards of abnormality as assessed by a trained observer.

For both self-perceived and observed morbidity, static or functional measures may be used. Static measures describe deviations from an accepted norm or healthy state defined by the subject in self-perceived morbidity and by an external party in observed morbidity. Functional indicators measure loss of performance, inability to perform certain tasks, or constraints in fulfilling certain expected roles.

Table 4-1 sets forth the classification of criteria for morbidity measures that we use to structure the following review.

Self-Perceived Morbidity

Self-perceived morbidity measures can be grouped into four categories: symptoms and impairments, functional disability, handicap, and health service use. The last category, use of health services, could be classified as either self-perceived or observed morbidity, but we have grouped it here because it fundamentally depends upon the recognition and behavior of clients of health services.

Morbidity surveys may depend upon the perception and reporting of *symptoms or impairments* by individuals. Typically, respondents are asked about the occurrence of illness or specific symptoms over a

Table 4-1   Classification of criteria for self-perceived and observed morbidity

Self-Perceived	Observed
Symptoms and impairments	Physical and vital signs
Functional disability	Physiological and pathophysiologic indicators
Handicap	Functional tests
Use of health services	Clinical diagnosis

defined time period — for example, "any illness in the past two weeks." Results from such surveys are the most common form of morbidity data in developing countries. Such information, while useful, is likely to contain serious biases and limitations, which we describe below.

Surveys *of functional disability* include questions on an individual's ability to carry out specific functions and tasks or on restrictions of normal activities. Questions may range from the general, such as inquiries about any restriction of normal activities," to the specific, such as those concerning the ability to perform a particular task. Common tasks of special interest in this context include dressing, meal preparation, shopping, climbing stairs, and physical movement. An extensive literature on disability, mostly related to surveys in industrialized countries, points up many conceptual difficulties in measuring functional disability (Manton, Dowd, and Woodbury, 1986; United Nations, 1986).

We define *handicap* as self-perceived functional disability within a specifically defined context. In other words, "handicap" attempts to measure the significance of a functional disability to an individual in a specific social setting. For example, if a violinist and a banker lose the use of their middle finger, the functional disability is the same, but the degree of handicap is different. To a banker, the loss of a middle finger may be an inconvenience; to a violinist, it would be catastrophic. Very few surveys attempt to measure handicap according to this definition, despite its recommendation by international agencies (World Health Organization 1980; Manton, Dowd, and Woodbury 1986).

Because data on functional disability and handicap are rare in developing countries, levels of *health service use* are often employed to estimate the morbidity burden of a community. Use of health services, however, is likely to yield a very inadequate measure of morbidity. The use of health care services is related to many factors beyond the recognition of illness, including the perceived efficacy of available health care, the ease of access to such care, and the price of the available services. Thus, changes in service use cannot be automatically ascribed to shifts in the underlying burden of illness. Despite such obvious limitations of this measure, many studies equate changes in health service use with changes in morbidity (e.g., Arokiasamy and Chen 1980; Panikar and Soman 1984).

These four measures of self-perceived morbidity are complex conceptually and very difficult to apply with high validity and reliability. Symptom reporting, the most common measure of self-perceived morbidity, is highly sensitive to many factors, some of which relate to the survey methodology itself (notably, language and wording, length of the recall period, the timing of the inquiry, and reporting by proxy respondents). Various methods have been developed to improve the reliability and validity of symptom reporting, such as "salience" questions, tracer lists, the use of diaries, and diagnosis inquiries. These factors are reviewed in more detail in the Appendix.

Several examples of surveys of self-perceived morbidity illustrate some of the problems. As part of the National Sample Survey of India conducted in 1973-74 (28th round), heads of household were asked about morbidity among household members. Each rural household member was asked about acute illness occurring in the two weeks before the survey. For the country as a whole, one in three Indians fell ill annually, with similar rates in urban and rural areas. Noteworthy is the reported morbidity rate for Kerala State, which was the highest, nearly three times the all-India average, despite the fact that Kerala has one of the lowest levels of mortality among Indian states (India, National Sample Survey 1980). The survey also inquired about chronic conditions. Table 2 gives the prevalence of illness by state in rural India for five specific chronic conditions. As with acute conditions, Kerala has a much higher prevalence of self-perceived chronic disease morbidity than other Indian states.

The annual US National Health Interview Survey provides another example of self-perceived morbidity data (e.g., National Center for Health Statistics 1986). The survey employs strict salience criteria. Figure 1 shows that reported acute morbidity in children under 18 years of age rises with income; the relationship with income is reversed in the over-45 age group. Table 3 gives the prevalence of self-perceived chronic illnesses in the United States in 1985 for the same five illnesses as shown in Table 2 for rural India, but disaggregated by age and sex. The prevalence of self-perceived hypertension and arthritis in older Americans approaches 50 percent; among females it exceeds that figure. Although the rates presented in Tables 2 and 3 are not directly comparable, from the data presented in Figure 2 it is apparent that self-reported acute morbidity in the United States is much higher than in rural Kerala, where in turn it is several times higher than the Indian national average for rural India. For each of the five chronic conditions, prevalence in the United States is much higher than in any Indian state.

Table 4-2   Prevalence of reported chronic illnesses per 1,000 persons: rural India, 1973-74

		Selected Conditions		
States	*Epilepsy*	*Hypertension*	*Asthma*	*Rheumatism*	*Piles*
Andra Pradesh	0.17	0.54	2.55	1.83	0.15
Assam	0.11	0.49	1.90	1.55	0.42
Bihar	0.27	0.20	5.19	1.79	0.81
Gujarat	0.09	0.21	2.07	0.04	0.08
Haryana	0.22	0.19	3.83	1.14	1.04
Jammu & Kashmir	0.10	0.96	1.27	0.87	0.30
Karnataka	0.14	0.49	3.02	0.25	0.21
Kerala	1.21	1.48	10.57	23.89	3.69
Madhya Pradesh	0.34	0.20	2.05	1.78	0.22
Maharashtra	0.14	0.20	3.15	0.34	0.44
Orissa	0.08	0.38	0.02	3.97	0.42
Punjab	0.65	0.81	6.30	1.73	1.49
Rajasthan	0.22	0.11	3.57	1.02	0.33
Tamil Nadu	0.36	0.43	2.23	1.25	0.37
Uttar Pradesh	0.28	0.08	4.19	1.47	0.50
West Bengal	0.28	1.41	4.72	2.84	1.13
India	0.28	0.44	3.76	2.51	0.65

Source: India, National Sample Survey 1980

Figure 4-1   Incidence of reported morbidity, by age group and family income: U.S., 1985

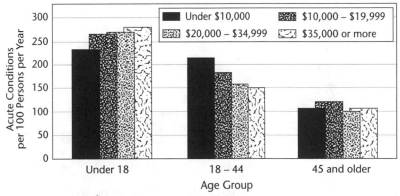

Source: NCHS (1986)

Table 4-3 Prevalence of reported chronic illnesses (selected) per 1,000 persons by age and sex in the United States, 1985.

	Age group			
Male	*under 45*	*45-64*	*65-74*	*75 and over*
Epilepsy	4.6	3.5	8.5	7.1
Hypertension	45.5	253.8	382.0	292.3
Asthma	35.9	27.4	42.4	21.9
Arthritis	21.6	205.9	342.2	398.5
Hemorrhoids	29.2	69.9	61.0	67.2
Female				
Epilepsy	4.4	1.9	9.6	—
Hypertension	34.9	263.5	461.7	453.8
Asthma	42.0	28.9	52.9	22.4
Arthritis	43.9	325.4	550.5	550.5
Hemorrhoids	38.9	72.0	71.2	46.1

Source: NCHS (1986).

Figure 4-2 Incidence of reported morbidity: Rural India (1973–74) and United States (1985)

Acute Conditions per 100 Persons per Year

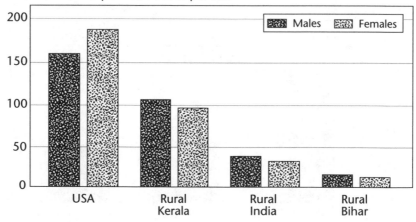

Source: NCHS (1986); India. National Sample Survey (1974)

Table 4-4   Morbidity as indicated by reported rates of bed disability and activity restriction by age and sex: United States, 1985.

Male	Bed disability: days per person	Work or school loss: days per person
Under 5	4.5	—
5-17	3.3	4.4
18-24	2.6	3.5
25-44	3.7	4.3
45-64	7.2	6.1
65+	13.4	8.4
All Ages	5.2	4.7
Female		
Under 5	4.3	—
5-17	4.4	5.3
18-24	4.8	5.4
25-44	5.8	5.9
45-64	9.3	6.9
65+	13.9	5.1
All Ages	7.1	5.8

Source: NCHS (1986).

Many of the limitations of self-perceived morbidity measurement apply equally. to functional disability. The specific tasks that individuals perform *at* each age would be expected to vary widely across cultures, making crossnational comparisons of limited value. Table 4 exemplifies results from a functional disability inquiry in the US National Health Interview Survey (National Center for Health Statistics 1986). The number of days restricted to bed or days lost from work or school are two commonly used measures. These rates of reported bed disability for the United States can be compared with self-reported bed disability from two longitudinal surveys in Kenya and Mexico (Murray et al. 1992). In those countries, adults in reproductive-age groups (15 to 55 years) reported 0.4 to 2.0 days of bedridden morbidity per year; in the United States for similar age groups, reported disability totalled 2.6 to 9.3 bed-days.

Observed Morbidity

Observed morbidity measures can be divided into four categories: physical and vital signs, physiological and pathophysiological indicators, functional tests, and clinical diagnosis.

Physical and vital signs include aspects of disease or pathology that can be detected by physical examination and vital signs like blood pressure. Surveys that collect such information require trained health professionals and are expensive and often logistically difficult. The validity and reliability of results depend upon the clinical skill of the health professionals conducting the examination (Cochrane, Chapman, and Oldham 1951). Not surprisingly, only a few such surveys have been conducted in developing countries (e.g., Colombia, Ministerio de Salud Pública 1969; Egypt, Ministry of Health 1989; Belcher et al. 1976).

Physiological and pathophysiological indicators include laboratory examinations of blood, urine, feces, and other body fluids, and diagnostic imaging such as radiography. Examples of physiological surveys include tuberculin skin sensitivity surveys and mass miniature radiography surveys. Surveys of body measurements, or anthropometry, may be classified as a physiological indicator, although body composition may reflect many factors, including heredity, diet, stress, and the social and physical environment. To the extent that their measurements are well executed, anthropometric results can yield highly reliable measures. Their interpretation, however, is fraught with hazards (Gould 1981).

One limitation of physiological and pathophysiological indicators is that any particular parameter may be defined as abnormal with respect to an arbitrary standard. For anthropometry, as an example, the cutoff point defining malnutrition is often two standard deviations below the mean of a reference population. The functional significance of such a definition is uncertain.

For infectious diseases, it is important to distinguish asymptomatic infection from a clinical disease with observable pathology. Most epidemiological studies on infectious diseases use pathophysiological surveys to measure the prevalence of infection. For example, the data on the presence of Ascaris eggs in stool examinations contain no information on clinically significant Ascaris infection. Similarly, a positive tuberculin skin test means that an individual was previously exposed to Mycobacterium tuberculosis, but only 6 to 8 percent of tuberculosis infections ever progress to clinical disease (Murray, Styblo, and Rouillon, 1990).

Functional tests assess an individual's ability to perform specific functions, such as running, lifting weights, and blowing up a balloon, or to perform intellectual tasks. Functional tests have been advocated by some as the gold standard of disability assessment. Assessments employing functional tests in developing country populations are exceedingly rare.

Clinical diagnosis may be made by a physician or a health worker based upon a constellation of evidence-symptoms, signs, and laboratory results. Together, these may lead to a probabilistic diagnosis. In most surveys, the clinical diagnosis is based only on symptoms and signs without the benefit of laboratory tests.

The distinction between self-perceived symptoms and a personal history as taken by a physician helps illustrate some of the differences in morbidity data. Hampton and colleagues (1975) found that 80 percent of diagnoses could be offered by physicians in a general outpatient clinic on the basis of case history alone. Because of their knowledge base and skills, physicians who are familiar with local patterns of illness can deduce and extract information from a patient that can lead to a clinical diagnosis that a patient cannot make alone. The dependence of clinical diagnosis on a history and physician skill, however, makes this form of observable morbidity less reliable and comparable.

Clinicians' diagnostic skills vary widely. Elinson and Trussel (1957) compared clinical diagnoses by two physicians examining the same patients. For some diseases, they found a two-fold discrepancy in the number of conditions diagnosed in the same group of patients. Also, in many surveys, diagnoses are often made without laboratory confirmation. For example, fever and an enlarged spleen in an area where malaria is endemic would probably be diagnosed as acute malaria. Additionally, symptoms that are self-perceived, most notably pain and neuroses, are a key input to clinical diagnosis. Finally, there are local and regional patterns in how physicians diagnose similar constellations of signs and symptoms. Clinical diagnosis can be less reliable than other observed measures of morbidity.

How comparable are the results of surveys dependent upon self-perceived morbidity compared with those based on observed morbidity? Several studies in the United States examined the relationship between self-reported morbidity and clinical examination (Krueger 1957; Elinson and Trussel 1957; National Center for Health Statistics 1967). Data from the Baltimore Health Survey of 1953-55 (Krueger 1957) reveal the large discrepancy between self-reported morbidity and clinical examination. Even more critical is the variance in correspondence by cause of morbidity — 2 percent for syphilis but 100 percent for rheumatoid arthritis. Krueger (1957) concluded that "the evidence from this study is that though some improvements in content and technique of interviewing can be made, the lay interview is not now or likely to soon become a valuable tool in the measurement of the prevalence of diagnosable chronic disease" (p. 960). Belcher et al. (1976) conducted an analogous comparison of self-perceived morbidity versus clinical diagnosis in Ghana. Their results show a similar variation in correspondence by cause (see Table 4-5). Missing extremities, for example, were rarely self-reported; perhaps because the individuals had adapted and no longer perceived the loss of a limb as morbidity.

These comparative studies suggest that self-perceived morbidity and observed morbidity may be measuring fundamentally different aspects of illness and disease.

An Approach to Measuring Morbidity

Why do measures of self-perceived morbidity and observed morbidity correspond so poorly? Why are the results of morbidity surveys so difficult to compare? In this section, we explore some of the reasons for the distinction between self-perceived and observed morbidity.

Morbidity, that is to say illness, is a type of knowledge. How do we obtain knowledge of ourselves or of others? Throughout history, philosophers have advanced theories of knowledge and perception. They have raised difficult challenges to those who seek to distinguish subjective knowledge from objective knowledge. For example, Protagoras said that "man is the measure of all things"; some have interpreted this to mean that each man is the measure of all things (Russell 1945). Thus, one's own perceptions are just as valid as another's. Observed morbidity in this school of thought is subject to the same limitations as self-perceived morbidity. In this article we do not attempt to address complex epistemological issues.

There are, however, some straightforward explanations for the difference between self-perceived and observed morbidity. Morbidity experiences, we propose, may be categorized into three groups: self-perceived pain and suffering; bodily changes that can be both perceived

Table 4-5   Comparison of prevalence of conditions reported in interviews and indicated by clinical examination in 3,653 patients: Selected conditions, Ghana, 1975.

Condition	Interview	Prevalence (per 1,000) Examination	Ratio
Tracer conditions			
Poliomyelitis	2.4	3.0	0.8
Pyoderma	103.0	156.0	0.66
Conjunctivitis	17.6	38.8	0.45
Diarrhea	8.9	32.4	0.27
Skin Ulcer	1.3	37.0	0.04
Malnutrition	8.1	321.0	0.03
Pediculosis	0.2	32.2	<0.01
Intestinal parasites	1.9	550.0	<0.01
Splenomegaly	0.0	284.0	<0.01
Anemia	0.0	117.0	<0.01
Chronic conditions or impairments			
Blindness	5.3	4.1	1.29
Leprosy	2.1	2.1	1.0
Poliomyelitis	2.4	3.0	0.8
Inguinal Hernia	5.6	19.4	0.29
Malignancy	0.3	1.6	0.19
Missing Extremity	0.3	5.3	0.06
Varicose veins	0.0	7.4	<0.01
Hypertension	0.0	6.2	<0.01
Other conditions			
Low back pain	44.8	2.7	16.6
Yaws	11.7	3.0	3.9
Pregnancy	48.0	30.0	1.6
Fever	51.8	139.4	0.37
Upper respiratory infection	5.0	351.0	0.1
Injuries	1.0	40.7	0.02

Source: Belcher et al. (1976)

and observed; and bodily changes that can only be observed but not perceived. Self-perception is the only source of knowledge about pain and suffering. Pain and suffering cannot be externally observed unless an individual chooses to express them. Self perception can also detect some bodily changes, coinciding with external observations. Other bodily changes, however, such as hypertension or certain malignancies, cannot be perceived at all since they are occult processes. In other words, we propose that to characterize a full range of morbidity, both self-perception and external observation are essential.

Why, then, do self-perceived and externally observed measures of discernible bodily changes (the middle-category morbidity) so often differ? Why are perceptions of pain and suffering so difficult to compare across communities or even within communities? The answer is complex but must include at least the following five factors:

(1)   "I am ill" is a comparative statement. It has meaning only with reference to some idealized state of health (Johansson 1991, 1992). An individual's health ideal, consciously or subconsciously, is shaped by individual and community factors. Individual knowledge and experience may shape personal health ideals. One would expect to find a relationship between a person's education, his or her contact with health services, and his or her health ideals, because all of these directly interact with knowledge and perception of health. The collective community experience may also influence health ideals. If everyone in a community has diarrhea most of the time, the health ideal for that community may not recognize diarrhea as abnormal.

(2)   In addition to varying idealized states of health, there may be, as Mechanic (1986) argues, personal predispositions in the perception of illness. For example, some people when asked to maintain a health diary refuse because the very act of maintaining a record makes them recognize more illness. This phenomenon led Mechanic and Newton to further investigate the link between introspection and illness perception (Mechanic and Newton 1965; Mechanic 1986). One could argue that such a phenomenon may exist at the conununity level as well. Increasing contact with health services may heighten a community's introspection on matters of health, leading to increased perception of morbidity.

(3)   Illness is a social and cultural phenomenon, shaped by culturally defined parameters of illness recognition and behavior. Kleinman (1988) and Kleinman and Tsung-Yi (1981) have written extensively on the phenomenon of illness as a culturally bound concept. Also, Veith (1970)

reports that while hysteria was once common in Western societies, it is now rare, suggesting changing social and cultural influences on health perception. The willingness of an individual to acknowledge sickness depends on social acceptance of particular types of illness and disability (Mechanic 1986).

(4) Stress and psychiatric illness may be expressed as physical symptoms (Kleinman and Tsung-Yi 1981; American Psychiatric Association 1987). For example, depressive disorders can be manifested by weight change, insomnia, fatigue, loss of energy, or change of appetite. This translation of mental to physical processes has been termed somatization.

(5) Conscious misreporting of morbidity to achieve other goals is another factor affecting self-perceived morbidity. Improved sickness compensation systems, especially in industrialized societies, may have led to increased frequency in the reporting (and misrepresenting) of illness.

If self-perceived morbidity is a function of both the burden of pathology and the individual's social and cultural context, then patterns of self-perceived morbidity analyzed by socioeconomic factors may well vary from those expected for observed morbidity. Earlier we noted that self-perceived morbidity rates in India were considerably higher for Kerala than for other Indian states. Yet, Kerala also has the lowest mortality rate in India and enjoys international recognition for its mortality decline (Panikar and Soman 1984; Panikar 1985; Nag 1985). Kumar and Vaidyanathan (1988) argue that Kerala may experience lower mortality at the price of poorer health. However, morbidity rates in Kerala, while high for India, are considerably lower than for the United States. Are Indians healthier than Americans? Are Biharis healthier than Keralites? We think probably not. The evidence is inconclusive. The World Bank's Living Standards Measurement Study provides reported rates of morbidity for Ivory Coast, Ghana, and Peru (Murray et al. 1992). In all three countries, rates of self-perceived morbidity rise with income. The case of Ghana is illustrated in Figure 3. Are the rich suffering a greater burden of pathology than the poor, or do they have more demanding health ideals and a social situation less willing to tolerate illness?

Self-perceived morbidity may be due to the burden of pathology or to variations in illness perception. Patterns of self-perceived morbidity by socioeconomic class are virtually impossible to attribute to either one interpretation or the other. We cannot simply conclude that intuitively

Figure 4-3   Incidence of self-perceived morbidity by economic group and age: Ghana, 1988.

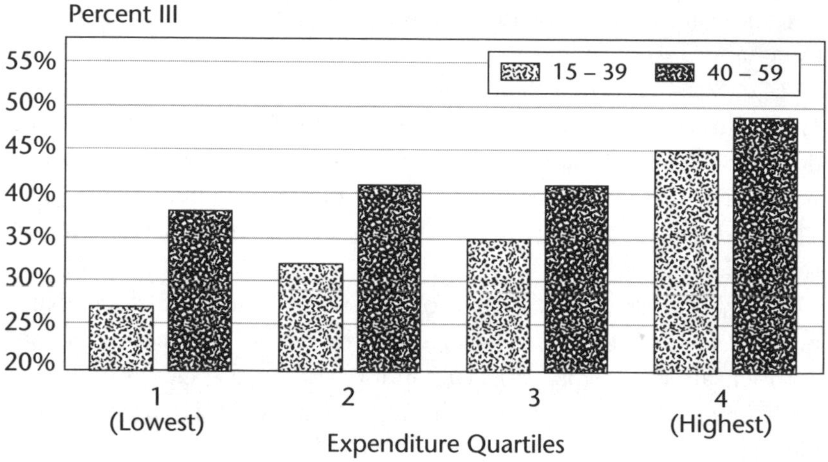

Percent Ill

Legend: 15 – 39, 40 – 59

Y-axis: 55%, 50%, 45%, 40%, 35%, 30%, 25%, 20%

X-axis: 1 (Lowest), 2, 3, 4 (Highest)

Expenditure Quartiles

Source: Murray, Yang, and Qiao 1992.

plausible patterns (that is, higher morbidity in poorer families) are due to real differences of pathology, while counter-intuitive patterns are due to differences in illness perception.

If the interpretation of self-perceived morbidity is so problematic, of what use are measures of self-perceived morbidity? First and perhaps most importantly, perceived illness is by itself a major social phenomenon. If more and more people in a society feel ill, this would be important to anyone concerned with well-being. Second, self-perceived morbidity provides critical information on the relevance of disease to the individual. Only through the individual can we learn about the true burden of pain and suffering. For a health planner concerned with community health, such information is vital. Many would agree that priority-setting should reflect both patterns of observed morbidity and the community's ranking of health problems. Third, in special circumstances, self-perceived morbidity can be a useful tool for monitoring changes in the burden of disease. Sudden changes in self-perceived morbidity probably reflect changes in the burden of pathology. Longer term changes, on the other hand, could equally be due to changing pathology or to social and cultural factors affecting illness perception.

Interactions of Morbidity and Mortality

What happens when changes in morbidity and mortality are considered together as central aspects of health transitions? *Health transition* is a convenient concept that is meant to capture the changing pattern of morbidity and mortality, the socioeconomic determinants of such change, and the response of the health care system. The interactions between morbidity and mortality may have significant effects on the pattern of health transitions. We review some of these interactive processes here. Many are speculative but serve, nevertheless, to illustrate the complexities of simultaneous change in morbidity and mortality.

Selection effect. Several authors (Shepard and Zeckhauser 1980; Feldman 1983; Manton 1982; Alter and Riley 1989) have proposed that as mortality falls, genetically weaker individuals survive longer and in turn are subject to higher rates of disease incidence. Over time, this selection effect would be expected to increase observed morbidity levels. Data presented by Alter and Riley (1989) for the period from 1846 to 1848 to 1893 to 1897 for persons in Manchester, England who were members of the Odd Fellows Society showed a 50 percent rise in reported morbidity even as mortality declined.

How would observed morbidity increase while mortality declines? In nineteenth-century England and Wales, most of the reduction in mortality was due to declines in infectious disease mortality (McKeown 1976). In the absence of effective medical interventions to reduce the case-fatality rate, declines in infectious disease mortality were probably due to decreases in disease incidence. For Alter and Riley's hypothesis of increasing frailty to be valid, individuals who survived because of lower rates of infectious disease must have had higher subsequent risk of acquiring chronic disease. This model of frailty extending across all diseases does not seem plausible, except in extreme cases such as major genetic disorders. Medical experience is more consistent with models of balance: susceptibility to one disease may be balanced by resistance to another. For example, carriers of the sickle-cell trait are apparently more resistant to malaria than non-carrier counterparts (Kan and Dozy 1980).

Riley (1990, 1991) has proposed a novel variant of the frailty model. He has observed in the records of various English Friendly and Sick Societies for the second half of the nineteenth century that the incidence of self-perceived morbidity does not change, only the prevalence. Prevalence increases owing to an increased duration of illness. According to Riley, this phenomenon may be due to the frailty of weaker individuals who survive because of reductions in the case-fatality rate. But he does not provide a biologically plausible explanation of increasing duration in the absence of increasing incidence of illness. Nor does he offer a realistic explanation why case-fatality rates are supposed to have declined in nineteenth-century England. Riley's more subtle argument should not be confused with the direct effect of a declining case-fatality rate on the prevalence of morbidity, which we discuss below.

Cohort effect. A cohort effect is almost the opposite of a selection effect. In this model, each individual is born with a health stock. Childhood infections, malnutrition, and risk factors all reduce the individual's health stock over time, leading to increased observed morbidity incidence and higher mortality risk as persons age (Grossman, 1972). Decreases in the incidence of infectious diseases will lower the incidence of observed morbidity and mortality for a cohort throughout life. Hepatitis B provides an excellent example of a cohort effect. In West Africa and China, early incidence of hepatitis B is followed several decades later by higher rates of hepatocellular carcinoma and cirrhosis (Beasley, Lin, and Hwang 1981). Other examples of the cohort effect include the decline in acute and chronic nephritis following malaria control in Guyana (Giglioli 1972).

Whether one finds a selection effect or a cohort effect depends on the balance of changes between incidence and the case-fatality rate. Pure declines in the case-fatality rate may allow weaker individuals to survive, leading to increased observed morbidity. Alternatively, declines in incidence may leave the population generally stronger, causing reductions in future observed morbidity and mortality.

Reverse cohort effect. Megan Murray (personal communication, 1990) has suggested a reverse cohort effect. Improved nutrition may increase immune system competence, leading to a decrease in the incidence and case fatality from acute infectious diseases. Improved nutrition, however, may also increase immune activity such that autoimmune disease incidence may actually increase. Autoimmune processes are now considered relevant to a wide range of chronic diseases, such as myasthenia gravis, Graves' disease, thyroiditis, some forms of diabetes, asthma, pernicious anemia, rheumatoid arthritis, and primary biliary cirrhosis. If this speculative hypothesis of a reverse cohort effect were true, it would explain some of the tradeoff between reductions in the incidence of infectious diseases and increases in chronic diseases. This theory is given some indirect support by studies showing that undernourished rats have lower levels of morbidity and live nearly twice as long as well-fed rats (McCay et al. 1939)

Delay of death. Gruenberg (1977) and Kramer (1980) have pointed out that in low-mortality countries such as the United States, the life expectancy of individuals with chronic diseases has increased faster than that of the rest of the population, leading to rising prevalence of disability. For example, the life expectancy of some individuals with Down's syndrome has been extended from early adolescence to 70 years. The net effect has been a doubling or quadrupling of the prevalence of Down's syndrome in the population. Gruenberg (1977) argues that these delay-of-death effects are significant for other disorders as well, such as arteriosclerosis, schizophrenia, diabetes, and spina bifida.

Compression of morbidity. Fries (1980, 1983) has proposed that rates of morbidity will decrease faster than mortality, so that chronic disease may be compressed into the final years of life. In this model, life expectancy is already near the highest possible level, meaning that health gains can only be achieved by reducing age-specific incidence rates while case-fatality rates remain constant or increase. There are, however, few examples of the compression of morbidity effect in populations.

Health service effect. Increasing use of health services could lower the case-fatality rate of diseases against which effective technologies exist, especially infectious and parasitic diseases. The use of health services can also increase sclf-perceived morbidity, for two reasons. First is the direct effect of increased numbers of individuals being diagnosed with conditions such as hypertension that are not directly perceivable. Second, increasing knowledge of health processes and health ideals may raise community and individual health standards to more exacting levels. The example of Kerala, described above, suggests that the health service effect may be a dominant theme in the health transition.

Recent Health Transition Experience in the United States

Recent changes in morbidity and mortality in the United States illustrate many of these issues. Between 1950 and 1985, mortality in the United States has declined dramatically at almost all ages (see Figure 4-4).

Figure 4-4 Percent reduction in the age-specific probability of death: United States, 1950-85

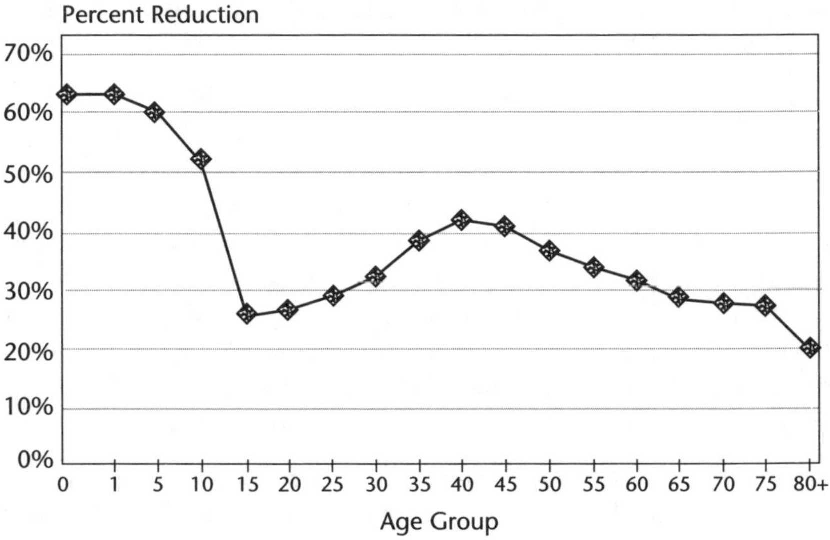

Percent Reduction

Age Group

Source: NCHS (1986)

Over the same period, information on self-perceived morbidity has been collected through the National Health Interview Survey and various assessments of institutionalized populations. Of the many analysts who have examined changes in morbidity and disability (Verbrugge 1984; Colvez and Blanchet 1981; Rice and Laplante 1988; Newacheck, Pudetti, and Halfon 1986; Feldman 1983; Chirikos 1986; Crimmins, Saito, and Ingegneri 1989), all report rising rates of disability in virtually every age group, except perhaps for those over age 75 (Crimmins 1987; Manton 1982).

No consensus exists concerning the interpretation of the pattern of morbidity change in the United States. Shepard and Zeckhauser (1980), Feldman (1983), Gruenberg (1977), and Chirikos (1986) argue that these changes are due to shifts in observed disability as well as in self-perceived disability. Chirikos (1986) and Chirikos and Nestel (1984) also argue that some of the increase in reported morbidity is due to expanded coverage and higher benefits in sickness compensation, which have made disability easier to sustain financially and more socially acceptable. As the methods used in collecting these data have changed over time, Wilson and Drury (1984) see the increase in morbidity as a statistical artifact. Finally, several authors (Colvez and Blanchet 1981; Verbrugge 1984; Crimmins, Saito, and Ingegneri 1989) find it difficult to ignore changes in illness perception. Verbrugge (1984) concludes that "Overall, the most plausible reasons for increased morbidity are people's greater awareness of their diseases, due to earlier diagnoses, lower population mortality rates, and, possibly, earlier accommodations for disease" (p. 509). Crimmins, Saito, and Ingegneri (1989) recognize the difficulty in distinguishing between changes in illness perception and observed morbidity. They note, "What is clear is that more people are reporting themselves as disabled" (p. 254). People also report that they have adapted to their condition by restricting their activity.

Transitions in Morbidity and Mortality

The preceding section reviewed possible patterns and explanations of simultaneous changes in morbidity and mortality. A conceptual analysis of the dynamics of health change, however, must address changes in both perceived and observed morbidity in relation to mortality change. Scarcity of empirical data constrains our analysis. In this section we outline a theoretical approach to interpret potential changes in morbidity and mortality.

Measuring three components of change, we propose, is necessary to describe a health transition: (1) self-perceived morbidity, (2) observed morbidity, and (3) mortality. Four basic mechanisms can, in various combinations, account for the observed changes: population age structure, disease incidence, illness perception, and the case-fatality rate.

As fertility and mortality decline, *a population's age structure* shifts toward later years. With this shift, a larger proportion of deaths will result from the chronic diseases of old age, such as cardiovascular diseases and neoplasms. The impact of this shift may be considerable. For example, in 1990 an estimated 4.8 percent of Africa's population was over 60 years of age while in Latin America the figure was 7.2 percent and in industrialized countries 17.1 percent (United Nations, 1991). A shift from Africa's age structure to an industrialized country's age structure would result in roughly a four-fold increase in the absolute numbers of deaths due to diseases of older age. From a health service provider's perspective, the combination of continued population growth and a shifting age structure can translate into a markedly increased burden of noncommunicable disease morbidity and mortality (e.g., Frenk et al. 1989, on Mexico; World Bank 1989, on Brazil).

A decrease in *disease incidence,* other things equal, should lead to a decline in observed morbidity and a parallel reduction of mortality. Self-perceived morbidity may decrease, remain the same, or even increase. Declines in observed morbidity incidence may be due to reduced infectious disease transmission, improvements in resistance to infections, or reductions in the prevalence of risk factors for noncommunicable diseases. For example, disease incidence could be reduced by vector-control programs, a decline in smoking, or improved personal hygiene. Disease incidence could also increase, leading to the converse change of increased observed morbidity and elevated mortality.

Changes in individual, social, and cultural determinants of *illness perception* can affect levels of self-perceived morbidity without any change in observed morbidity or mortality. We postulate that health ideals tend to be raised in all populations, since once knowledge is obtained it is hard to lose. Declines in self-perceived morbidity due to changes in illness perception may be possible for specific illnesses, but perceived morbidity as a whole is unlikely to decline without major concomitant declines in observed morbidity.

Changes in the *case-fatality rate* alone will lead to changes in mortality, but may have little direct effect on the incidence of observed or self-perceived morbidity. Health service provision and improved nutrition are probably the major mechanisms leading to better survivorship among those who have disease. A classic example is oral rehydration therapy, which can prevent diarrheal mortality without lowering the incidence of disease. Few social, economic, or health technology interventions, however, will operate through only one of these mechanisms. For example, maternal education may increase self-perceived morbidity by raising health ideals, decrease observed morbidity through lower incidence of infectious diseases, and decrease the case-fatality rate through more timely recourse to effective medical care. Each group of causes should be analyzed separately because groups of causes may change in different directions. A change that decreases the case-fatality rate of one disease may increase the incidence of another. A simple example is radiation therapy to treat certain cancers, which can lead to increased incidence of other cancers in later life.

Given the three components of change in health — self-perceived morbidity, observed morbidity, and mortality — a priori, we can postulate eight potential patterns of change. The eight patterns represent all possibilities of rising or falling self-perceived morbidity, observed morbidity, and mortality. Our discussion of the four basic mechanisms of the health transition suggests that some patterns of change are more likely than others. A common pattern would be a decline in observed morbidity and mortality in tandem with an increase in self-perceived morbidity. If declines in observed morbidity outpaced increases in illness perception, then all three components of health could decline through the health transition. Proponents of the selection effect would expect increases in observed and self-perceived morbidity as mortality declines. With some modification, this would also be the pattern observed with pure case-fatality interventions in which mortality is reduced without affecting the incidence of morbidity. Some patterns exist, such as found in the island nation of Nauru, where smoking, obesity, alcohol consumption, and other types of risk-taking behavior have led to rising morbidity, observed and self-perceived, and higher mortality. A potential pattern in which self-perceived morbidity declines while observed morbidity decreases would be similar to the pattern expected on the basis of the compression-of-morbidity argument, for which no empirical evidence yet exists.

Conclusion

This article has illustrated the complex task of defining and measuring morbidity in human populations. We lack adequate conceptual frameworks to approach an understanding of the dynamics of morbidity and mortality change. Because of the limitations of data and our primary reliance upon self-perceived morbidity data, there is a tendency to conclude that morbidity is likely to rise during health transitions. But such a conclusion is wrong; it runs starkly counter to observed health conditions in developing countries. Diseases such as tuberculosis, onchocerciasis, filariasis, trachoma, leprosy, polio, and many others that cause significant disability are much more prevalent in developing countries than in industrialized countries. Other parasitic diseases such as intestinal nematodes and malaria may be major causes of undetected morbidity and disability through mechanisms such as anemia and growth retardation. We should not ignore the greater burden of observed morbidity in developing countries simply because morbidity is difficult to monitor.

Analysis of the complex and confusing patterns of change in mortality, causes of death, self-perceived morbidity, and observed morbidity that characterize health transitions requires a multi-disciplinary approach. For example, understanding of changes in illness perception will most likely come from the fields of anthropology and psychiatry rather than epidemiology or public health. The patterns we have examined suggest to us that the wisdom of many fields-including demography, epidemiology, economics, anthropology, public health, education, medicine, psychiatry, politics, and philosophy-will be needed to illuminate the complex dynamics of health transitions.

Appendix

Biases and limitations of measures of self-perceived morbidity

Many factors influence the outcome of assessments of self-perceived morbidity from survey instruments, including:

Language and wording. The wording of questions can have a significant effect on the reported burden of illness. Subtle differences, especially when translated into other languages, can lead to altered meanings and reported levels of morbidity. In some cultures, for example, there are different terms for diarrhea depending on the season, age of the child, and character of the stool.

Salience. The concept of salience was developed to overcome the apparent lack of comparability between self-perceived and reported morbidity (Mechanic and Newton 1965). Individuals are asked to report only on illness that results in specific action-for example, change in activity, change in diet, or consultation with a health care provider. The particular salience criterion may vary from survey to survey. In the United States, the salience criteria of the National Health Interview Survey (NHIS) are whether the illness caused a reduction of customary activity for one or more days, or whether a physician was contacted (National Center for Health Statistics 1986: 3). In several developing countries, the following salience criteria were used in recent morbidity surveys: unable to perform usual routine for at least 24 hours, unable to take normal food for at least 24 hours, or requiring bed rest for at least 24 hours (Pakistan, Federal Bureau of Statistics 1986; Thailand, National Statistics Office 1983). Clearly, when salience criteria are used, the rate of self-perceived morbidity will decline, and salience cannot probe for some illnesses (for example, a migraine headache is not counted in the NHIS unless it leads to the loss of a day's activity or a visit to a doctor) that are not related to the criteria employed. Salience criteria are not universally used. For example, the World Bank's Living Standards Measurement Studies in Ivory Coast, Ghana, and Peru had no such criteria (Murray et al. 1992).

Recall period. The length of the recall period may have an effect on reporting error (Linder 1965; Kroeger 1983; Ross and Vaughan 1986). Recent events are usually reported more frequently than distant illness. The resulting loss of accuracy over time is more pronounced for acute than chronic conditions. Results from the 1954-55 California Health Survey illustrate the effect of the length of recall period on reported morbidity rates (Linder, 1965).

Tracer lists. Lists of symptoms may be used to increase the yield of reported morbidity. Data from the US NHIS illustrate how the use of probing questions or tracer lists can more than double the amount of illness reported (Linder, 1965). Kroeger's (1983) review of developing country morbidity surveys found tracer lists to be infrequently used.

Diaries. Another method that can increase the reporting of morbidity is longitudinal maintenance of diaries by the respondent (Mechanic and Newton 1965; WHO 1967). For acute conditions, diaries are more sensitive than cross-sectional recall surveys.

Proxy respondents. When an adult in the household is asked to report on illness of another member, often a child, two independent sources of bias may exist. First, individuals tend to report less illness for others than for themselves. For example, Linder (1965) shows a 4 to 20 percent error generated by proxy respondents. Not all studies, however, have confirmed this bias (Enterline and Capt 1959). Second, some proxy respondents appear to report generally more morbidity for themselves than for other household members (Mechanic and Newton 1965). These problems may be an especially important source of bias in parental reporting of morbidity in children.

Diagnoses versus symptoms. Some surveys use tracer lists to ask respondents about specifically diagnosed diseases. This method presumes respondents' knowledge of disease diagnosis. Also, diagnosis surveys may be influenced by contact with health services that provide people with medical information on disease diagnosis and processes.

Timing. Seasonal variability in morbidity, particularly acute morbidity, means that surveys covering only a brief time period may misrepresent the average annual rates of illness.

Acknowledgement

This article is reprinted with permission of the Population Council, from Murray, C.J.L. and L.C. Chen, 1992, "Understanding morbidity change." *Population and Development Review,* 18(3): 481-503.

References

Alter, G., and J.C. Riley. 1989. "Frailty, sickness, and death: Models of morbidity and mortality in historical populations." *Population Studies,* 43: 25–45.

American Psychiatric Association. 1987. *Diagnostic and Statistical Manual of Mental Disorders, III.* Washington, DC: American Psychiatric Association.

Arokiasamy, J.T., and P.C.Y. Chen. 1980. "A comparison of morbidity patterns in Peninsular Malaysia 1959 and 1979." *Medical Journal of Malaysia,* 34: 336–342.

Beasley, R.P., C.C. Lin, and L.Y. Hwang. 1981. "Hepatocellular carcinoma and hepatitis B virus: A prospective study of 22,707 men in Taiwan." *Lancet,* 2: 1129–1133.

Belcher, D.W., A.K. Neumann, F.K. Wurapa, and L.M. Lourie. 1976. "Comparison of morbidity interviews with a health examination survey in rural Africa." *American Journal of Tropical Medicine and Hygiene,* 25: 751–758.

Chirikos, T.N. 1986. "Accounting for the historical rise in work–disability prevalence." *Milbank Memorial Fund Quarterly: Health and Society,* 64: 271–301.

Chirikos, T.N., and G. Nestel. 1984. "Economic determinants and consequences of self-reported work disability." *Journal of Health Economics,* 3: 117–136.

Cochrane, A.L., P.J. Chapman, and P.D. Oldham. 1951. "Observer's error in taking medical histories." *Lancet,* 1: 1007–1010.

Colombia, Ministerio de Salud Pública. 1969. *Estudio de Recursos Humanos Para la Salud y Educación Medica en Colombia: Investigación Nacional de Morbilidad: Evidencia Clinica.* Bogota: Ministerio de Salud Pública.

Colvez, A., and M. Blanchet. 1981. "Disability trends in the United States population 1966–76: Analysis of reported causes." *American Journal of Public Health,* 71: 464–471.

Crimmins, E.M. 1987. "Evidence on the compression of morbidity." *Gerontologica Perspecta,* 1: 45–49.

Crimmins, E.M., Y. Saito, and D. Ingegneri. 1989. "Changes in life expectancy and disability-free life expectancy in the United States." *Population and Development Review,* 15: 235–267.

Egypt Ministry of Health. 1989. *Final Report: The Health Examination Survey. Morbidity, Nutritional and Dental Status in Cairo*. Ministry of Health Publication No. 38/4.

Elinson, J., and R.E. Trussel. 1957. "Some factors relating to degree of correspondence for diagnostic information as obtained by household interviews and clinical examinations." *American Journal of Public Health*, 47: 311–321.

Enterline, P.E., and K.G. Capt. 1959. "A validation of information provided by household respondents in health surveys." *American Journal of Public Health*, 49: 205–212.

Feldman, J. 1983. "Work ability of the aged under conditions of improving mortality." *Milbank Memorial Fund Quarterly: Health and Society*, 61: 430–444.

Frenk, J., et al. 1989. "Health transition in middle-income countries: New challenges for health care." *Health Policy and Planning*, 4: 29–39.

Fries, J.F. 1980. "Aging, natural death and the compression of morbidity." *New England Journal of Medicine*, 303: 130–135.

Fries, J.F. 1983. "The compression of morbidity." *Milbank Memorial Fund Quarterly: Health and Society*, 61: 397–419.

Giglioli, G. 1972. "Changes in the pattern of mortality following the eradication of hyperendemic malaria from a highly susceptible community." *WHO Bulletin*, 46: 181–202.

Gould, S.J. 1981. *The Mismeasure of Man*. New York: Norton.

Grossman, M. 1972. "On the concept of health capital and the demand for health." *Journal of Political Economy*, 80: 223–255.

Gruenberg, E.M. 1977. "The failure of success." *Milbank Memorial Fund Quarterly: Health and Society*, 55: 3–24.

Hampton, J.R., et al. 1975. "Relative contributions of history-taking, physical examination, and laboratory investigation to diagnosis and management of medical outpatients." *British Medical Journal*, 2: 486–489.

India, National Sample Survey. 1980. "On morbidity: National sample survey twenty-eighth round. Schedule 12; October 1973–June 1974." *Sarvekshana*, 17–20: S137–S180.

Johansson, S.R. 1991. "The health transition: The cultural inflation of morbidity during the decline of mortality." *Health Transition Review*, 1: 39–68.

Johansson, S.R. 1992. "Measuring the cultural inflation of morbidity during the decline of mortality." *Health Transition Review*, 2: 78–89.

Kan, Y.W., and A.M. Dozy. 1980. "Evolution of the hemoglobin S and C genes in world populations." *Science*, 209: 388.

Kleinman, A. 1988. *The Illness Narratives: Suffering, Healing and the Human Condition*. New York: Basic Books.

Kleinman, A. and T. Lin, eds. 1981. *Normal and Abnormal Behavior in Chinese Culture*. Dordrecht: Reidel.

Kramer, M. 1980. "The rising pandemic of mental disorders and associated chronic diseases and disorders." *Acta Psychiatrica Scandinavica*, 62(Suppl): 285.

Kroeger, A. 1983. "Health interview surveys in developing countries: A review of methods and results." *International Journal of Epidemiology*, 12: 465–481.

Krueger, D.E. 1957. "Measurement of prevalence of chronic disease by household interviews and clinical evaluations." *American Journal of Public Health*, 47: 953–960.

Kumar, B.G., and A. Vaidyanathan. 1988. "Morbidity in India: Some problems of measurement, interpretation and analysis." Paper presented to 6th annual convention of the Indian Society for Medical Statistics, National Seminar on Statistics in Medicine, Health, and Nutrition, October 27–29.

Linder, F.E. 1965. *National Health Interview Surveys*. Geneva: World Health Organization. Public Health Papers; v. 27.

Manton, K.G. 1982. "Changing concepts of morbidity and mortality in the elderly population." *Milbank Memorial Fund Quarterly: Health and Society*, 60: 183–244.

Manton, K.G., J.E. Dowd, and M.A. Woodbury. 1986. "Conceptual and measurement issues in assessing disability cross–nationally: Analysis of a WHO–sponsored survey of the disablement process in Indonesia." *Journal of Cross-Cultural Gerontology*, 1: 339–362.

McCay, C.M., L.A. Maynard, G. Sperling, and L.L. Bames. 1939. "Retarded growth, lifespan, ultimate body size and age changes in the albino rat." *Journal of Nutrition*, 18: 1–13.

McKeown, T. 1976. *The Modern Rise of Population*. London: Edward Arnold.

Mechanic, D. 1986. "The concept of illness behavior: Culture, situation and personal predisposition." *Psychological Medicine*, 16: 1–7.

Mechanic, D., and M. Newton. 1965. "Some problems in the analysis of morbidity data." *Journal of Chronic Diseases*, 18: 569–580.

Murray, C.J.L., K. Styblo, and A. Rouillon. 1990. "Tuberculosis: Burden, interventions and costs." *Bulletin of International Union against Tuberculosis and Lung Diseases*, 65(1): 626.

Murray, C.J.L., R.G.A. Feachem, M. Phillips, and C. Willis. 1992. "Adult morbidity: Limited data and methodological uncertainty." In R.G.A. Feachem, et al., eds. *The Health of Adults in the Developing World*. New York: Oxford University Press.

Murray, C.J.L., I.G. Yang, and X. Qiao. 1992. "Adult mortality: Levels, patterns, and causes." In R.G.A. Feachem, et al., eds. *The Health of Adults in the Developing World*. New York: Oxford University Press.

Nag, M. 1985. "The impact of social and economic development on mortality: Comparative study of Kerala and West Bengal." In S.B. Halstead, J.A. Walsh, and K.S. Warren, eds. *Good Health at Low Cost.* New York: Rockefeller Foundation.

National Center for Health Statistics (NCHS). 1965. "Health interview responses compared with medical records." *Vital and Health Statistics,* Series 2. Data Evaluation and Methods Research, no. 7.

National Center for Health Statistics (NCHS). 1967. "Interview data on chronic conditions compared with information derived from medical records." *Vital and Health Statistics,* Series 2. Data Evaluation and Methods Research, no. 23.

National Center for Health Statistics (NCHS). 1986. "Current estimates from the National Health Interview Survey, United States, 1985." *Vital and Health Statistics,* Series 10, no. 160.

Newacheck, P.W., P.P. Pudetti, and N. Halfon. 1986. "Trends in activity-limiting chronic conditions among children." *American Journal of Public Health,* 76: 178–184.

Pakistan, Federal Bureau of Statistics. 1986. *National Health Survey 1982–83.* Karachi: Government of Pakistan.

Panikar, P.G.K. 1985. "Health care system in Kerala and its impact on infant mortality." In S.B. Halstead, J.A. Walsh, and K. S. Warren, eds. *Good Health at Low Cost.* New York: Rockefeller Foundation.

Panikar, P.G.K., and C.R. Soman. 1984. *Health Status of Kerala: The Paradox of Economic Backwardness and Health Development.* Trivandrum: Centre for Development Studies.

Rice, D.P., and M.P. Laplante. 1988. "Chronic illness, disability and increasing longevity." In S. Sullivan and M.E. Lewin, eds. *The Economics and Ethics of Long-Term Care and Disability.* Washington, DC: Brookings Institution.

Riley, J.C. 1989. *Sickness, Recovery and Death: A History and Forecast of Ill Health.* Iowa City: University of Iowa Press.

Riley, J.C. 1990. "The risk of being sick: Morbidity trends in four countries." *Population and Development Review,* 16: 403–432.

Riley, J.C. 1991. "The prevalence of chronic diseases during mortality increase: Hungary in the 1980s." *Population Studies,* 45: 489–496.

Ross, D.A., and J.P. Vaughan. 1986. "Health interview surveys in developing countries: A methodological review." *Studies in Family Planning,* 17: 78–94.

Russell, B. 1945. *A History of Western Philosophy.* New York: Simon and Schuster.

Shepard, D., and R. Zeckhauser. 1980. "Long-term efforts of interventions to improve survival in mixed populations." *Journal of Chronic Diseases,* 33: 413–433.

Thailand, National Statistics Office. 1983. *Health and Welfare Survey 1981.* Bangkok: National Statistics Office.

United Nations. 1986. *Development of Statistics of Disabled Persons: Case Studies.* New York: United Nations.

United Nations. 1991. *World Population Prospects 1990.* New York: United Nations.

Veith, L. 1970. *Hysteria: The History of the Disease.* Chicago: University of Chicago Press.

Verbrugge, L. 1984. "Longer life but worsening health? Trends in health and mortality of middle-aged and older persons." *Milbank Memorial Fund Quarterly: Health and Society,* 62: 475–519.

Wilson, R.W., and T.F. Drury. 1984. "Interpreting trends in illness and disability: Health statistics and health status." *Annual Review of Public Health,* 5: 83–106.

World Bank. 1989. *Adult Health in Brazil: Adjusting to New Challenges.* Washington, DC: World Bank.

World Health Organization. 1967. "Morbidity statistics: Twelfth report of the WHO expert committee on health statistics." *Transactions of the World Health Organization 389.*

World Health Organization. 1980. *International Classification of Impairments, Disabilities and Handicaps: A Manual of Classification Relating to the Consequences of Disease.* Geneva: WHO.

5

Objectivity and Position:
Assessment of Health and Well-Being

Amartya Sen

Introduction

Objectivity is central to scientific knowledge. It is important also for practical reasoning, ethics and jurisprudence. While I have been concerned with these broader issues elsewhere (Sen 1982, 1983a, 1983b, 1993), in this paper I concentrate on a much more limited range of methodological issues, related to the assessment of health and well-being.

That objective knowledge can be deeply threatened by the subjectivity of observations has been often discussed and emphasized (in my judgment rightly so). The observer's personal prejudices and leanings can leave a lasting imprint on observation and analysis. The fear of such "subjectivity" has bred a deep suspicion of the influence of the observer's position on what is observed.

I argue that the idea of objectivity requires explicit acceptance and extensive use of variability of observations with the position of the observer. Positionality can be fruitfully seen as a parametric feature of objectivity, and has to be distinguished from subjectivity. Being subjective is, in a deep sense, a denial of — or a challenge to — objectivity of observations and assessments. In contrast, the recognition of the influence of observational position is part and parcel of the objectivity of observations, and its influence has to be acknowledged and scrutinized in arriving at generalized objective assessments.

In this context, it is important to distinguish between "positional objectivity," which is a claim regarding the objectivity of observations from a certain position, and "transpositional objectivity," which takes us beyond that. The latter has to build on the former. I also argue that both positional objectivity and transpositional objectivity have their own relevance, and even though they link with each other in many different ways, neither can supplant the other. Some practical examples are discussed to illustrate the concrete relevance of the issues outlined. The illustrations deal with the assessment of health and well-being.

Observations, Presumptions and Impersonality

We have to distinguish between the objectivity of *specific observational statements* and that of *generalized presumptive claims* (dealing with such matters as observational inferences, causal connections, descriptive assessments and evaluative affirmations). Observational objectivity is, in an important sense, prior to the objectivity of generalized presumptive claims. The latter admits more freedom of conclusion, consistently with objectivity, than does the former, given the need to go more deeply into assessment and generalization. This is not to deny that what we believe we have actually observed may also depend on our theories regarding what to expect. There is a two-way relation between observations of object and theories regarding them. Observations are influenced by preexisting concepts, and these concepts in turn can be influenced by the results of observations. The acceptance of the former direction of influence does not entail a rejection of the latter.[1]

Two central features of objectivity are (1) *observation dependence,* and (2) *impersonality.* These issues are captured well by the standard *Oxford English Dictionary* characterizations of "subjectivity": (i) "having its source in the mind", and (ii) "pertaining or peculiar to an individual subject or his mental operations". The first feature relates to the inward-looking nature of subjective judgments or theories. The second feature is one of *interpersonal variance.* Objectivity demands taking observations seriously and also demands that there be some *invariance* vis-à-vis the subject who is doing the observation and assessment.

A central problem in understanding objectivity concerns the contrast between "subjectivity" and "positionality". A person's observations and reflections may be influenced not only by what may be described as the observer's subjectivity, but also by his or her objective "positional" characteristics.

For example, an object may look larger or smaller depending on our position vis-à-vis the object. This is a variability that is patently related to the person's actual position vis-à-vis the object studied. It would be odd to say that a person is "being subjective" in reporting that an object — positioned at a great distance — looks small from where he stands. If he were to insist that the object is, in fact, simply tiny, that would, of course, be a different matter. It would be a departure from objectivity due to his failure to take adequate note of the particularity of the objective position from which he made his observation. But that does not make the first statement — constructively dependent on the position of the observer — any less objective.

Variations and Positional Parameters

One part of the search for an optimal combination of objectivity and subjectivity (as Thomas Nagel describes it in his *The View from Nowhere,*1986) may possibly be conveniently seen as the pursuit of the relevant kind of objectivity in different contexts. Nagel points out that objectivity is a characteristic of which we can have more — or less. It is not just a matter of either being objective or not being objective. Nagel presents the issue thus:

> A view or form of thought is more objective than another if it relies less on the specifics of the individual's makeup and position in the world, or on the character of the particular type of creature he is. The wider the range of subjective types to which a form of understanding is accessible — the less it depends on specific subjective capacities — the more objective it is (p. 5).

There are some ambiguities in interpreting the criterion of greater or lesser reliance on the specifics of the individual and his or her position. The troubling issue is the possible relevance, referred to earlier, of the specifics of a person's "position", broadly defined, as part of the objective analysis. This depends, of course, on the subject matter. Some observations or assessments are irreducibly "positional" (e.g., how large an object looks), whereas others are not (e.g., how large the object is).

There are two rather different types of questions involved in assessing objectivity of claims, and both are closely connected with the relevance of positionality. One is that of "accessibility" on which Nagel focuses in the quoted passage, and the other is that of "priority" among different accessible and understandable views. Greater accessibility can be one criterion in assessing priority, but other standards must also be used. Taking note of positional parameters makes it easier to understand why certain observations took the form they did and makes those observations — and remarks and theories based on them — that much more accessible. But we may have to choose between accessible views from different positions, and there we might need other criteria to supplement that of accessibility to determine what may be taken to be more objective than the rival views.

Positional and Transpositional Objectivity

There is a sense in which there can be no view from nowhere. What can be taken as a view from nowhere must be, in some ways, a constructed and scrutinized derivation based ultimately on the views from particular positions. On this interpretation, a non-positional view must be a transpositional view. There is a clear sequential priority of the positional observation.

The articulator can either make specifically positional utterances, or transpositional statements. Correspondingly, there are issues of *positional objectivity* and the bigger question of *transpositional objectivity*. In assessing how large an object looks from somewhere, the primary concern has to be with the views of that object from that position (no matter where the articulator happens to be). The fact that the object looks different from *elsewhere* is not counterevidence to the truth or to the positional objectivity of that statement (though that fact is central to making *comparative* positional statements, e.g., that an object looks small*er* from a more distant position). That the moon looks small *from where I am* is not contradicted by the actual size of the moon, or the fact that it looked big enough to Neil Armstrong.

On the other hand, in assessing how large the object "in fact is", or how large the object can be said to be *without* a positional characterization, it is very relevant to take critical note of the views from different positions (related to space as well as other parameters). Criteria would, then, have to be found for discriminating between different objectively positional views to arrive at appropriate transpositional statements. The appraisal of *transpositional* objectivity calls for rules of assessment — of "priority" — that have to go beyond what is needed in examining the demands of objectivity of observations from an amply *specified position*.

The contrast between "positional"and "transpositional" objectivity is not, however, as sharp as it may first appear (see also Sen 1993). Positional specifications tend to be typically incomplete, and some implicit transpositional assessment is standardly involved in examining objectivity from some specified — but not exhaustively specified — position.

The simplest criterion of transpositional acceptability may be one of congruence of *all* the relevant positional views. A view can, then, be taken to be *transpositional* because of its being *omni*-positional. Sometimes "the view from nowhere" may be based on the existential quantifier rather than the universal quantifier, and can refer to the existence of a position from which that statement could be truthfully made. To say that "Leonardo da Vinci's 'Adoration of the Magi' looks beautiful" is not a claim that it is attractive from everywhere (e.g., ten miles away from the observer, or one inch from her nose), but that there exists a position (or many positions) from which it does look beautiful.

In other cases, some distinguished positional views may be taken to be particularly important and decisive in the scrutiny for an appropriate transpositional assessment. For example, in checking the time, the view presented by some special nuclear clock may well be taken as decisive, and any alternative observation, say, that according to my own perfectly ordinary watch, might be outweighed in the critical scrutiny (even when the assessment and articulation are done by me). The idea of transpositional objectivity incorporates ideas of coherent reasoning accessible to others and not anchored on positionally peculiar observations.

A particular positional view may get priority because it might help to "tie up" other positional observations in a coherent way. A special nuclear clock could serve as such an anchor piece, helpful in cogently explaining variations of the observations made with other clocks. Similarly, a close observation of an object may reveal something about its shape that can be used to explain other observations made from greater distance. Persons at different distances from the object may all see the advantage, in this case, of the close view, and can accept how their own — more distant — positional observations may all fit well with that closer diagnosis. And so on.

The interpositional scrutiny of different positional observations need not be isolated or inward-looking, and may involve related observations and their connections. For example, the clinical observation of malaria, in a particular case, based on a blood test by a qualified medical practitioner, may command attention precisely because of the regularities of connection established through accumulated evidence, and this may contrast with an alternative observation, proffered by the local "wise man" (e.g., that it looks to him like a transparent case of kal-azar). The exact criteria of discrimination for transpositional objectivity may vary with the nature of the subject matter, but the principles underlying the criteria would have to incorporate *inter alia* certain general characteristics of accessibility and cogency (including coherence over an extensive domain).

Position-selected Objectivity and Its Relevance

If we take a fully deterministic view of causation, it can be argued that anyone's actual observation of any object can be entirely accounted for by an adequate specification of his or her positional parameters vis-à-vis the object. If those parameters were all to be specified as part of the positional identification, then the observation based on those parameters would be potentially fully explainable to others. In this sense, any actual observation can be seen as positionally objective for some appropriately thorough specification of positional parameters. So-called subjective features influencing an observation would, then, be *included* in the specified positional parameters.

If a person who is scared and uncritical mistakenly sees a rolled umbrella in the hands of another person as a gun, the (transpositional) unobjectivity of the observation that the other person had a gun does not contradict the *positional objectivity* of his seeing what seemed to him to be a gun. By bringing in all the positional parameters (including his being scared and hurried), his observation can be made accessible to and understandable by others, given the extensive specification of circumstances and mental states. On the other hand, if we do not specify the position with all those parameters, and simply ask whether a person encountering another with a rolled umbrella in good light would be objective in taking that umbrella to be a gun, the answer could certainly be "no".

The belief in women's inferiority in particular skills may be statistically associated with living in a society that partly or wholly reserves those skilled occupations for men (let us call such societies S-societies). That association does not make that belief objective — either transpositionally, or even from the position of living in an S-society. The positional specification in the form of living in such an S-society is, of course, incomplete. In denying the positional objectivity of the *observation* of women's inferiority from that underspecified position, the relevant point is not the *transpositional unobjectivity* of the alleged feminine inferiority, nor the fact that in other societies women are not viewed as being inferior in these ways. The immediate issue is the nonnecessity of taking such a view of feminine inferiority even for those living in an S-society. Contrary views can be taken consistently with living in an S-society, and the critique of that view can be "internal" (rather than arising from outside that society).[2]

However, if the specification of the position is extended in particular ways (including, for example, specifying particular types of conservative social conditioning, closed-minded schooling, the absence of knowledge outside the boundaries of the local society, nonreading of scientific or political literature, intellectual inability to consider counterfactual possibilities, and so on), it is possible to arrive at a thoroughly specified position such that the perception of women's inferior skill would be positionally objective from that particular *thoroughly specified position*. In a transpositional assessment ("Are women inferior in these skills?"), that view, though positionally objective from that exhaustively specified position ("Do women appear to be inferior in these skills in these societies when viewed with all these positional characteristics?"), would not be very influential because of the peculiar and partisan nature of that thoroughly constrained position.

Subjective Probability and Positional Objectivity

Positional objectivity often has interest of its own (in terms of understanding of attitudes, beliefs, actions) without being necessarily a ticket to transpositional eminence.[3] For example, in taking prudential decisions about how to act, the special relevance of one's own position can hardly be ignored. It may be useful to note that while the so-called "subjective probabilities" are *defined* in terms of degrees of belief or credence (and are thus personal), the vast decision-theoretic literature on how to *form, modify or adjust* these beliefs makes extensive use, implicitly, of considerations of positional objectivity. Indeed, the relationship between so-called "subjective" and "objective" probabilities can be helpfully seen in terms of the distinction between positional and transpositional objectivity.

To illustrate, consider a case in which you have tossed what we both accept as an even coin and you can see whether it is head or tail that has come up, but my view is obscured by your palm. You ask me what bets would I take, and thus enquire about my so-called "subjective probabilities" (as they are defined in the literature).

It is easily seen that I cannot sensibly take either a purely subjective view or a transpositionally objective view in deciding on what bets to take. It would be silly of me to take, say, a 1-to-10 bet that it is a head (even if I feel tempted by that suggestion), since I should know that for an even coin the "chances" don't favor that bet. I can, of course, be as subjective as I like without straining the meaning of "subjective probability" (that term, as explained before, refers only to the defining of probabilities in terms of bets I am willing to take, rather than going into the basis of the bets that I am willing to take), but it would not be sensible for me to be so subjective in choosing the actual bets I take.[4]

On the other hand, what I have to seek is not objectivity that ignores the relevant peculiarities of my own position. Either head or tail has definitely come up and you actually know what it is. In any transpositional assessment of truth of the kind used in science, your view — based on seeing the coin — will get understandable priority. But in my position, I don't know what your view is any more than I can observe which way the coin has come up. In deciding on bets, if the sensible view to take by me — or by anyone else in my position — is to act on the basis of a reading of a 50-50 chance, then the claim must be that that view is indeed unprejudiced and objective from my position. Positional objectivity is, in this context, exactly what is being sought, and it has to be distinguished both from subjectivity and from general transpositional objectivity.

Illness and Management of Health Care

In the analysis of ill health and morbidity, the subject's perceptions are obviously of central importance. The doctor's need to inquire into the patient's feelings, sensations and concerns can hardly be overemphasized.

In medical management and health care there are different observational positions with their own peculiar relevance. The self-perception of the patient can differ from the assessment of the doctor; observations by doctors can contrast with those by other health workers; the perspective of the general practitioners can diverge from that of specialists; and so on. It is critical to see the importance of each of these observational positions, without attempting to subsume one in another. The positional objectivities can clash with each other, and while transpositional assessment is ultimately important, that need does not do away with the relevance of the respective positional observations.

The issue of positional objectivity is important not only from the point of view of the patient, but also that of the health practitioner. Arthur

Kleinman (1986) notes the alienating effects of various influences (what I shall call "positional parameters") that can affect the observation of patients by health practitioners, including "the gallows humor that journeymen in health care develop to manage the anxieties and frustrations they experience in the exigent difficulties of their trade," "institutional demands for technical efficiency," "insurance demands that the intervention be technologized for purposes of reimbursement," and also "the not-so-covert values of the biomedical discourse," all of which mould "their clinical construction of reality".

These influences may well make their "construction of reality" non-objective in a transpositional sense, but the force of the positional objectivity (given the specified positional parameters) deserves serious recognition for medical reform. That force depends crucially on the objectivity of those observations in the limited positional context. The reclassification of "the patients" into types such as "con men", "socio-paths" or "deadbeats" may reflect a failure of transpositional objectivity, but to see such practice merely as examples of personal subjectivity would be to ignore the powerful positional influences that make these distortions look real and insightful.[5] Positional objectivity has to be given a central place in the science and practice of medicine not only from the point of view of the patients, but also that of the health practitioners.

Assessment of Morbidity

Turning to the issue of assessment of morbidity, positional objectivity from the point of view of the patients themselves can be very important in some cases. In many contexts, the perception itself is part of the ailment. Having a headache, or experiencing nausea or dizziness, can be seen as a disease in itself and not just a symptom of one. In these cases the priority of the self-perceptual view would seem to be hard to escape in a transpositional assessment.

But in other cases, self-perception can be a difficult basis for transpositional appraisal and diagnosis of medical conditions and health status. Perception-based empirical analysis can be plagued (1) by perceptual variability both interpersonal differences and intertemporal volatility, and also (2) by systematic social influences that may make interpersonal comparisons particularly problematic.

Self-perceptions can be enormously affected by one's general mental outlook. The problem is not so much that a hypochondriac is not ill — he may well be very ill — but that his more frequent and more insistent complaints do not indicate that he is more ill than the cheerful patient who is always reassuring his doctor that he is fine ("Never felt better, but tell me, doctor, are you well and full of job satisfaction?").

A particularly difficult problem relates to systematic social influences. Understanding of morbidity is often associated with education, and the privileged frequently report higher incidence of illness. There is another connection that deserves more attention than it has tended to get. Systematic use of medical services both (1) reduces one's morbidity, and (2) increases the self-perception and reporting of morbidity. A population that goes to see doctors regularly may enjoy better health, but at the same time will have a clearer awareness of health problems and will be seen as making more frequent use of medical services. This connection makes international or interregional comparisons of health conditions based on questionnaires and on observed use of medical services not only misleading, but sometimes perversely so.

Interregional Contrasts of Morbidity

Take the different states of India. The state, Kerala, that has the highest level of longevity (a life expectancy now well over 70 years in comparison with the Indian average of 58 years), also has incomparably the highest rate of reported morbidity. Even in age-specific comparisons, Kerala has remarkably higher rates of reported morbidity than any other Indian state, so that the difference is not just a reflection of the higher age pattern of the Kerala population. This has sometimes been seen as a bit of a mystery. It does superficially seem odd that a population that is so plagued by illness and disease, needing so much medical care, should be exactly the one that lives the longest and escapes premature mortality so successfully.

To disentangle the picture, what is needed is not so much to ignore self-perceptions. Quite the contrary. It is to see that the position of having an enormously higher literacy rate than elsewhere in India and having the most extensive public health facilities in the country make the Kerala population perceive illnesses and do something about them in a way that does not happen in the rest of India. It is also important to see that seeking more medical attention is not only a sign of the awareness of health condition, it is also a way of seeking remedy (presumably one goes to the doctor to get medical help rather than to influence medical statistics). There is no real mystery here once the positional conditions are woven into the interpretation of medical statistics.

The fact that this is a likely explanation of the higher morbidity level in high-longevity Kerala is supported also by comparing the reported morbidity rates in Kerala and India, on the one hand, and in the United States, on the other. These comparisons have been made by Murray and Chen (Chapter 4, this volume). In disease by disease comparison, it turns out that while Kerala has much higher reported morbidity rates for most illnesses than the rest of India, the United States has even higher rates for the same illnesses. If we went by self-reported morbidity, we would have to conclude that the United States is the least healthy in this comparison, followed by Kerala, with the rest of India enjoying the highest level of health (led by the states most backward in education, such as Bihar and Uttar Pradesh).

The conclusion to emerge is not the irrelevance of self-perception of illness for an objective analysis of morbidity. It is rather the need to see the self-perceptions in terms of positional analysis, relating self-perception and seeking of medical help, on the one hand, and levels of education and public health facilities, on the other.

Gender Inequality and Perception Biases

Nowhere, perhaps, is the importance of positional interpretation as basic as it is in understanding gender inequality. This is partly because the perceptions of individuals in family living have a decisive part to play in the cohesion and success of the family. The issue of what Marx called "false consciousness" is central to gender inequality. The relevant perceptual issues apply to self-assessment of well-being and also to the understanding of who is being how "productive" and who is "contributing" how much to the family's joint benefits.[6]

There is also a dissonance between the ranking of perceived morbidity and that of observed mortality of men and women, similar to that between the Indian states. Indian women have tended to have a higher mortality rate than Indian men for all age groups (after a short neo-natal period of some months) up to the ages of 35 to 40 years. And yet these reported morbidity rates of women, rates which are parasitic on self-perception (for reasons discussed earlier), often tend to be systematically lower than that of men. This is not only a reflection of women's deprivation in education, but also of the acceptance of greater discomfort and illness as a part of the prevailing mode of living. On an earlier occasion, I have discussed the remarkable fact that in a study of postfamine Bengal in 1944, widows had hardly reported any incidence of being in "indifferent health" whereas widowers complained massively about just that (Sen 1985, Appendix B).

The perception of seriousness of diseases and of the need to seek professional medical attention also affects actions. There is evidence of systematically less use of hospital facilities by women vis-à-vis men (and by girls vis-à-vis boys) in India, even in major cities (see Kynch and Sen 1983; Sen 1985, Appendix B). Less frequent use of the medical services simultaneously decreases reported morbidity and increases vulnerability to disease.

By constraining the positional parameters very thoroughly, it would be possible to attribute positional objectivity to the Indian rural women's lack of sense of relative deprivation in health or well-being (in the way already discussed). That positional objectivity has importance in understanding self-perceptions of Indian women, and also in explaining various actions and non-actions. On the other hand, this positional objectivity, achieved through extensive constraining, would not readily translate into transpositional objectivity of women's relative deprivation, nor into positional objectivity from the general position of being an Indian rural woman.[7]

I have confined my comments on gender inequality here to India only, but similar statements can be made about most of the developing countries in South Asia, West Asia and North Africa, and about China. At a different level — dealing not so much with health and nutrition but with the general distribution of benefits, opportunities and chores — a similar analysis would have relevance to gender inequalities in the richer countries of Europe and America as well.

A Concluding Remark

Transpositional assessment of interregional or intergroup contrasts of health conditions cannot be based just on — or even primarily on — comparisons of the respective self-perceptions of health. At the same time, the positional data on self-perceptions have importance of their own. In particular, they even help to explain differential rates of progress in improving health conditions (assessable by transpositional criteria).

It is important not only to distinguish positional objectivity from transpositional objectivity, but also to see their respective, distinctive relevance, and to take note of their interconnections (even when the interrelations look apparently perverse). A subjective observation or assessment may well be made positionally objective through suitably specific constraining of positions, but that would not make that observation or assessment particularly relevant for transpositional objectivity. On the other hand, that limited positionally objective view may be enormously important in explaining behaviors, decisions and outcomes, e.g., why a region with less education and less public health facilities may be characterized both (1) by worse health conditions and higher mortality, and (2) by a lower recognition of morbidity and a less acute perception of being ill. The rejection of the evaluative eminence of heavily constrained positional views may go hand in hand with the endorsement of their explanatory and predictive relevance.

Acknowledgements

This article draws extensively on my Storrs Lectures entitled "Objectivity," given at the Yale Law School in September, 1990, and on a paper based on those lectures (Sen 1993). For helpful comments on earlier versions, I am most grateful to Lincoln Chen, Arthur Kleinman, Christopher Murray, Thomas Nagel, Emma Rothschild, and Thomas Scanlon.

Notes

1 To illustrate, consider the case (much discussed in ancient Indian philosophy) of a person seeing a rope as a snake. The perception of the snake is based, as Nyaya philosophers had emphasized, on the person's past experience and his acquired "snake-concept" which influences his anticipation (see Bimal Matilal, *Perception*, Oxford: Clarendon Press, 1986, pp. 204-5). But there would still be a distinction between the person's claims regarding what he has *observed* (viz., something fitting his snake-concept), and what he comes to believe *is* there (viz., a snake). If, for example, the observation of the rope seems to fit the "snake-concept" used for identification, without having other observable characteristics that may emerge to be importantly relevant to being a snake, that would indicate the inadequacy of the "snake-concept" used by the observer. The relationship between concepts and observations must work both ways.

2 On related matters, see Nussbaum and Sen (1988); Walzer (1988); Geertz (1989).

3 Indeed, I have elsewhere tried to argue that in ethical analysis *positional* objectivity must be of central importance even when *transpositional* considerations are also relevant. In judging how one should live or what one should do, the peculiar relevance of one's own position cannot be obliterated despite non-discriminatory concerns about universalist principles.

4 The Bayesian rules regarding rational behavior in betting, including how to revise the bets in light of further observations, leave little room for personal subjectivity, and this is, of course, quite consistent with probabilities being

defined in terms of bets and thus being called "subjective probabilities" in that specified sense.

5 On the case studies and the related general issues, see Kleinman (1986), pp. 235-6, and the literature cited there.

6 Elsewhere I have tried to analyze intrafamily distributions in terms of "cooperative conflicts", with elements of conflicts superimposed on congruence of interests. The outcomes that may emerge on the basis of implicit acceptance of some distributional norms - regarding divisions of benefits and chores - can be deeply inegalitarian. But the aspects of conflict and inequality may be systematically obscured by the nature of the respective perceptions, and these perceptual biases can have a major influence on the survival and stability of the inegalitarian outcomes. On this, see my "Gender and Cooperative Conflict," (1990).

7 For a more extensive discussion of this question, see Sen (1993).

References

Geertz, C. 1989. "Outsider Knowledge and Insider Criticism." Unpublished ms. Princeton University: Institute for Advanced Study.

Kleinman, A. 1986. "Uses and misuses of the social sciences in medicine." In D.W. Fiske and R.A. Shweder, eds. *Metatheory in Social Science: Pluralisms and Subjectivities.* Chicago: University of Chicago Press.

Kynch, J., and A. Sen. 1983. "Indian women: Well-being and survival." *Cambridge Journal of Economics,* 7: 363–380.

Nagel T. 1986. *The View from Nowhere.* Oxford: Clarendon Press.

Nussbaum, N., and A. Sen. 1988. "Internal criticism and Indian rationalist traditions." In M. Krausz, ed. *Relativism: Interpretation and Confrontation.* Notre Dame, IN: University of Notre Dame Press.

Sen, A. 1982. "Rights and agency." *Philosophy and Public Affairs,* 11: 3–39.

Sen, A. 1983a. "Evaluator relativity and consequential evaluation." *Philosophy and Public Affairs,* 12: 113–132.

Sen, A. 1983b. "Accounts, actions and values: Objectivity of social science." In C. Lloyd, ed. *Social Theory and Political Practice.* Oxford: Clarendon Press.

Sen, A. 1985. *Commodities and Capabilities.* Amsterdam: North-Holland.

Sen, A. 1990. "Gender and cooperative conflict." In I. Tinker, ed. *Persistent Inequalities.* New York: Oxford University Press.

Sen, A. 1993. "Positional objectivity." *Philosophy and Public Affairs,* 22(2): 126–46.

Walzer, M. 1988. *The Company of Critics.* New York: Basic Books.

6

An Anthropological Perspective on Objectivity: *Observation, Categorization, and the Assessment of Suffering*

Arthur Kleinman

The reader of this volume may rightly ask why a collection of papers representing the intersection of the health and social sciences should address conceptual questions concerning the measurement of health status. The reason, as Chapter 4 by Murray and Chen should make clear, is that the measurement of morbidity necessitates both the assessment of subjective complaints and a recognition of health indices as positioned knowledge. Both requirements challenge a straightforward positivist approach to measurement. While their chapter indicates the need and even the necessity of taking into account patient reports and practitioner interpretations, they nonetheless conclude that objective measures are primary. Objectivity, it is argued, is an essential prerequisite for reliable intra- and intersocietal comparisons of the sort required to underwrite claims about health and social change.

It is not that objectivity is not an understandable goal. It is, however, a goal whose theoretical grounds and implications are all too often taken for granted by epidemiologists, public health experts, and even many social scientists. One social science discipline which does not take this objective for granted is anthropology.

Critiques of positivism and objectivism in the health sciences are central to the intellectual program of medical anthropology (Good 1994; Kleinman 1988). Inasmuch as several of the editors and contributors to this volume are medical anthropologists, it is appropriate to engage the argument the objectivist position seeks to advance. The fact that objectivist epistemology currently dominates research and thinking in international health makes it all the more important that an alternative, "culturalist" point of view also be recognized. This point of view is intended as an important complement to objectivism, not a replacement. The critique that I offer does not attempt to represent all relevant culturalist responses to the challenge of objectivism. Rather it is one that has emerged from my own work over two and one-half decades as a medical anthropologist engaged in cross-cultural research on illness and care.

Reliability Versus Validity or the Primacy of Categories in Observation

Objectivism emphasizes the observational basis of verification. In research parlance, we refer to the verification of observations as reliability. A finding is considered reliable when it is verified with a high degree of confirmation. For example, different raters may observe whether or not a patient demonstrates weakness in the performance of a task, or exhibits unsteady gait when asked to walk in a straight line, or reports feeling sad. Their degree of agreement after observing the same patient sample is frequently quantified as a correlation coefficient of the reliability of their assessment of a particular feature of morbidity.

But observations presuppose concepts of what is being observed. The act of measuring ischemic heart disease begins with a concept of what constitutes the condition. This concept is operationalized as clinical criteria — chest pain, narrowed coronary arteries, stress-induced or other causes of insufficient oxygenation of heart muscle. The concept — be it a professional or lay category — precedes and guides the observation. Thus, both symptoms (complaints) and signs (observable indications) of disease are in fact interpretations. Conceptual categories shape our interpretation of observed states, whether those observations are subjective or objective. Validity — that is, the verification of the conceptual categories that organize our observation — is both different from and a more fundamental aspect of verification (measurement) than reliability.

The following example is drawn from psychiatric nosology but applies equally to any other kind of conceptualization of health.[1] Ten trained observers are asked to interview the same ten adult American Indian informants who have experienced the death of a spouse, parent, or child in the previous month. The interviewers will determine with a high degree of agreement that these informants report the experience of hearing and/or seeing the recently deceased family member beckoning them to the afterworld. This experience is very common among adult

American Indians. Yet it is distinctly uncommon among other adult North Americans. If nine of the observers agree that the same eight American Indian informants have had this experience, they will have achieved a high degree of reliability. We can have a high degree of confidence in this observation. But if they describe the observation as a "hallucination," that is, a pathological percept (which it would be for adult non-Indian Americans), they would have an empirical finding that was reliable but not valid. Validity requires the qualifying interpretation that the percept is not pathological, but rather both normative and normal for American Indians. Since it is neither culturally inappropriate nor a predictor or sign of disease, it cannot be labelled a hallucination. It requires some other designation, perhaps a pseudohallucination or a culturally appropriate, personally normal percept, in order for the observation to be both reliable and valid.

Thus, when measuring morbidity of any sort, reliability is necessary but not sufficient to assess verifiability. If measurements lack validity, then morbidity has not been adequately assessed. The problem with findings that have reliability but not validity is by no means limited to mental health; it is a serious and frequently encountered problem in clinical evaluations of outpatient complaints and behaviors.

Context, Interpretation and the Experience of Suffering

Unlike epidemiologists and economists, anthropologists conducting studies in international health focus on individuals and small groups in local worlds: a village, a group of villages, an urban neighborhood, a social network. Ethnographic research usually involves relatively long periods — often months, sometimes a year or more — living together with the people one is studying, observing daily activities, and interviewing and reinterviewing a relatively small group of key informants. Ethnography seeks to describe indigenous categories of the body, the self, health, illness, and healing, and to interpret their relationship to the social structure, the political economy, and their historical changes. Those descriptions are understood, in current cultural theory (Kleinman 1992), as positioned interpretations of positioned interpretations. In other words, the ethnographer establishes his own position as a usually nonindigenous field worker who possesses a certain conceptual orientation and focused problem framework from which he encounters members of the community who are themselves positioned (on account of gender, class, caste, etc.) participants in local worlds. The empirical result of this utterly human — because uncertain and changing — though professionally disciplined and controlled engagement is positioned knowledge; that is, a view from somewhere. Context and interpersonal dialogue are understood to shape the knowledge so that it is always particular to a local world. So qualified, however, it can be compared across cultural worlds.

From an objectivist perspective, the ethnographer's account carries a positioned validity.[2] But the ethnographer does not regard this validity as "objective," because it is never a "view from nowhere" — some transpositional domain of ultimately real nature — nor is it verified straightforwardly as an observation or series of observations. Rather the ethnographer constructs a professional category based on the interpretation of local popular or expert categories; he interprets a field of interpersonal experience as he narrates (forms a story of) the felt flow of that interpersonal world which he encounters as stories told to him — stories of illness, disability, and therapy.

Ethnographic knowledge is never impersonal. It represents not only the public, focused account of informants, but also the subsidiary, tacit knowledge that is part of the practical life activities of both informants and ethnographer (Polanyi and Prosch 1975: 22-45). Thus, the anthropologist's ethnography cannot be objective, because it is embedded in subjective and interpersonal understandings. The anthropologist strives for interpositional knowledge of a local world by comparing understandings of positioned participants. At the same time he struggles to place his findings in a constrained, multipositional professional discourse of academic writings, one that is external both to the local world of his informants and to his own institutional and cultural settings. What the anthropologist seeks to achieve is not objectivity of observation, but controlled interpositionality of interpretation in an academic discourse. Translation of findings into the interpositional context of scholarship is the final stage of the work, not a precommitment or initial move.

The anthropologist in international health credits the knowledge of local informants concerning everyday health practices, illness episodes, and therapeutic actions. Is he mistaken in doing so? Objectivism defines this practice as epistemologically unsound. After all, patients do not have privileged access to objective knowledge about their underlying conditions that can be verified through measurement with a high degree of probability. The patient's subjective knowledge is less reliable than the medical researcher's objective knowledge. Doubt is cast on the informant's (and the ethnographer's) constructions.

Two comments need to be made here. First, the researcher's knowledge — that of the epidemiologist, the economist, the public health physician as much as the ethnographer and clinician — is a construction not so very different in kind, though often quite different in degree of systemization and control, from that of the informant. The histologist interpreting a surgical pathology slide or autopsy specimen of tissue presumed to be cancerous constructs the object of his inquiry (Canquilhem 1989). He or she works with a historically derived and continuously changing set of categories that defines malignancy. These categories distinguish malignant from premalignant or borderline cases. They delineate stages of invasiveness and spread in different systems. And they require the focal and tacit knowledge of the interpreter for diagnosis. Anyone who has ever confronted the task of differentiating malignant melanoma from dyplastic cells under a high resolution microscope knows that the categorization, with its operationalized diagnostic criteria, has to be learned. Once learned, "experience" is required to feel confident one is making an objective assessment. The same can be said of "reading" a chest X-ray, interpreting a CT scan of the skull, listening to abnormal heart sounds, examining a rash, and conducting an epidemiological survey based on such interpretations. That practical sense, the experienced feel of mastery of a field, is of the same order as practical competence in everyday life, a learned sensibility — a subjective knowledge essential to rationality (Bourdieu 1990).

Second, informants actually can at times be shown to possess privileged knowledge of the body that predicts at least certain health outcomes. That is to say, "subjective" knowledge may sometimes be more valid and useful than "objective" knowledge.[3] For example, Lazarus and Launier (1978) have demonstrated that subjects' "self-appraisal" of stressful events can predict what will be experienced as stressful. More impressively, Idler and colleagues (1990) have found that elderly persons' "subjective" self-assessment of their health is a better predictor of mortality than "objective" biomedical measures. Similarly, Yelin et al. (1980) have demonstrated that subjects' assessment is a better predictor of return to work among disabled chronic pain patients than more objective clinical or radiological tests. Working with informants in Mexico who believe they suffer or are believed by others to suffer from a "culture-bound condition," *susto* (soul loss), Rubel et al. (1984)

determined that even though biomedical measures could not diagnose the condition or determine the pathology, sufferers had higher mortality rates than matched community control subjects. This indicated to them that subjective complaints and lay interpretations were sensitive to disease processes that biomedical methods could not measure.

Another way in which subjective knowledge contributes to health outcomes is through the application of that knowledge to make health-relevant choices. Informants use their tacit health knowledge to decide whether to smoke, wear a condom, wash their hands, or strengthen social ties when in crisis. The health consequences of such decisions are very real.

Murray and Chen, in this volume, refer to surveys in which populations with more education living in more affluent surroundings that had higher indices of general health (and that were therefore presumed to be healthier) utilized health care services more frequently. These populations were found to have reported more symptoms than poorer, less well-educated groups, who utilized services less frequently and who lived in locations with lower indexes of general health. This finding, which seems widespread, should not diminish interest in the pertinence of personal complaints.[4] It is well known in the social survey literature that perceptions of the relative significance of a problem increase with rising expectations. It is also well known that members of disadvantaged groups tend to suppress complaints of misery, especially when interviewed by members of dominant groups, if they feel there is little that can be done or that their complaints may cause trouble (Guarnaccia et al. 1990; Scott 1990).

The positioned place of patient and family reports of symptoms, then, does not make those interpretations erroneous; it only qualifies that local knowledge. Some patients with peptic ulcer craters in their stomachs may not complain of pain; other individuals with the "classical" abdominal pain associated with peptic ulcer disease may have no pathology. This does not mean that such patients are not conveying valid information about their experience of bodily processes; it only demonstrates a gap between experience and biology. Social expectation, cultural priority and personal response fill that gap. Why should the materialistic determination of pathology and its projection onto predictions about the future be considered more authentic than the always culturally and personally positioned human expression of suffering in the exigency of the here-and-now? The sufferer's interpretation of suffering needs to be taken into account in the assessment of pain, distress, or dysfunction in order for such assessments to have validity in the experience of real people in real worlds.

Suffering is, moreover, not only a "subjective" phenomenon, but also an interpersonal one. The distress of an Alzheimer's patient is part of a micro-context of distress in which the family becomes the locus of suffering and indeed even of the illness experience. We do not dwell in worlds where dichotomies between real and unreal disease, objective and subjective health problems, valid versus reliable diagnoses, or distinctions of mind from body are part of everyday experience. These are professional constructions that are imposed on local worlds. Many chronic pain patients, for example, experience serious, disabling pain in the back or the head with objective evidence of only very modest if any "real" pathology on the CT-scan or MRI. Pain for them is certainty, whereas for their health professionals it is doubt (Scarry 1985). Telling a chronic back pain patient not to worry because there is no evidence of "real" disease infuriates many because it disaffirms their experience. This is the logical outcome of the overvaluing of the usual biomedical understanding of objective measures and the devaluing of subjective ones — a characteristic of high-technology biomedicine. It has been shown repeatedly to have a disastrous result on care (Good et al. 1992). By delegitimizing the interpersonal experience of suffering, this approach manages to be simultaneously inhumane and scientifically invalid.

In this volume, Das criticizes the response of health professionals to the plight of the victims of the chemical poisoning at Bhopal. Her criticism turns on the insistence by those physicians that objective measures replace self report and experience to determine the consequence of exposure. When objective indexes are used, they measure biological change as if it were fungible, separable from the experience of distress and the bearing of suffering. Indeed, "objectivity" in medicine is formulated so as to require such an artifactual, context-independent metric. Yet, can such an objective health index validly measure the consequence of poisoning on the person, and on the processes that mediate the cognitive, affective, interpersonal, and neurobiological changes that together constitute suffering?

In one sense, ethnography comes closer than other methodologies to crossing positional boundaries, because it requires specification and analysis of multiple (including self-) perspectives. Yet objectivists may argue that ethnography does not provide objective knowledge at all, inasmuch as the knowledge it constitutes remains positioned (or at best interpositional and experiential), even if the ethnographer seeks a framework independent of position. Sophisticated objectivists do not require that objectivity leave out human experience. Yet that may well be the unintended result when the quest for transpositional objectivity requires a leap from interpositional to extrapositional grounds and from intersubjective to objective claims. In this sense, the "best" of measurements may become obstacles to the advancement of international health objectives.

Defined this way, a search for position-independent objectivity may lead the researcher to reject positioned knowledge. When this happens, for example in relying solely on HIV sero-status and AIDS fatality rates to measure the AIDS pandemic, something fundamental to the human experience of suffering is lost, namely, its grounding in greatly different local worlds and local lives (Farmer and Kleinman 1989).

Calls for the rejection of a narrow definition of human suffering are beginning to be heard among researchers in the field of international health. When infant mortality rates obscure other aspects of child "health", such as survival followed by malnutrition, disability, and mental health problems, a new epistemology is required. Perhaps the goal of international health studies should be to combine just that degree of transpositionally objective reliability which can be achieved while still making feasible a high degree of interpositional, experiential validity.[5] To raise this question is one of the purposes of this volume.

The chapters in this collection show clearly that classical metrics of mortality and morbidity are necessary but not sufficient to describe health transitions. They need to be supplemented by measures of disability, behavioral and social pathologies, and suffering. These measures will differ in a fundamental way from standard assessment techniques. The same degrees of reliability and validity should not be required. Or, if they are, different kinds of measures should be employed reciprocally to assure that both features of illness and care are assessed.

If these cautions are pertinent to the measurement of health changes, they are even more significant for the assessment of social changes and the mediating processes that lead from particular social processes to health outcomes. An understanding of the health consequences of urbanization in a developing society such as Kenya, for example, cannot be achieved by treating urbanization as a unified variable that can be objectively operationalized, inquired about, and assigned a quantitative value for any population. Rather, urbanization as a concept needs to be unpacked — that is, broken down into microprocesses and understood in the historical context of particular local worlds. Consider, for example, a marginalized woman who migrates with her children from a disintegrating rural community to a big city slum without support from husband or kin. Her experience of urbanization is very different from that of a woman and her children who migrate from a vital rural community where they retain social ties to a market town where husband and maternal kin have already made a home in a neighborhood of fellow villagers and are engaged in a thriving business. The characteristics of the rural-urban migrants, the community from which they come, their resources, the type of uprooting (voluntary, forced), the forms of migration, the situation into which they migrate — all contribute to qualify the "variable" of urbanization. Measuring the mediators that transform social processes into health outcomes requires parsing urbanization as a social category into those components that are locally valid. No social change can be validly assessed without assessment of its contextual meaning for those who experience it. That meaning will mediate between social world and the person's processes of body and self. Measurement will need to canvass meaning, context, process, and their relationship to health indexes. Such relational measures will require both objective and subjective information. Clearly, the requirements for this type of research, which loom large in the chapters that precede and follow this one, cannot be met unless we move beyond the objectivist and subjectivist dichotomy toward interdisciplinary, interpositional forms of assessment that combine quantitative and qualitative evaluations. We must broaden the scope of objectivist measurement to make room for what is at stake for real human beings.

Notes

1 This example also appears in Kleinman (1988:10-14), where its implications for psychiatric diagnosis are discussed at length.

2 The reliability of an ethnographic account is often untested.

3 Amartya Sen, writing in this volume, would seem to differentiate immediate awareness of bodily conditions — body knowledge — from subjective knowledge in the strict sense, whose source is the mind. Body knowledge is a positioned objective knowledge in his formulation.

4   Surveys in the U.S., however, show that blacks, low income persons and the elderly generally rate their health status lower than do whites, higher income and younger persons. Thus, in these studies, subjective complaints are in keeping with objective measures (Barker et al. 1991:10).

5   On the relation of positionality and objectivity, see Sen, this volume. On this particular point concerning the problem of positioned knowledge in the search for the supra-positional or trans-positional, we are in agreement.

References

Barker, D.C. et al., eds. 1991. *Challenges in Health Care. A Chartbook Perspective.* Princeton, NJ: Robert Wood Johnson Foundation.

Bourdieu, P. 1990. *The Sense of Practice.* Stanford: Stanford University Press.

Canquilhem, G. 1989. *The Normal and the Pathological.* N.Y.: Zone Press.

Farmer, P., and A. Kleinman. 1989. "AIDS as human suffering." *Daedalus,* 118(2): 135–160.

Good, B.J. 1994. *Medicine, Rationality and Experience.* Cambridge: Cambridge University Press.

Good, M.J., et al., eds. 1992. *Pain as Human Experience: An Anthropological Perspective.* Berkeley: University of California Press.

Guarnaccia, P., et al. 1990. "A critical review of epidemiological studies of Puerto Rican mental health." *American Journal of Psychiatry,* 147(11): 1449–1456.

Idler, E., et al. 1990. "Self-evaluated health and mortality among the elderly." *American Journal of Epidemiology,* 131(1): 91–103.

Kleinman, A. 1988. *Rethinking Psychiatry: From Cultural Category to Personal Experience.* New York: Free Press.

Kleinman. A. 1992. "Pain and resistance: The delegitimation and relegitimation of local worlds." In M.J. Good, et al., eds. *Pain as Human Experience: An Anthropological Perspective.* Berkeley: University of California Press.

Lazarus, R., and R. Launier. 1978. "Stress-related transitions between persons and environment." In L. Pervin and M. Lewis, eds. *Perspectives in International Psychology.* New York: Plenum.

Polanyi, M., and H. Prosch. 1975. *Meaning.* Chicago: University of Chicago Press.

Rubel, A., et al. 1984. *Susto, A Folk Illness.* Berkeley: University of California Press.

Scarry, E. 1985. *The Body in Pain.* New York: Oxford University Press.

Scott, J.C. 1990. *Domination and the Arts of Resistance.* New Haven: Yale University Press.

Yelin, E., et al. 1980. "Toward an epidemiology of work disability." *Milbank Memorial Fund Quarterly:Health and Society,* 58: 386–445.

7

Moral Orientations to Suffering:
Legitimation, Power, and Healing

Veena Das

What is the meaning of suffering? In a sense one may say that this is the classic problem of philosophy and anthropology. In its classical mould, the existence of suffering poses an existential and cognitive problem of loss of meaning which results in a common human address to religion as a source for the resolution of this question. We need not rehearse all the arguments of Weber in his essays on the problem of theodicy and the systematization of religious thought in various attempted resolutions to this contradiction.[1] It is enough to notice the continuity and stability of the framework provided by Weber as testified, for instance, in an essay by Geertz (1973), who states that the problem of suffering is an "...experiential challenge in whose face the meaningfulness of a particular pattern of life threatens to dissolve into a chaos of thingless names and nameless things." Therefore, "as a religious problem, the problem of suffering is, paradoxically, not how to avoid suffering, but how to suffer, how to make of physical pain, personal loss, physical defeat, or the helpless contemplation of other's agony something bearable, supportable — something, as we say, sufferable." Pain and suffering, however, are not simply *individual* experiences which arise out of the contingency of life and threaten to disrupt a known world. These may also be experiences which are actively created and distributed by the social order itself. Located in individual bodies, they bear the stamp of the authority of society on the docile bodies of its members. Thus we are in need of examining the social mechanisms by which the manufacture of pain on the one hand, and the theologies of suffering on the other, become means of legitimating the social order rather than being threats to this order. This, at any rate, is how I interpret Durkheim's concern with the manner in which totemic symbols are inscribed on individual bodies through a series of painful mutilations in initiation rituals or the self inflicted lacerations on the body in piacular rituals.[2] Let me immediately add that I do not adhere to the view that individuals simply submit to these experiences without any resistance, but I do wish to affirm that a theory of suffering must break from the traditional mode of conceptualizing it as an intellectualist problem of theodicy and instead look at the way in which the dialectic of the individual and the collective develops in the context of pain and suffering. Finally, I see no reason for privileging religion as the domain in which theories of theodicy and soteriologies are located over other domains such as that of family, bureaucracy, law, and medicine.

I would like to begin by making a distinction between two important formulations of the place of suffering in human life and then to illustrate by two ethnographic examples how these orientations give direction to the meaning of suffering. The first direction creates an elaborate discourse on the meaning of suffering that essentially legitimizes the producer of the discourse rather than the victim; the second allows the possibility of the rise of novelty and the creation of a healing discourse.

The first orientation to suffering, which I shall characterize as an internal orientation, creates a movement out of two distinct but related moments. In the first moment, the injustice of life in which meaningless suffering occurs is recognized; in the second moment suffering is converted into an accusation against life — thus making life itself something which must be justified. This orientation, embodied in the discourse of power, insists that responsibility for suffering must be acknowledged by the sufferer himself or herself. Thus it not only masks from the powerless the manner in which their suffering may have been manufactured and distributed by an unjust society , but further disallows them to exorcise their suffering by holding that they are personally responsible for what has befallen them. Thus while the cosmologies of the powerless may hold the capriciousness of gods and sheer contingency of events to be responsible for the disorder of their lives — which at the very least has the potential of freeing them from having to take personal responsibility for their fate even as it masks the real sources of their oppression from them — there is no place in the cosmologies of the powerful for chaos. If the contingent and chaotic nature of the world were to be acknowledged it would have the potential of dismantling the structures of legitimacy through which suffering is imposed upon the powerless. Clothed in a language of responsibility, the discourse of power ends up with the equation that pain is equal to punishment, and the injustice of life testified to by suffering can only be redeemed by further suffering. This discourse is to be found not only in the attempts at rationalization and systematization of religious thought but also in bureaucratic and judicial discourse. In an unsystematic way it may be found scattered in the everyday discursive practices of the family.

The second orientation to suffering, which I shall call an external orientation, holds existence to be blameworthy, but points to the capriciousness of gods, the inexplicability of the world, the contingency of events and accidental nature of our lives to be the reason for suffering. Thus it does not make the sufferer internalize his or her suffering — nor does it posit a meaningful world or a just god who can be made responsible. Dare one say, it gives irresponsibility a positive sense? By renouncing a search for meaning it affirms the suffering person; rather than accusing life, it affirms existence.[3] I shall first show how these two discourses of suffering are woven into the discursive practices of the family and then proceed to a demonstration of their transformation in judicial and bureaucratic discourse through rationalization and system-atization.

The Family and its Discourse on Suffering

In this section, I describe a case in which the constant refrain of suffering, the split references to the sufferer as both a victim and the one responsible for her own fate, the construction of a world in which suffering must have meaning struggled with an opposite voice. This was the voice in which the world was sought to be constructed as chaotic, represented as nothing but the irresponsible play of gods; a world in which it was the capriciousness of the gods and not the actions of humans that was held responsible for the suffering which befell them. The voice articulating chaos could not be sustained in this case and the victim finally internalized her pain completely; she took the pain itself as evidence of guilt so that in asserting the meaningful nature of the world she herself was extinguished.

I shall give a brief description of the case, since I have discussed some of these issues elsewhere (Das 1990). In 1984 I became involved in the process of rehabilitation of some of the survivors of the anti-Sikh riots which followed the assassination of Indira Gandhi, the Prime Minister of India. One of the families of survivors with whom I worked very closely was that of Shanti, whose husband and three sons had been burnt alive by a mob as they hid in an abandoned house. Shanti and her two daughters escaped death because women had not become a target of violence in these riots. They had, however, been compelled to watch the actions of a murderous crowd, as they were hiding on a terrace of a house in the street in which the crowd had gone on a rampage. It seemed that the crowd had come to know of the whereabouts of Shanti's husband and sons. After hurling abuses at the hidden men, the crowd had doused the abandoned house with kerosene and set fire to it.

At one stage Shanti's elder daughter had even tried to save her baby brother who was hiding in the house with his father by running into the crowd and imploring them to spare the child even if they were going to set fire to the house and kill the older men. I have described elsewhere how the actions of the crowd were not random and chaotic; in these riots there seems to have been an implicit contract that the death of Indira Gandhi was to be avenged by a kind of ritual killing of adult men (Das 1989; Das and Bose 1987). Children and women had remained safe from the crowds even when they were not hiding. It was tragic that Shanti was the only woman in the locality to have lost a young child to the murderous crowd and she blamed herself excessively for having been unable to save the child.

Let me first give a brief account of how Shanti described the fate of her family during the riots and then show the organizing images through which these events came to be articulated within the family. Following are extracts from Shanti's descriptions of the events:

> My husband had expected that the riots would remain confined to another block in the locality because people of that block had been locked in a conflict with the faction of the Congress party that was instigating and organizing the violence. We thought some *goondas* may loot our houses. But what did we have to do with the assassination of Indira Gandhi? Why should we have thought that anything would happen to us?

In response to my question about how, then, her husband and children had died, she said:

> Some people, the neighbors, one of my relatives, said that it would be better if we hid in an abandoned house nearby. So my husband took our three sons and hid there. We locked the house from outside, but there was treachery in people's hearts. Someone must have told the crowd. They baited him to come out. Then they

poured kerosene on that house. They burnt them alive. When I went there that night the bodies of my sons were on the loft — huddled together.

It was my own *mama* (mother's brother) who had advised my husband to hide. He revealed the hiding places of the Siglikar Sikhs to the leaders of the mob. He bartered their lives for his own protection. Go and see his house. Not even a broken spoon has been looted.

They hurled challenges upon my husband to come out. If he had been brave he would have come out and then my little child would have been spared. But he remained mute. The crowd burnt the house.

In this initial formulation of the narrative, in which the fragmentation and jerkiness of the style somehow mirrors her own fragmentation, we see that Shanti saw the violence as stemming equally from her own kinsmen as from the "mob" (*bhida*). The general and vague characterization, "some people, the neighbors, one of my relatives," came to be particularized later to her mother's brother. That the betrayal should have come from the mother's side is poignant, for in contrast to the mother's brother, Shanti's own mother, as we shall see, made every effort to save her from the devastating consequences of this violence, and from the pathological mourning which finally claimed her life.

One of the organizing images through which Shanti communicated her pain and her sorrow was her search for a way to end her life. To people like me who represented the outside world, she would say, "I want *sukha* (peace) — can't you give me *sukha?*" These were almost the first words that she uttered to me when I went to her house. She often left it to the other women who were always around her, including her mother, her sister, and her two young daughters, to explicate the meaning of these enigmatic words. They would often join in to explain that Shanti was asking for an injection to end her life. For instance, when she uttered these words to me, her mother immediately rebuked her, saying, "I keep telling her, 'Daughter, do not talk so,' but does she listen, does she care?" This would be followed by soulful laments from Shanti that since she had lost her child, what was there for her to care for? The structure of lament and consolation resembled that of mourning laments, but it is important to note that the other women around her were trying to shift the burden of guilt from her to the inexplicable forces that had overtaken the fate of the community. They were also trying to make her acknowledge the fact that though her sons had died, she had two daughters who could provide a reason in favor of life.

The first theme in the conversation of the women, then, pertained to the question of Shanti's guilt. Shanti herself spoke in several voices — sometimes blaming her husband for having insisted on taking the baby with him in his hiding place rather than leaving it with Shanti; sometimes blaming him for not having the courage to face the crowd (loudly lamenting that in a similar case another man had come out to face the crowd and though the crowd had doused him with kerosene and killed him, they had been honor-bound to spare his child); at still other times she blamed her daughter for not having been successful in preventing the crowd from burning down the house. All these were, however, demands upon others which she herself felt were of a fantastic storybook character. In the final analysis, almost in recognition of this fact, she gathered all this guilt upon herself and held herself responsible for the death of her child. "Everyone used to say I was mad, and they were right — if my husband had trusted me with the baby he would have lived." Or, "Every woman knew that children were not being killed. Only I was stupid. Only I lost a child."

The response of the women to these laments was to move responsibility from known and identifiable people to the impersonal forces and the events that had unleashed this violence in the first place. For instance, one old woman repeatedly iterated that it was a *storm* that had come — and who could have saved anyone from the fury of that storm? Other women blamed the crowd (*bhida*), for it was they who had suddenly shattered their world. "If they wanted to take revenge they should have killed those guards who were the assassins. What had we done that such devastation was wrought upon us?"

The second theme in the women's discourse in relation to Shanti was that Shanti had not lost all her children. After all, her two daughters were alive. Shanti, however, rejected the daughters as *counterfeit* children (*nakli bacche*). She had so internalized the patriarchal discourse of the family that to her, all sense of worth came from being the mother of sons. In failing to protect her son, she had failed as a woman; the greatest duty of a woman, she repeatedly told me, was to ensure the continuity of men. In other words, continuity beyond death was to be found only for men in the generations of patrilineal succession. She would lament that her husband and his ancestors would have no sons to perform ancestral rites and that the dead would roam like homeless spirits in the absence of future male progeny to continue the line. It is important to note that her mother, her sister, and her daughters, along with the other women of the neighborhood, repeatedly tried to contest this construction of reality. They would try to make her see her connectedness with her daughters. "Are they not born of your womb, the same as your sons? Then why do you treat them like this?" Even her five-year-old daughter understood the mother's quest for a son and tried to assure her that she herself would never marry but would stay with her mother and be "like a son". Neither the words nor the close body contacts with which the women tried to make her sorrow flow among them were successful in shaking Shanti from her obsessive guilt of having failed as a mother of sons, even if she had not failed as a mother of daughters. It is my contention that Shanti was not able to take the path offered by the women, to 'forget' her place in the male genealogies within which she constituted herself as 'guilty' and 'blameworthy', and to forge new female genealogies within which she could have created a new life for herself. The path of positive 'irresponsibility' that I postulated in the introduction to this paper, which was there as a possibility in the discourse of women, for whom such devastation attests the chaotic nature of the world, the irresponsibility of gods rather than the failing of human beings, was not taken by Shanti.[4] I now attempt to show the manner in which the male members of the extended family and the surrounding male community sought to fix the blame of the tragic deaths upon Shanti so that their bitter recriminations and her own sense of worthlessness as a woman began to mirror each other in a way that led to her tragic end.

I mentioned earlier that Shanti was constantly surrounded by women, especially her mother and sister. Shanti had slipped into a kind of infantile behavior in relation to her mother, who performed all the maternal functions ranging from feeding her to accompanying her during her morning ablutions. Although the mother's presence was a nourishing presence for Shanti, it was against the patrilineal norms of this society which do not allow the natal kinsmen or kinswomen of a woman to visit her for any prolonged periods of time in her conjugal home. After the tragic deaths of her husband and sons, Shanti had been persuaded by her brothers to come and live with them in Alwar, a small town in Rajasthan. However, she was deeply disturbed by the normalcy of everyday life there, and had yearned to come back to her house in Delhi where the whole neighborhood had suffered in a manner similar to hers. Not trusting her to be able to look after herself, Shanti's mother had come with her and was caring for her. This was accepted as normal and necessary by the women in the local community, for, as they said, who can be closer to a woman than her mother?

After a month or so, Shanti's husband's father came to live with her on the grounds that she needed the protection of a male member. This old man presented a picture of tragedy at the close of his life, for, as he would say, *"hum to ghar se beghar ho gaye"* — we have been made into homeless people. However, along with his sorrow there seemed to have been a great need on his part to hold Shanti as blameworthy for the death of the male members of the family. He was also resentful of her because as next of kin of the dead husband and the three sons, Shanti had received Rs.40,000 as compensation. He felt that this money rightly belonged to him, as he was the male survivor.

After his arrival in Delhi, the old man began to first comment subtly on the inappropriate behavior of Shanti's mother in staying in her daughter's conjugal home for such a long period of time. Nothing was said directly, but he would often say how difficult it must be for Shanti's mother to stay with her daughter, abandoning her own sons and grandsons for such an inordinately long time. "Circumstances have compelled her to stay here, otherwise, which woman can stay on in her married daughter's house like this? If nothing else, the world would say, 'What a shameless woman!'" *"Halaat se mazbur hai nahin to kaun aurat byahi beti ke ghar itne din reh sakti hai? Aur nahin to duniya kahegi kitni behaya aurat hai."* After a while he began to imply through various subtle forms of innuendo that Shanti's mother was making her more helpless and dependent day after day because she wanted to grab the money that Shanti had received from the government. Faced with these subtle but unmistakable insults, Shanti's mother found it impossible to stay on in her daughter's house. Before she left, I remember, she held me by my shoulders and implored that my friend Mita, who was working in the community and was very close to Shanti, and I must look after Shanti. "I am very fearful for her, and I leave her to your care *(Mujhe us ke liye bahut shanka ho rahi hai— mein use tumhara bharose chod rahi hun)*."

After the departure of Shanti's mother, the space in and around the house came to be defined more and more as a male space, and Shanti's inability to engage in life was seen as malingering. Friends of her husband's father and men of the community would sit and recreate the events of the riots and bemoan the fact that the old man had been left without any heir. Slowly the theme of Shanti's responsibility in the whole matter came to be woven into this discourse. "My son was happy in Calcutta, where we had lived. It was Shanti who wanted him to come to Delhi." "Old though I am, I have to take on the responsibility of looking after this household. Shanti, as everyone knows, poor thing, is half-witted. If she was not so, would Tehal (Shanti's husband) not have trusted her with the baby? Why would the baby have had to die?" Shanti's response to all this was to sit immobile on a string cot the whole day and repeat over and over again that all she wanted was to die.

It was not that the old man actively encouraged her to die. In fact one day, in a dramatic gesture, he fell on her feet in my presence and implored her that she must live. The next moment, however, he shook his head, and vaguely addressing everyone who was there, said, "But how can she live? It is the dead who call her. It is the dead who do not let her live in peace."

At one point of time a near confrontation occurred between Shanti and her husband's father. The old man wanted to hold an expensive and elaborate religious ceremony to ensure peace to his dead son and grandsons. Shanti said that if so much were to be spent on the ceremony out of the money she had received as compensation, what provisions could she make for the future of her daughters? After all, she said, they did not have a father or older brothers any more who would look after them. How would she find money to arrange their marriages? The old man expressed great shock that Shanti wanted to stand in the way of a ritual that would give peace to the departed souls. There is a touch of tragedy here, for even a fleeting concern for her daughters, barely given voice by Shanti, was construed by her husband's father as a betrayal of the male line.

In the end, it seems that the bitter recriminations of the old man — "it's your fault, it's your fault" — could no longer be resisted, and Shanti completely internalized this accusation. The women, who had struggled for female connectedness to be established, to make Shanti acknowledge her daughters in the same way that she was acknowledged by her mother, failed in the task of establishing this connectedness. To be connected to the past and the future, Shanti's husband's father had continually implied, was a male prerogative. The women's laments had tried to articulate the idea of a chaotic world — a world in which gods mocked men and made them their playthings. The constructions of meaning, the elaborate rituals to ensure relations between men beyond death, stood mocked in the presence of such happenings as the riots. How was this a meaningful world? And in such a world, devoid of all meaning, why should a woman take upon herself the responsibility of creating order when even god was not so much a lover of justice as a spectator who amused himself with the lives of men and women? But such constructions were resisted by the community of men who began talking of martyrdom, the long tradition of martyrs in Sikh history, the obligation to remember one's responsibilities to the dead, and above all, the refusal to let a new construction of self and of life emerge for the surviving woman.

In the end, Shanti gave in to the "superior" male constructions and rejected that healing which could only have come if she had acknowledged the meaningless and absurd nature of the deaths of her husband and sons rather than finding ways of blaming herself for having been unable to save them. One day when her daughters had gone to school, her husband's father had gone to get groceries and her sister had gone to the fields to relieve herself, Shanti "did her work," as her elder daughter put it. When the sister came back she found Shanti hanging from the ceiling fan. Her husband's father arranged a proper funeral — and thus, in attempting to assert the meaningful nature of the world, a life was extinguished.

In the face of sudden calamity, anthropological wisdom tells us, one searches for meaning, and the elaborate theodicies of every religion attest to this meaning. In contrast, I have suggested elsewhere and here that in India the male discourse and the female discourse take opposite paths in the face of calamity (Das, 1986). The male discourse insists upon holding on to meaning. It makes linear connections with the past. Deaths in war, riots, and feuds are meaningful, and even heroic, deaths. In male discourses even women are made to articulate the heroism of men and of children who face their executors with a smile; as mothers of martyrs they are given places of honor in male narratives. Struggling with this is often a different narrative — a narrative that is given voice by women in moments of loss. This narrative asserts the precious quality of life over and above every abstraction — be "honor," "heroism," "preservation of community" or "threat to the nation". It resists with force the idea that deaths and calamity are means by which mankind is elevated through a spectacular display of heroism. Simultaneously it refuses to acknowledge the failure of the victim as the source of suffering. When Shanti would lament, "Why did I not *understand* that the killers were not after children?", she would be reassured by the women, "Don't you know how many pretexts death can find to attack human beings? When such times come, one's judgment does not function (lit., one's judgment is killed)." The contrasting narrative of her husband's father was that she had failed to save her child because she was stupid, because she had insisted that the family move to Delhi from Calcutta, because she did not know how to read the signs correctly. It was as if a telos was being posited in which every move of Shanti had been a slow but definite move towards the destruction of her husband and sons.

I hope it is clear from this discussion that the attempt to create meaning in the face of suffering functioned here as simply a discourse to legitimize the power of the male patriarchal head over the female members of the family. Too often in my earlier work, I have been influenced by the dominant anthropological models in which one equates the search for meaning as the defining feature of the moral actor and of the moral universe. I would now like to stress the hidden dimensions of power that inform the theodicies of suffering and serve to block any paths through which an individual like Shanti could have related to her suffering by being allowed to renounce the search for meaning and thus transform this suffering. As Shanti hugged the shadows in the household, taking on the role of a kind of magical malingerer hanging on to the peripheries of life, I feel her return to the world perhaps could have been accomplished, if only she would have been allowed to reconstitute herself, so as not to discover what she *was* but to become, *what she was not* in her earlier life.

Reflecting on Shanti's case we see that events that may seem remote and distant to a family in a slum, such as the assassination of a national leader, can lead to calamity in their personal lives, but so absurd are the connections through which this happens that they can only testify to the chaotic nature of the world in which they inhabit. Would it not be better for this chaos to be articulated rather than for people to extinguish themselves in the so-called search for order? It is only the powerful who have the luxury of assuming that life has meaning, for they can exercise the kind of control over events that would connect their personal, social and political lives. For the rest, I endorse the works of a good friend, a truck-body-builder who lived in the same community as Shanti and who succinctly summarized the meaning of death: "Our deaths mean nothing. Alive, we are hostages in the hands of the government against the terrorists, and dead, we become numbers in the hands of the militants."

Am I then saying that Shanti's life and her death were meaningless? Why was her death described by her young daughter as her "work?" In my understanding, the passive posture of the malingerer that Shanti had undertaken, her physical immobility corresponded to a fantastic mental search to find out why she had "failed" to save her son. In the world of women, this failure was given a particular place. The women watched over her, all the while encouraging her to redefine herself as a mother of daughters. Shanti's own personal quest to understand why she had "failed" and how she was to construe this failure, was sought to be given a particular interpretation in the world of women. That interpretation, in my view, was grounded in a theory of disorder, which itself is a prepotent orientation of the powerless to a world that seems so out of reach. Instead of making Shanti the passive recipient of the cultural oppression which disallowed both the private working out of her experience and a new sense of connections, it could have come to constitute an active orientation to the world. This is why I cannot bring myself to interpret her death through a master symbol, not even the master symbol of resistance. Her death must forever remain elusive to me, a testimony to the unequal dialectic between the norm giving, powerful male society and the attempts to resist those norms by the constant reconstruction and kaleidoscopic organization of memory in the inner lives of the individual.

Bureaucratic and Judicial Transformation of Suffering

In the diffused verbal and non verbal practices of the family, described in the last section, suffering was allowed a place, but only to legitimize the position of the male head. My second example shows that in the practices of the state, the suffering of the people may also undergo a judicial and bureaucratic transformation that secures the power of the state but does nothing for the amelioration of the condition of the victims of calamity. I propose to show this with the example of the Bhopal disaster, generally acknowledged to be the worst industrial disaster in human history.

Before I describe this disaster and the judicial and bureaucratic appropriation of the suffering of the victims, it may be useful to make some general observations on chemical disasters and the public response to these. In an excellent paper on the subject of chemical disasters, Reich (1982) has observed:

Chemical disasters appear by surprise. They represent an extraordinary event that disrupts the normal flow of social life. But paradoxically such crises in society create windows on normality. Through the windows of a chemical disaster, one can peer at political and social processes not usually accessible or visible.[5]

One of the most important aspects of these political and social processes as described by Reich is that despite the pervasive uncertainty arising from the fact that the impact of toxic chemicals in the environment on human beings cannot be described in mechanistic terms, bureaucratic decisions are presented as if they were grounded in certainty. Toxic victims and their representatives often contest these bureaucratic defini-tions of illness and safety and also try to expand the scope of the event from private suffering to the political issue of public policy. Reich's characterization of what happens in the case of chemical disasters, and especially the difficulties encountered by victims in bringing these issues into the domain of public consciousness, is lucid and clear. However, due to the nature of the chemical disasters that he has analyzed (contamination of cooking oil in the case of Japan, and animal feed in the case of the United States), his emphasis is on the understanding of the transformation of private trouble into public issue. He also shows how bureaucratic rationality resists this transformation. In the Bhopal case, however, the disaster was experienced right from the start as a *collective disaster*. Yet bureaucratic and judicial rationality, coupled with the exercise of power by the multinational, operated in a manner that denied victims their suffering. The denial did not occur through repression and censorship alone, but rather through a manner of talking about their suffering so that it came to be constituted purely as a verbal object, dissolving the concrete and existential reality of their being.

The Event

Sometime in the night of December 2–3, 1984, between 30 to 40 tons of methyl isocyanate (MIC) escaped from a huge storage tank at the Union Carbide factory located in Bhopal, the industrial capital of Madhya Pradesh. The earliest descriptions of the gas were of a creeping, deadly, yellow, choking vapor which was intensely irritating to the eyes and the lungs. Between December 3 and 6, about 2500 people died as a result of inhaling this deadly vapor.[6]

At the time of the leakage, it is possible that very little was known about MIC. In the earliest stages, the Union Carbide officials repeatedly claimed that MIC was not more potent than tear gas, and that it caused only surface damage.[7] Since the leakage, however, much more has become known about MIC. Of all the known industrial isocyanates, MIC is the most potent pulmonary irritant and the second most potent sensory irritant. Its toxic hazard is related to the fact that the vapor pressure of MIC is exceedingly high: hence, even a short duration of exposure is likely to result in severe effects (Alarie et al. 1987). Among the acute effects of MIC is immediate death due to profound hypoxia resulting from blockage of airways, by necrotic epithelial cells, mucus, fluid and fibrin. Experimental research on animals as well as clinical observations on survivors have confirmed that there is a complex response to varying degrees of exposure to the gas. At higher dose levels, there were life threatening manifestations of pulmonary damage among the survivors, reflected in the clinical conditions of bronchi-constriction, pulmonary oedema, etc. At the intermediate levels of exposure there was eye damage, including corneal opacity, and high risks of cataract. At relatively low doses, sensory and neurological responses have been found (Anderson, Kerr Muir, Mehra and Salmon 1985; Gassert et al. 1987). Although Union Carbide scientists have tried to maintain that MIC has no long-term effects, other research seems to make it almost certain that there are several long-term effects, including chronic respiratory conditions, development of corneal opacity, and involvement of the immune system. It is not only likely that local immunity gets altered, but as experimental research with animals has shown, there is persistent bone marrow suppression, and suppression of lympho-proliferative responses.[8]

My purpose in drawing attention to these studies is simply to point out that experimental research and clinical experience in the last five years have confirmed what the survivors of the Bhopal tragedy were constantly asserting: their condition was not improving, they were compelled to run after different kinds of medical personnel, they were unable to work and hence found it difficult to sustain themselves, and their children were constantly falling ill and were subject to enormous suffering. The population of more than 300,000 that resided in the 36 wards near the factory, and which were identified as gas-affected on the basis of incidence of mortality in these localities between December 3 and 6, 1984, was generally poor and did not, therefore, have the resources to deal with a tragedy of this gigantic proportion which had suddenly shattered their lives. They had the experience of total and abject suffering but they did not have the language to transform this experience into forms that would make sense in the political domain within which it came to be addressed.

Within one month of this tragedy, suits were filed by many American lawyers in courts in America on behalf of several victims. Within a week of the tragedy, several American lawyers had flown into Bhopal and obtained powers of attorney from victims to pursue cases against the Union Carbide Corporation and its Indian subsidiary. These lawyers were described by many as "ambulance chasers" since their fees were said to be based on a contingency sharing of the obtained damages. In any case, in view of the difficulties of pursuing the case by such a large number of poor victims against one of the most powerful multinationals, the Government of India passed the Bhopal Gas Leak Disaster (Processing of Claims) Act in March 1985. With this act, the government of India, in accordance of its *parens patriae* function, took upon itself the responsibility of the conduct of the case and welfare of the victims.

The legal and litigational issues arising out of this case are important[9] and will surely become part of the ongoing debates on toxic torts (Elliot 1988; Rosenberg 1984; Royce and Callahan 1988). Here I shall only describe those events that are necessary for the understanding of *one* judicial text, *viz.* the judgment of the Supreme Court of India, delivered on December 22, 1989, on the constitutional validity of the Bhopal Act. This is a text in which we can see clearly the professional transformation of the suffering of the victims of Bhopal and the window it opens towards the understanding of how suffering has become a means for the legitimation of the state in India today.

The major events in the litigational history of this episode that need to be kept in mind are the following:

1. The Bhopal Act was passed by the government of India in March 1985, consolidating all claims arising out of the Bhopal disaster and making the government the only competent authority on the basis of the *parens patriae* function of the state to represent the victims.

2. In the initial pursuit of the case in 1985 in a New York District Court, the government of India represented that its judicial system was not competent to deal with the complex legal issues arising out of this disaster. The government of India's strategy was to either force Union Carbide to submit to U.S. laws on environmental protection, safety regulations, and liability of hazardous industry, and thus secure compensation for the victims in accordance with law and standards of compensation in the United States, which Union Carbide seemed anxious to avoid; or to ensure that Union Carbide was brought under the jurisdiction

of the Indian courts. This was important since the strategy of Union Carbide was to deny that any entity other than its Indian subsidiary, with far lower assets, was liable. Judge Keenan, in whose court this was adjudicated declared faith in the Indian judiciary and bound Union Carbide to the jurisdiction of Indian courts (Baxi and Paul 1985; Baxi 1990).

3. Hearing of the case began in 1986 in the district court of Bhopal. An application for interim relief was filed on behalf of several victim organizations in 1987, and the judge ruled that Union Carbide should pay Rs.350 *crores* as interim relief, which would be adjusted against final settlement. Union Carbide appealed against this ruling in the High Court, where the quantum of interim relief was reduced to Rs.250 *crores.*

4. Union Carbide appealed to the Supreme Court against the Madhya Pradesh High Court order. It was while hearing the petition for interim relief that the Supreme Court, to the surprise and dismay of victims, made a judicial order on February 15, 1988, asking the government of India and Union Carbide to settle at 470 million dollars. Part of the settlement deal was immunity granted to Union Carbide and its subsidiaries against any criminal or civil liability arising from the Bhopal disaster at present and in the future.

5. There were widespread protests against the settlement, although it received the support of some important jurists.[10] It was widely believed that the courts had been pressured or influenced by the Congress government, which was then in power, to issue the order and that the government had made a private deal with Union Carbide. Regardless of the truth of these allegations, the order was challenged on several legal grounds. One of these was a challenge to the constitutional validity of the Bhopal Act, since it took away from victims the right to be heard.[11]

6. The court gave its judgment on the Bhopal Act, holding it to be constitutionally valid, on December 22, 1989. The court was not required to pronounce on the settlement since that was to be heard by another bench; nevertheless, the court made several pronouncements defending the settlement. This particular text is what we shall analyze in detail in this section. To the extent that a judgment creates a master discourse in which the various voices are appropriated in a kind of monologic structure, it is important to see how these voices represent the suffering of the victims to which references abound.

Of the several issues that this case raised, we shall take up only one. How did the government use its *parens patriae* functions, and what did it understand by the act of being surrogate victim as implied by this function? In normal circumstances, *parens patriae* refers to the inherent power and authority of a legislature to provide protection to the person and property of persons *non sui juris*, such as minors, insane and incompetent persons. The victims of the Bhopal disaster had been assimilated to the category of *non sui juris*, even when in the normal course of events they would not be considered judicially incompetent because it was evident that they did not have the resources to pursue the case themselves. However, the act was challenged on the grounds that by its enactment, the government had constituted itself as surrogate of the victims and taken away their right to be heard. Certain sections of the act, it was argued, amounted to a naked usurpation of power. The implication of this argument and the timing of the challenge was that having usurped power in this manner, the government had used it to compromise the rights of victims by unilaterally arriving at a settlement and granting immunity to Union Carbide against the expressed wishes of the victims. Thus guardianship in this case amounted to a pretext through which the issue was sought to be resolved against the interests of the victims.

The counter argument to this plea was presented by the then Attorney General, who had represented the government in February 1988 and defended the settlement with Union Carbide in court and outside. In defense of the Bhopal Act he argued that the disaster had been treated as a national calamity by the government of India. The government had a right, and indeed a duty to take care of its citizens in the exercise of its *parens patriae* jurisdiction or in a principle analogous to it. He reminded the court that they were not dealing with one or two cases, but with a large class of victims who, because they were poor and disabled, could not pursue the case against a powerful multinational. In the course of the arguments he maintained that:

Rights are indispensably valuable possessions, but the right is something an individual can stand on, something which must be demanded or insisted upon without embarrassment or shame.

When rights are curtailed — permissibility of such a measure can be examined only upon the strength, urgency, and pre-eminence of rights and the largest good of the largest number sought to be served by curtailment.

If the contentions of the petitioners are entertained... rights may be theoretically upheld — but ends of justice would be sacrificed... the consent of victims should be based upon information and comprehension of collective welfare and individual good.

Here I must make a digression and point out that the issues arising out of the necessity for the government to act as surrogate to people who because of disease or handicap (e.g., comatose patients, patients with serious mental trauma) are unable to make their own decisions have been widely debated in recent years. It is generally agreed that the surrogate has to apply a "best interest" standard in making decisions on behalf of people declared to be judicially incompetent (President's Commission Report 1983). However, the interpretation of "best interest" standard has varied. According to one interpretation, the best interest standard requires "a surrogate to do what, from an objective standpoint, appears to promote a patient's good without reference to the patient's actual supposed preferences." Such a view has been challenged on the ground that a surrogate is acting in the best interest of the patient only if he tries to replicate the decisions that a patient would have made if he was capable of doing so.[12] Evocation of objectively determined interests as against subjectively expressed preferences can simply mask power in the name of doing good.

The same question now presented itself before the Supreme Court. In its earlier judicial order, the Supreme Court had claimed that it had acted in the best interest of the victims. But the victims were contesting this. How could the court defend the actions of the government and its own actions in promoting the settlement, when victims themselves were protesting against it? It is in this context that the "suffering" and the "agony" of victims seems to have found its *raison d'etre* of allowing the judiciary to create a verbal discourse which would legitimize the position of the government as the guardian of the people, and the judiciary as the protector of the rule of law.

In their judgment, the judges upheld the constitutional validity of the Bhopal Act. In a stirring statement they declared, "Our Constitution makes it imperative for the State to secure to all its citizens the rights guaranteed by the Constitution and when the citizens are not in a position to assert and secure these rights, the State must come into the picture and protect and fight for the rights of the citizens." This is a principle that expands greatly the power of the state to act as guardian and deprive people of their normal constitutional rights including the right to petition a court of law. Aware of this contradiction the judges further stated, "It is necessary for the state to ensure the fundamental rights in conjunction with the Directive Principles of state policy to effectively discharge its obligations and for this purpose, if necessary, to deprive some rights and privileges of the individual victims in order to protect these rights better and to secure them further." But in what way had the meager settlement served to secure the rights of the victims or led to "greater good of greater numbers" — the utilitarian principle formulated by the attorney general and the judges at several times in the course of the argument?

The judgment stated that the Court had, in its earlier judicial order which instructed both parties to settle on the conditions described earlier in the paper, acted in the interest of the victims. "The basic consideration the court recorded, motivating the conclusion of the settlement was the compelling need for urgent relief, and the Court set out the law's delays duly considering that there was a compelling duty both judicial and humane, to secure immediate relief for the victims." Here is the first invocation of the suffering of the victims; since there was a compelling need to provide immediate relief, the Court had been moved by humane considerations to instruct parties to settle. The Court simply neglected to mention that the urgent need for immediate relief was precisely what the victims had asked for in their petition for interim relief, which had been upheld by lower courts! Further, immediate need for relief was simply stated as the motivation behind settlement, but there was nothing in the judicial order that would instruct government to provide this immediate relief — neither the procedure for dispersal of money nor any timetable having been formulated by the Court. One would not, therefore, be incorrect in concluding that the suffering of the victims was more a verbal ploy than a condition that caused serious concern to the judiciary or the government.

On the question as to why the Court had not found it fit to invite the opinion of victims themselves, at least through some representative organizations, about the proposed settlement before passing the judicial order, the judges noted that this had been because of a certain degree of uneasiness and skepticism expressed by the learned counsel of both parties "at the prospects of success in view of their past experience of such negotiations when, as they stated, there had been uninformed and even irresponsible criticism of the attempts to settlement." Thus the first imperative to arrive at a meager settlement was the "suffering" of the victims. The second imperative to do this with complete secrecy and present victims with a *fait accompli* was the irresponsibility and inability on the part of victims to understand the issues.

Thus the situation was as follows: A multinational corporation was engaged in the production and storage of an extremely hazardous industrial chemical for which it had been given the license to operate by the Indian government. Despite the known hazards of industrial isocyanates and diisocyanates, neither the multinational corporation or its Indian subsidiary, nor the government of India had considered it important or necessary to inquire into the nature of hazard to the people posed by the activities entailed in its manufacture and storage at the various times between the setting up of the factory and the spillage of the gas. The people of Bhopal, especially those staying around the factory, had not been warned of the dangers posed to them by these industrial activities, nor had any regulations been made and implemented about the placement of such factories.[13] The result of all these activities geared towards the "development" and "industrialization" of India was that more than 300,000 people were suddenly one night blighted by crippling disease and more than 2,500 died horrible deaths. Yet the people to be declared incompetent and irresponsible were neither the multinational nor the government, but ironically the sufferers themselves.

How had the Court arrived at the particular sum of 470 million dollars as adequate compensation for the 300,000 victims already known to have been affected? Were the victims right in alleging that there was no evidence of the application of judicial mind behind this order? The fact was that medical examination of only half the claimants out of the 600,000 claimants had been completed at the time that the court-ordered settlement, through procedures that were highly questionable.[14] Similarly, the medical folders that recorded the basis on which a victim's status was determined for purposes of compensation were not made available to them or their representatives on grounds of medical secrecy. Thus bureaucratic decisions could not be contested by victims.

Incidentally, it should be noted here that since the December 22 judgment, the victim groups have been able to secure some primary documentation on the procedures through which extent of victimization was estimated. It has been found that even the figures produced in the Supreme Court during the hearing by Madhya Pradesh Council were arrived at after the settlement, and therefore could not have been the basis for the settlement. Further, the procedure by which the status of a claim was determined was based on a kind of scoring system by which each symptom was given a score and finally the scores were aggregated. Despite the fact that the medical journals have constantly used the rhetoric of MIC being the most lethal gas known to man, the scoring system used the analogy of organ by organ injury rather than systemic damage as a result of toxic insult. To compound it all, patients who could not produce documentary evidence in the form of records of hospital admission or proof of having been treated in the first few days of the gas disaster were declared to be "uninjured" regardless of the state of their health at the time of examination.[15] This disregard of all human and medical ethics is appalling, for anyone familiar with mass disaster would know that the immediate task at the time of disaster is to reach help and not to keep meticulous individual records. All this has been justified on the grounds of bureaucratic and legal necessity. The macabre quality of this discourse can be seen in the fact that Union Carbide has repeatedly tried to present itself as the real "friend" of the victims whose offer of "the best medical treatment for victims" was rejected by India. In making such arguments Union Carbide lawyers simply fail to mention the fact that at the same time that these offers were being made, the medical scientists flown into Bhopal by Union Carbide were declaring that MIC was not a dangerous gas at all and that if victims had died, it was their own fault. To take just one example of this attitude, consider the statement of Dr. Peter Halberg, one of the three doctors sent by UCC as part of its 'relief efforts' to Bhopal. According to the learned doctor, "MIC created a heavy cloud, which settled very close to the earth, killing children because of their immature lungs, the elderly because of their diminished lung capacity, those who ran because their lungs expanded too rapidly."[16] The transformation of healers into merchants and touts of death unfortunately has always been a possibility inscribed into the medical discourse, as the labors of Robert Lifton have proved. How was this potential to be resisted?

Here we can see that disabled though the victims were they did not let this particular construction of their reality go unchallenged.[17] In response to the question as to how the Court at the time of settlement had arrived at the judgment that the sum was reasonable, it had been stated in the clarificatory orders that the reasonableness of the sum was based not only upon independent quantification, "but the idea of reasonableness for the present purpose was necessarily a broad and general estimate in the context of a settlement of the dispute and not on the basis of an accurate assessment of adjudication." In other words, victims were irresponsible and uninformed when they inquired about the basis on which the Court had arrived at the estimate of the victimization or the principles by which compensation was being determined, but the Court itself had only been motivated by humane considerations when it refused to divulge any of the medical information about the nature and extent of damage caused by MIC.

In its final transformation then, the suffering of the victims was considered sufficient reason to justify the settlement and to uphold the usurpation of power by the government on the principle that the Bhopal Act could be upheld if it had proved to be in the interests of the victims (the proof of the pudding is in the eating — as the learned judges stated). Therefore, although the judges conceded that justice did not *appear* to have been done (since the victims were not given a hearing), they also argued that justice was, nevertheless, *done* on the principle that a small harm can be tolerated for a larger good. The judges were concerned to signal their own humanity and to protect the legitimacy of the judicial institution of which they were a part. The "suffering" of the victims was a useful narrative device which could be evoked to explain why victims had not been consulted; why their protests over the settlement could be redefined as actions of irresponsible and ignorant people; and above all, why the judges had not felt obliged to ask the government and its medical establishment to place for public scrutiny what it had accomplished by way of providing relief and help to the victims, and in the process, what was the knowledge that had been generated on the impact of the deadly isocyanate on the health of people; and finally, that they had completely failed to fix responsibility for the accident and thus had converted the issue of multinational liability into that of multinational charity.

In the course of the judgment, it was evident that there was no lack of concern for the impact of hazardous industry on *society in general;* it was only the interests of these particular victims that could not be fully protected. Thus there were acute reflections on the dangers arising from hazardous technology. The judges stated that there were vital juristic principles that touched upon problems emerging "from the pursuit of such dangerous technologies for economic gains by multinationals." The judges also noted the need to evolve a national policy to protect national interests from such ultra-hazardous pursuits of economic gain. However, the sufferings of the people clearly came in the way of evolving these juristic principles. To quote the judgment on this issue:

In the present case, the compulsions of the need for immediate relief to tens of thousands of suffering victims could not wait till these questions, vital though these may be were resolved in due course of judicial proceedings; and the tremendous suffering of thousands of persons compelled this Court to move into the direction of immediate relief, which, this Court thought, should not be subordinated to the uncertain principles of law…

In all these discussions at the judicial and bureaucratic levels, "victim" finally became a totally abstract category. The judges did not seem to have any clear idea about how many victims there were or the havoc caused by MIC poisoning on their bodies and minds. In a moving speech protesting the settlement, one illiterate woman stated: "We only ask the judges for one thing — please come here and count us." In the judicial discourse, however, every reference to victims and their suffering only served to reify suffering, and to dissolve the real victims so that they could be reconstituted again into nothing more than verbal objects.

The Sequel

Life sometimes redeems itself by allowing historical truths to mimic narrative truths rather than the other way around. The judgment of December 22 had concluded on a note of humility on the part of the judges. "It is well to remember…time has upset many fighting faiths…and one must always wager one's salvation upon some prophecy based on uncertain knowledge…Our knowledge changes: our perception of truth also changes…"

Almost in response to this grudging recognition that the "judicial truth" that the judges had pronounced might alter if circumstances altered, the Indian people, in the general elections held in late December 1989 and early January of 1990, voted the Congress Government out of power. A new government came into power and showed the possibility of a humane approach to the problem of Bhopal victims. While submitting itself completely to the rule of law in the fight against Union Carbide, it nevertheless decided that it would support the victims in the various review petitions challenging the settlement that were to be heard. Further, it took its role as guardian of the victims with great seriousness, stating that there could be no conflict of interest between victims and government. Recognizing their urgent need for succor, the government evolved a scheme for interim relief that was not dependent upon litigational uncertainties or bureaucratic rationality. Thus it offered to support every one of the 106,000 households by granting them the minimum of Rs.750 per month for the next three years. The sum of Rs.360 *crores* (amounting to a little more than half the settlement amount) that was required to support the scheme was to come out of the government's own coffers and was adjustable only against final settlement. The motive behind this was to do away with the kind of rationality by which victims, who are already destroyed by disease, are again victimized in the process of acquiring appropriate certificates to satisfy the bureaucrats. Further, representatives of victim groups were actively associated in the evolution of the scheme and would continue to help in the dispersal. At one stroke the victims were transformed from incompetent, irresponsible people to ones whose subjective preferences were to be taken into account even when the government acted as surrogate for them due to the enormous legal complexities of the case. Above all, the limits of judicial and bureaucratic rationality were recognized by the state, and it decided to absorb the uncertainties itself rather than make victims bear the costs. The resolution of legal issues will only unfold itself over a period of time, and that is a story that will have to be told at another time. But there is no doubt that the government proved its humanity by simply putting aside the humiliating procedures that had been evolved by the bureaucracy and the medical establishment to make victims prove beyond reasonable doubt their victimage — as if their debilitated condition was not attested already by the attacks of chronic cough, difficulty of breathing, constant watering of the eyes, listlessness, inability to work, grief at the loss of children — could only be proven by the code numbers and certificates that the bureaucrats controlled. This is what finally set it apart from Union Carbide, who will no doubt use the massive research it has conducted on animals in the last five years to argue that MIC causes nothing more than simple injury.

Concluding Comments

In considering orientations to suffering, we have seen how suffering may be appropriated by the discourse of the powerful both within the family and the state. The presence of paradox, self-concealment, plural connotations, distensions of metaphor act as shears through which suffering is sought to be cut off from the victim to become the child of the pronouncer of this discourse. In both the cases we examined, the more suffering was talked about, the more it was to extinguish the sufferer. We saw the transformation of protector into perpetrator, leading to a double victimization of the victims. Thus the patriarch of the family sacrificed the women for the connections between men, and doctors were transformed from healers into bureaucrats whose job was more to sort out people into slots rather than to heal them.

In each case those who suffered were transformed into malingerers. Whereas in literature and poetry, the malingerer lives on the peripheries of society, and his or her melancholy and physical disability become a sign of all that is wrong with *society*, in the case of modern medical science, bearing the stamp of industrial discipline, malingering becomes a moral fault. In the case of Bhopal, especially, victims whose suffering and disease challenged the certainty of a bureaucratically defined medical science came to be themselves stigmatized. "If we cannot understand your disease by the tools of our discipline, then you must be at fault;" this was the message by which the magical melancholy malingerer of poetry became the slothful sinner against industrial and bureaucratic discipline.

Both the cases described here are important signs of our times. They both represent the capacity of society to inflict terrible disease and ill-being on its vulnerable and weak sections such that their whole world may be destroyed in one stroke. With changes in industrial technology, including the technology of violence, traditional conflicts are amplified and new unpredictable disorders are let loose upon people. This is why we must be wary of all evolutionary schemes for description and analysis of disorder. Even such innocuous terms as "health transition" may have a dangerous potential in that they assume that diseases are distributed on some kind of an evolutionary scale. In societies such as India, one can find the oldest of diseases and the newest of diseases. The tragedy is that it is the same population which suffers from both kinds of diseases. In the Bhopal case, it was the poor who were compelled to live near the factory in open spaces or broken *jhuggis* (shanties), and who suffered the worst consequences of the exposure to the lethal gas. In the case of the riots also it was the slum dweller who had to pay the costs of urban disorder and who was most vulnerable to death by violence. All that Indian society could evolve by way of a response was a bureaucratic construction of suffering. In such cases, the very notion of health becomes a contested site and disasters become an opportunity for the exercise of new kinds of power over victims. A radical discourse can only be fashioned if we discard all paternalistic notions by which health is handed down to the poor through a paternalistic and bureaucratically defined rationality and allow for people to demand health, as they define it, as a basic human right. As I have argued elsewhere, it is necessary to evolve a communicative morality rather than an imperative one, if the very state of ill-being is not to be used as a means of stigmatizing a person or a class of people.[18]

For the victim, life may be understood backwards, but it must be lived forwards, and a discourse on suffering is worth having only if it helps the victim to live forwards. Perhaps it is now the turn of the anthropologist to pay heed to the terrible warning contained in these two cases, lest we too become a part of the tribe that creates discourses of power on the pretext of understanding suffering, or that uses the suffering of the people only as occasion for professional interventions and transformations.

Acknowledgement

I am grateful to Upendra Baxi for many insightful discussions on the general issues raised here and to Radha Kumar, Prashant Bhushan and again Upendra Baxi for much help in formulating the legal and medical issues concerning the Bhopal disaster. During my work on the riot victims described in this paper I was helped considerably by the assistance of the Indian Express Relief Committee, and my colleagues and students in the Delhi University. Ranendra Das and Jishnu Das worked for long hours over the statistical materials contained in ICMR reports. Arthur Kleinman provided detailed comments which helped towards greater clarity. The victims of these disasters continue to bear the burdens of modern Indian society and as their scribe I struggle with the hopeless inadequacy of my conceptual tools to give them voice. But to everyone who has helped in this, I am more grateful than I can say.

Notes

1 Theodicy, sin, and salvation were three key terms in Max Weber's sociology of religion. See, Max Weber, *The Sociology of Religion*, Beacon Press, 1963, (translated by Ephraim Fiscoff). Also see his "Social psychology of world religions," in Hans Gerth & C. Wright Mills (ed.) *From Max Weber*, Oxford, New York, 1946.

2 I have developed this argument in an essay entitled, "What do we mean by health?," presented at the Health Transition Workshop, held in Canberra, 15 – 19 May, 1989. In J.C. Caldwell, S. Findley, P. Caldwell, G. Santow, W. Cosford, J. Braid, and D. Broers-Freeman. 1990. *What We Know About the Health Transition: The Cultural, Social and Behavioural Determinants of Health,*

Health Transition Series, No. 2, Volumes 1 and 2. Canberra: Health Transition Centre, Australian National University.

3 These two approaches are lucidly presented in Gilles Deleuze, *Nietzsche & Philosophy,* The Athlone Press, London, 1983.

4 I realize that such a discourse leads to a displacement of responsibility and cannot, therefore, be described as radically critical in nature but at the very least it does not make the victim bear all the costs of a calamity. I must acknowledge here a gap in my thinking but also an inability to accept the kinds of arguments currently proposed by several radical thinkers in India who find the unintended function of such calamities, to be the raising of consciousness.

5 See also his, "Environmental politics and science: The case of PBB contamination in Michigan," *American Journal of Public Health,* 73: 302–313, 1983.

6 See the report on the Bhopal disaster in *The Lancet,* Dec.15, 1984.

7 Thus L.D. Loya, medical officer, Union Carbide India Ltd. stated at the time of the disaster on December 3rd 1984 that "The gas is non-poisonous. There is nothing to do except ask patients to put a wet towel over their eyes". Quoted in David Dembo et al., eds., *Nothing to Lose but Our Lives,* Council of International and Public affairs, Delhi: New York and Indian Law Institute, 1987, p.40. See also Veena Das, "What do we mean by health?" (1990) for a discussion of how Union Carbide consistently misled and misinformed public opinion, and the theoretical issues involved in a definition of health that is arrived at through bargains struck between the State, its medical establishment and forces of capitalism.

8 The long term effects are lucidly summarized in N.Anderson, "Long term effects of methyl isocyanate," *The Lancet,* June 3, 1989. See also Daya R. Verma "Hydrogen cyanide & Bhopal," *The Lancet,* Sept.2, 1989, for an account of how the long term effects of methyl isocyanate were sought to be obscured by a clever manipulation of the suggestion that the deaths had been caused by hydrogen cyanide, which is much less lethal than methyl isocyanate.

9 For a clear and concise picture of these issues, see Upendra Baxi, "The Bhopal victims in the labyrinth of the law: An Introduction," in U. Baxi and A. Dhanda, eds., *Valiant Victims and Lethal Litigation: The Bhopal Case,* Delhi: Indian Law Institute, 1990: i–lxix. This book puts together in one place all the legal records necessary for an understanding of the issues.

10 Among those who defended the settlement was the eminent jurist and human rights worker V.M.Tarkunde who defended the settlement on grounds of pragmatism and in the interest of securing speedy relief for the victims. As many of his critics have noted, this abstract concern was not translated into any concrete action. Tarkunde, who is no stranger to the use of courts for securing human rights, did not, for instance, use this institution for securing interim relief for the victims or demanding any mechanism for disbursal of the amount to reach victims. On the inadequacy of the settlement, see for example, the letter of the reputed tort lawyer Melvin Belli, characterizing the settlement as the most

"unethical" in his fifty year experience of dealing with tort law. *Times of India*, March 7, 1989. My own calculations show that even if half the claims were only valid, the sum was just enough to sustain the affected households at the minimal income of Rs.700 p.m., and a minimal subsidy for risk to life, for a maximum period of ten years. I have not included costs of medical care in these calculations. Thus without even going into questions of rights, the sum is not even adequate to ensure the survival of severely affected households for the next twenty years - the normal life span, given the age distribution of victims.

11 Writ Petition No.268 of 1989, no.164 of 1986, No.981 of 1989, and No.1551 of 1986.

12 See especially Chapter 4 of *Deciding to Forego Life Sustaining Treatment.*

13 Incidentally it would be difficult for anyone to believe that Union Carbide did not have any inkling about the nature of methyl isocyanate as claimed by them, for its production had been discontinued in England and only small amounts were stored in Carbide plants in such countries as Germany!

14 To mention only one fact, although clinical studies with survivors showed development of small airway and large airway obstructions which worsened with the passage of time, tests of pulmonary functions were done on a minuscule number of claimants. Mostly it was assumed that survivors were exaggerating their symptoms.

15 For a reasoned critique of the procedures of evaluation of health status of victims by the Directorate of Claims, see C.Sathyamala, N.Vohra and K.Satish, *Against all odds: The health status of the Bhopal survivors.* Delhi:1989.

16 Quoted in David Dembo, C.J.Dias, Ayesha Kadwani and Ward Morehouse, eds., *Nothing to Lose but our Lives.* See note 7, above.

17 In public meetings or demonstrations in Bhopal, the audience can always hear the 'folk' poetry and songs composed by victims in which such doctors come in for scathing attacks; even bodies ravaged by toxic gas and bureaucratic insult, can produce their own poetry after all.

18 I am grateful to Madam Gopal for the formulation on malingering.

References

Alarie, Y., et al. 1987. "Sensory and pulmonary irritation of methyl isocyanate in mice and pulmonary irritation and possible cyanide-like effects of methyl isocyanate in rats and guinea pigs." *Environmental Health Perspective*, 72:159-67.

Anderson N., M.D. Muir, V. Mehra, and A.G. Salmon. 1985. "Exposure and response to methyl isocyanate: Results of a community-based survey in Bhopal." *British Journal of Industrial Medicine*, 45:469-75.

Baxi, U. 1990. "The Bhopal victims in the labyrinth of the law: An introduction." In U. Baxi and A. Dhanda, eds. *Valiant Victims and Lethal Litigation: The Bhopal Case.* Delhi: Indian Law Institute.

Baxi, U., and T. Paul. 1985. *Mass Disasters and Multinational Liability: The Bhopal Case.* Delhi: Indian Law Institute.

Das, V. 1986. "The work of mourning: Death in a Punjabi family." In I. Merry White and S. Pollak, eds. *The Cultural Transition: Human Experience and Social Transformation in the Third World and Japan.* Boston: Routledge & Kegan Paul.

Das, V. 1989. "Voices of children." *Daedalus*, 118(4):263–294.

Das, V. 1990. "Our work to cry: Your work to listen." In V. Das, ed. *Mirrors of Violence.* Delhi: Oxford University Press.

Das, V., and M. Bose. 1987. "The legacy of despair." *Illustrated Weekly of India.* Bombay, (February 1–7): 32–33.

Elliot, S. 1988. "The future of toxic torts: Of chemophobia, risk as a comparable injury and hybrid compensations systems." *Houston Law Review*, 25.

Gassert, T., et al. 1987. "Long-term pathology of lung, eyes and other organs following acute exposure of rats to methyl isocyanate." *The Lancet*, 72:95–103.

Geertz, C. 1973. *The Interpretation of Cultures.* New York: Basic Books, Inc.

President's Commission for the study of ethical problems in medicine and biomedical and behavioral research. 1983. *Deciding to Forego Life Sustaining Treatment: Ethical, Legal and Medical Issues in Treatment Decisions.* Washington, DC: U.S. Government Printing Office.

Reich, M.R. 1982. "Public and private responses to a chemical disaster in Japan: The case of Kanemi Yusho." *Law in Japan: An Annual*, 15:102–109.

Rosenberg, D. 1984. "The causal connection in mass exposure cases: A public law vision of the tort system?" *Harvard Law Review*, 97(4):849–929.

Royce M.D., and J. Callahan. 1988. "Isocyanates: An emerging toxic tort." *Environmental Law*, 18(2): 293–319.

Section III

Rediscovering the Social Nature of Mortality Change

8

Child Mortality Differences, Personal Health Care Practices, and Medical Technology: The United States, 1900-1930

Gretchen A. Condran
Samuel H. Preston

Discussions of the factors responsible for mortality decline in the past century have emphasized the relative importance of economic development and public health programs (e.g., McKeown 1976; Preston 1980). Focus on these broad, systemic factors has until recently directed attention away from personal health care practices as a factor in mortality variation. However, recent studies of microlevel data in developing countries have shown that child mortality levels are typically closely associated with mothers' literacy and ethnicity, findings that suggest a strong role for unmeasured child care practices that vary among groups differentiated on these dimensions (United Nations 1985). More specific investigations into behavioral differences between well-educated and poorly educated mothers appear to support this suggestion (e.g., Clelland and van Ginneken 1988). Ethnographic studies in a variety of settings have shed light on how women's education affects the relations between generations and between sexes in ways that are pertinent to child care practices (e.g., Caldwell, Reddy, and Caldwell 1988).

This paper examines the role of behavioral factors in child mortality in the United States during the period 1900-1930. We first review cross-sectional differences in child mortality among social groups for evidence of behavioral influences. This section is based upon public use samples from the United States censuses of 1900 and 1910, each of which asked questions of ever-married women regarding the number of children they had borne and the numbers of them who had survived. We then examine the issue of whether behavioral changes played an important role in the large decline that occurred in U.S. child mortality during the period 1900–1930.

Cross-sectional Differences in Child Mortality, 1900 and 1910

The pattern of mortality differentials in the United States in 1900 was quite different from that typically observed in developing countries today (Preston, 1985; Preston and Haines 1990). A smaller mortality advantage was associated with mothers' literacy and much smaller advantage accrued to the professional classes. Controlling no other variables, literate women had 30 percent lower child mortality in the United States in 1900, compared to an average difference of 45 percent in 11 developing countries providing comparable data. Wives of professionals enjoyed only a 7 percent advantage in the United States but enjoy a 35 percent advantage in the developing countries today. Urban residents suffered a penalty of 28 percent in the United States, compared to a 23 percent advantage in the average developing country. When other social, economic, and residential variables are introduced, the contrasts remain. Mothers' literacy becomes insignificant in the United States, while typically remaining one of the most powerful predictors in developing countries. Residence in urban areas continues to be associated with very high mortality in the United States but not in developing countries.

The interpretation offered for these contrasting patterns is that infectious disease processes were poorly understood by physicians, public officials, and parents in 1900; that few effective techniques of disease prevention or treatment had been developed; and that the few effective techniques that were available had been slow to diffuse (Preston and Haines 1990; Chapter VI). In short, the upper classes had access to little in the way of technical expertise that they could use to turn their material advantages into longer life. As further evidence of this point, offspring of physicians had mortality levels only 6 percent below the national average, and children of teachers enjoyed no advantage whatsoever. The interpretation is buttressed by a review of the state of medical knowledge and practice in the late nineteenth century. The fact that urban residents had mortality so much higher than those in rural areas was additional evidence of the extent to which mortality remained in the grips of natural forces.

In contrast, the literate and professional classes and urbanites in developing countries today have access to a much superior body of medical and public health techniques. Microorganisms are recognized as the source of major childhood diseases and this recognition has led to the development of an array of preventive and curative methods that are available to the privileged classes through both private and public sources.

The other demographic arena in which behavioral differences in child mortality are manifest in developing countries today is ethnicity. For example, populations of Chinese origin have low child mortality wherever they are located, and Muslim minorities have high child mortality levels compared to other groups (United Nations 1985).

At the turn of the century, the United States was home to a wide array of immigrant groups, and this offers a unique opportunity to investigate ethnic mortality differences in a historical setting. But because of its small size, the public use sample from the 1900 U.S. Census is not an effective vehicle for investigating these differences. The public use sample from the 1910 Census, released in 1989 (Strong et al. 1989), is far more promising because it is 3.66 times larger and immigration to the United States was very rapid between 1900 and 1910.

Preston, Ewbank, and Hereward (1990) investigated the relative mortality levels of ten major foreign-born groups in the United States in 1910. Before any other variables were controlled, six of these ten groups (British, Irish, Eastern European, French-Canadian, Polish, and Italian) had child mortality levels that were significantly higher (at a 1 percent significance level) than that of native women of native parentage. The tendency of immigrants to live in large cities was the single most important factor in accounting for their excess mortality. However, after other social, economic, and residential variables were controlled, only three groups had significantly different mortality, and only two groups — French-Canadians and Jews — had levels that differed by at least 15 percent from that of natives of native parentage.

Even though few ethnic groups had anomalous child mortality levels, the two that did were spectacular. French-Canadians had 39 percent higher child mortality than native whites of native parentage and Jews had 45 percent lower mortality, once other variables such as literacy, husband's occupation, English-speaking ability, and size of place were controlled. Furthermore, these groups also had the highest and lowest mortality levels, respectively, among second generation women (women born in the United States of foreign-born mothers). They also maintained their relative positions in other countries. Quebec had by far the highest child mortality levels in Canada as late as 1926 (Nagnur 1980). A family reconstitution study in the Sanguenay region in northern Quebec finds exceptionally high infant mortality rates of 215-222/1000 in 1900-09 (Gauvreau 1990). Even within Montreal, French-Canadians had 50 percent higher infant mortality rates in 1859 than Protestants or Irish Catholics (Thornton and Olson 1990). And Jews had exceptionally low mortality nearly everywhere that they lived. A compilation of comparative infant mortality rates of Jews and non-Jews in 29 European countries or cities in the period 1819-1913 by Schmelz (1971:15-25) shows that Jews had much lower mortality nearly everywhere. Their median advantage in the 73 region-period combinations investigated was an astonishing 40 percent, very close to their advantage in the United States (Condran and Kramarow 1990: Table 1).

These two groups provide striking evidence of the importance of behavioral factors in child mortality before the advent of modern medicine. What were the specific factors responsible for the peculiar mortality levels of these two groups? The principal quantitative informa-tion is derived from Woodbury's (1925) classic prospective study of infant mortality for the Children's Bureau, based upon births in eight eastern cities during 1915-1917. This study also found French-Canadians to have exceptionally high, and Jews exceptionally low, infant mortality. Table 8-1 contains the levels of infant mortality for these groups in the Woodbury study, along with information on their distribution on certain variables that are relevant to mortality. These variables do not include mothers' literacy because its relation with mortality was so weak in the Children's Bureau study (as the large investigation in Baltimore revealed; Rochester 1923) that it was omitted in Woodbury's final report. But literacy could not have accounted for the mortality difference between the groups. Among the ten ethnic groups investigated in the 1910 census, Jewish mothers had the second lowest proportion literate at 66.5 percent, compared to 82.7 percent for French-Canadian mothers (Table 8-1). Whatever behavioral differences existed between the groups were not transmitted by schooling.

French-Canadians and Jews were located on opposite ends of the spectrum on many of the determinants of infant mortality shown in Table 8-1. Particularly important are breastfeeding differences, with Jews and French-Canadians at opposite ends of the distribution of the prevalence of artificial feeding. A standardization for type of feeding eliminates 29 percent of the raw difference in infant mortality rates between the groups

Table 8-1 Comparison of French-Canadians and Jews in the United States, 1910-1917, on Variables Related to Child Mortality

	French-Canadians	Jews
Infant Mortality Rate, 1915-17[a]	171.3 per 1000	53.5 per 1000
Infant Mortality Rate from Gastric and Intestinal Diseases, 1915-17[a]	64.2 per 1000	10.5 per 1000
Child Mortality Index, 1910[b]	143.1	62.3
Child Mortality Index, Controlling Social-Economic Variables, 1910[c]	139.0	55.2
Percentage of Children Born to Literate Mothers, 1910[c]	82.7	66.5
Percentage of Children Born to Mothers Who Spoke English, 1910[c]	65.7	60.9
Percentage of Births in Families Where Husband Earned Less Than $650, 1915-17[a]	43.2	44.5
Percentage of Births to Mothers Employed Away From Home During Infants' First Year of Life, 1915-17[a]	16.1	1.1
Percentage of Births to Mothers Employed Away From Home During Pregnancy, 1915-17[a]	27.2	2.1
Percentage of First Nine Months of Life In Which Babies Were Exclusively Artificially Fed, 1915-17[a]	44.0	11.3
Percentage of Births of Order Five or Higher, 1915-17[a]	42.6	32.9
Percentage of Births to Mothers Under Age 20 or Over Age 45, 1915-17[a]	29.1	20.3

[a] Woodbury (1925:103-124). Figures refer to eight cities.
[b] Preston et al. (1990: Table 6). Figures refer to child mortality among women married in the United States who appeared in the 1910 Census. The value of the index for the full sample is 100.0.
[c] Preston et al. (1990: Table 8).

in the Woodbury study. However, the infant mortality advantage of Jews relative to French-Canadians or to native whites cannot, for the most part, be traced to the specific mechanisms examined by Woodbury nor to high levels of literacy.

By the turn of the century, there was an immense interest in the child survival successes of Jews. Apart from Woodbury's study there was little quantitative information available on the sources of their superior performance. But the commentary of contemporaries is informative about the perceived bases of Jewish exceptionalism. As Condran and Kramarow (1990) point out, Jews often served as a screen on which commentators could project their own vision of the most important factors in child survival. Nevertheless, several recurring themes are very informative (Condran and Kramarow 1990).

One is the degree of devotion of Jewish parents to their children. Jews were described as especially caring and responsible parents, as manifest in low rates of desertion of Jewish men and low rates of labor force participation by Jewish mothers, a factor that facilitated longer periods of breastfeeding. Ashby's (1922) lengthy discussion of low Jewish infant mortality in Manchester, England in 1911 cites especially mothers staying at home and breastfeeding their babies, their strong love for their children so that they would make any sacrifice for their welfare, and their scrupulousness about providing wholesome and regular meals and good clothing.

A second recurring theme is cleanliness. While there was some dispute about whether Jewish homes were cleaner than those of others, there was widespread acceptance of the view that handwashing was unusually common and that adherence to strictures about food purchasing and preparation probably led to cleaner food being placed on the table.

A third emphasis is that Jews had better access to health care and were better informed about the nature of infectious disease. Especially in the United States, the Jewish immigrant population, in striking contrast to other immigrant groups, contained many physicians. There is evidence that Jews attended dispensaries more frequently and were less exposed to quackery than other immigrant groups (Davis 1921). Davis suggests that Jewish newspapers accepted fewer advertisements for health related products than did the other immigrant papers in the country. Jews were, according to most accounts, in the forefront of accepting the new medical technologies. There were no anti-vaccinationists among the Jews (Davis 1921, Fishberg 1911).

Fishberg argued that every physician knew that Jews were always ready to take advantage of any new measure to prevent or cure disease. This trait was not new among the immigrants in this country but applied to the Jews in Europe as well.

> It must be emphasized in this connection that the Jews in Eastern Europe, superstitious as they are undoubtedly, believe in infection as a cause in the transmission of certain diseases; they believe that disease may be transmitted by personal contact, by fomites, dwellings, and food, and are willing to follow the advice of medical men in these matters (Fishberg 1911:285).

> Adherence to the notion that important diseases were spread, interpersonally, while perhaps reinforced by the germ theory of the 1860s and beyond, did not necessarily rest upon it. Ideas about contagion were very old but had largely been repudiated by a nineteenth century emphasis on miasmata as the source of disease (Tesh 1988).

Cause of death figures lend credence to the notion that Jewish emphasis on breastfeeding and clean food was an important feature of their low infant and child mortality. Among major causes of death contained in the Woodbury study, the Jewish deficit was greatest in digestive diseases at 58 percent. Interestingly, the French-Canadians showed by far their highest excess mortality from this cause of death (Woodbury 1925:104). Both groups, however, maintained their pattern of deviation for nearly every cause of death.

The behavioral differences between Jews and French-Canadians that are reflected in their relative child mortality levels are likely to be related to relationships within the family. Jewish families appear to have been unusually child-centered. Among the twelve ethnic groups in the United States in 1910 investigated by Jacobs and Green (1990), only Jewish children were more likely to be in school at ages 14-18 than offspring of native white parents, once other variables were controlled. In contrast, French-Canadian children aged 10-19 were second least likely to be in school and second most likely to be at work among 10 ethnic groups, in both cases trailing Italian children (Preston, Ewbank, and Hereward 1990). The smaller families and long birth spacing among Jews are other features that have come to be identified with modern child-oriented families.

Furthermore, in a setting in which the child survival advantages of breast-feeding were widely acknowledged (e.g., Meckel 1990), breastfeeding cannot be simply treated as an exogenous biomedical variable unrelated to decisions about child care. Many French-Canadian women curtailed breastfeeding in order to return to work, typically in New England textile mills. Hareven (1982) and Hareven and Langenbach (1978) have documented domestic relations among French-Canadian families in Manchester, New Hampshire, around the turn of the century. They note the major contribution that mothers and children were expected to make to the family economy. In order to facilitate mothers' work, young children were not only taken off the breast but were also sometimes loaned out for the work week, sent back to Quebec, or placed in the hands of older siblings. As noted, they were less likely to attend school when they grew up, and more likely to work, than children of most other ethnic groups. Hareven (1982:109), though generally sympathetic to her subjects, notes a certain callousness towards children among this group. It seems plausible that child mortality differences between Jews and French-Canadians were related to these apparent differences in the direction of flow of intergenerational resources, a theme whose importance for child mortality has been stressed by Caldwell (e.g., 1988).

From this evidence, it appears that persistent behavioral differences in child care practices associated with "cultural" identity were prominent on the mortality landscape a century ago. In contrast to the present, however, these differences were not closely associated with mothers' literacy. They were associated with attitudes towards children and the role of children in the household economy. And they were certainly associated with practices affecting the incidence and fatality of the major infectious diseases of childhood. Whether by chance, group evolution of sensible practices through trial and error, or a better-informed view of the nature of infectious disease, Jews were the forerunners in child survival.

Ethnic differences in child mortality formed part of the evidence in support of the view that parental practices were a key to improving child mortality. Contemporary writers sought to uncover the specific factors that differentiated the mortality levels of different groups and bring them to the attention of a wider audience. Other factors that pointed towards personal behavior as a major factor in child mortality levels were new understandings in bacteriology and a perceived failure of public work and sanitation projects to reduce infant mortality. We now turn attention to the more difficult question of whether changes in parenting behaviors played a major role in the decline of infant and child mortality in the United States during the first three decades of the century.

Child Care Practices and the Decline in Child Mortality, *1900-1930*

The first three decades of the twentieth century witnessed the fastest absolute decline in child mortality in the history of most western countries. In the United States, the probability of dying before age 5 fell from .180 in 1895 to .077 in 1929-31 (Preston and Haines 1990; National Center for Health Statistics 1984:14). Surprisingly little has been written about this important episode. Obviously, public health reforms were responsible for some part of the advance, especially in cities. Improvements in medicines and drugs were at most a small part (less than 10 percent) of the story (McKeown 1976; McKinlay and McKinlay 1977). Standards of living were improving, but the United States in 1900 would rank in the top fifth of the international income distribution if it were transported to the present, and its population was exceptionally well fed as well as highly literate (Preston and Haines 1990). It does not seem likely that rising living standards could account for more than a quarter of the U.S. advance (see also Preston 1975).

The causes of death that were responsible for the rapid decline in infant and childhood mortality from 1900 to 1930 shed some light on the nature of the mortality decline. Table 8-2 contains the rates of mortality for infants, one to four year olds, and the entire group under age fifteen for the years 1900 and 1930. All rates refer to the 10 original registration states (plus the District of Columbia) in 1900. The rates for those under fifteen in 1930 were standardized to the age distribution of the population under fifteen in 1900. The table shows the percentage of the overall decline in mortality for each age group that is attributable to specific causes of death.

The causes of death shown in Table 8-2 were selected because they were both important sources of the mortality of children and traceable over the time period in question. Unfortunately, they account for only half of the decline at ages below 15. But among these causes, diarrheal diseases overwhelmed all other causes as a source of mortality decline. For infants, nearly a third of the mortality decline was due to the decrease

Table 8-2 Decline in U.S. Child Mortality by Age and Selected Causes
of Death, 1900-1930.

	Death Rates/10,000		Percent of Change Attributable To Causes
	1900	1930	
Age 0-1			
All Causes	1496.30	680.00	
Measles	16.31	3.75	1.5
Scarlet Fever	2.84	.36	.3
Whooping Cough	33.22	13.38	2.4
Diphtheria	8.83	1.44	.9
Diarrhea and enteritis	341.61	72.70	32.9
Tuberculosis	14.96	6.08	1.0
Pneumonia	164.74	105.75	7.2
Violent Death	23.79	10.06	1.6
Total of Listed Causes			*48.1*
Age 1-4			
All Causes	179.80	48.00	
Measles	8.92	2.15	5.1
Scarlet Fever	6.49	.98	4.2
Whooping Cough	6.08	1.74	3.3
Diphtheria	19.02	2.86	12.3
Diarrhea and enteritis	20.07	4.77	11.6
Tuberculosis	3.94	3.08	.6
Pneumonia	38.28	10.72	20.9
Violent Death	6.13	8.19	-1.6
Total of Listed Causes			*56.6*
Age under 15			
All Causes	184.90	74.79	
Measles	4.31	1.01	3.0
Scarlet Fever	3.14	.55	2.4
Whooping Cough	4.35	1.51	2.6
Diphtheria	9.45	1.51	7.2
Diarrhea and enteritis	31.41	6.91	22.2
Tuberculosis	3.62	2.06	1.4
Pneumonia	25.53	11.76	12.5
Violent Death	5.84	6.92	-1.0
Total of Listed Causes			*50.3*

Source: 1930 calculated from figures in Sydenstriker (1933), and U.S. Bureau of
the Census (1933, 1934). 1900 calculated from figures in Preston and Haines
(1990) and Glover (1921).

in the death rate from diarrheal diseases. Diarrheal disease contributed less to the mortality decline for children age one to four than for infants, where pneumonia was the leading source of decline and diphtheria was slightly more important than diarrhea. Diphtheria was even more important for older children, accounting for 16 percent of the overall decline in mortality for those aged 5 to 14. For all children under fifteen taken together, diarrheal diseases were the most important source of mortality decline, followed by pneumonia and diphtheria.

Despite its importance in the overall decline in childhood death, the decline in the death rate from diarrheal diseases among infants and young children has not been adequately explained. Diarrheal diseases took an enormous toll in young lives in the nineteenth century. Infants died from these diseases largely in the summer months, and the decline in the summer death rate was rapid during the first three decades of the twentieth century (Lentzner 1987; Lentzner and Condran 1985; Cheney 1984). Diarrheal diseases were attributed at the time to improper feeding practices: poor choice of foods, improper amounts, or food that was contaminated. They were often considered a problem of weaning or of failure to properly breastfeed an infant.

Attempts to link the decline in diarrhea to large scale public health activities have been only partially successful. Condran and Cheney (1982) were unable to relate the decline in diarrheal death rates in Philadelphia after the turn of the century to the installation of water filters. Changes in Philadelphia's milk supply were harder to track, but appeared too late to explain the large portion of the decline in the death rates from these diseases that occurred early in the twentieth century. Condran and Cheney did observe that child hygiene clinics, aimed primarily at the education of mothers, appeared to accelerate the decline in diarrheal diseases in the wards where they were established. Because they were both an important source of mortality decline for children and a cause of mortality that could have been affected by changes in hygienic practices, especially with regard to infant feeding, diarrheal diseases will be the focus of much of the discussion that follows.

In the rest of this chapter, we examine the possibility that changes in personal health care practices — including the use of physicians and hospitals — made a major contribution to child mortality declines during this period. Our basic strategy is to examine the efforts made to inform mothers about what were considered to be proper child care practices during the first three decades of the twentieth century. We outline the methods used to reach mothers and then examine the message that was being sent and the changes in it over time. We ask how the broad changes in the concept of disease that were occurring at the time altered the advice on child care and were transmitted to mothers. Advice on child care and actual practice are, of course, two different things. We have brought whatever evidence we could find to bear on the issue of who was receiving the message and whether they were acting upon it. Actual changes in behavior, unfortunately, remain largely undocumented and undocumentable. Increasingly enlightened child care advice is neither a necessary nor a sufficient condition for behavioral changes that would reduce child mortality. But in an era when such advice was eagerly sought and vigorously dispensed, we consider it likely to provide a useful clue about the sources of mortality change.

Changing Ideas About Disease[1]

The claim that infant and child mortality could be strongly influenced by mothers' behavior would have surprised neither American nor British health officials and physicians in the first two decades of this century. During this time extraordinarily heavy responsibilities were placed on mothers to secure their children's health and survival, and much of the emphasis of social and health reformers was directed to educating mothers. These efforts were stimulated in part by recognition of the importance of behavioral factors in child mortality, as revealed through mortality differences by ethnicity and breastfeeding practices. But a more important motive was the belief that the public health measures of the nineteenth century were not reaching young children and hence their mortality was not improving as rapidly as mortality at other ages (Winslow 1909; Hedger 1909). The American Academy of Medicine organized a Conference on the Prevention of Infant Mortality in New Haven in 1909 to focus public attention on the problem. At this conference, the first of its type, the great health statistician C.E.A. Winslow argued:

> I think that the main reason for our poor showing in the matter of infant mortality is precisely the fact that the campaign must be pre-eminently one of popular education. Typhoid fever and malaria can often be routed on a large scale by the engineer; but infant mortality must be met and conquered in the home. The intelligence of the individual mother is the only ultimate safeguard against the perils of infancy; and it is much harder to bring

education to the mothers of a community than to lead pure water into its houses (Winslow 1909:224).

Winslow's ideas echoed a refrain that had been articulated clearly in Britain a few years earlier in George Newman's extremely influential study (Aykroyd 1971), *Infant Mortality: A Social Problem*, published in 1906. Newman noted that, while the English crude death rate had declined by 28 percent between 1851-60 and 1901-05, the infant mortality rate had fallen by only 10 percent, with all the decline occurring in the five years after the turn of the century (Newman 1906:3). After reviewing a good deal of statistical evidence about infant mortality in Britain, he concluded:

> Wherever we turn, and to whatever issue, in this question of infant mortality, we are faced with one all-pervading primary need — the need of a high standard of physical motherhood... it becomes clear that the problem of infant mortality is not one of sanitation alone, or housing, or indeed of poverty as such, *but it is mainly a question of motherhood*. (Newman 1906:257; Newman's emphasis)

At the end of the nineteenth century and throughout the first three decades of the twentieth century, as disease and mortality increasingly were seen as within human control, the responsibility for children's health was placed firmly on mothers. A "good" mother could be the first line of defense against childhood disease. She managed the infant's and young child's immediate contact with an often hostile environment that could include filthy tenements, hot summers, exposed privies, and contaminated milk supplies. A mother was believed to have many opportunities to reduce her young child's exposure to infection and chances of death. Maternal instinct, however, could not be trusted in these matters; public health officials, physicians, and mothers themselves seemed to agree that as both child and health care became more "scientific," mothers needed education in proper child care practices. As a result, a variety of methods were used to disseminate information to mothers. The form and to some extent the content of these efforts varied by the audience to be reached, but the overall message was clear: mothers could positively affect the life chances of their children by following a set of rules.

The new focus on maternal responsibility coincided with increasing acceptance of the germ theory of disease in the decades following Koch's identification of the tubercle bacillus in 1882. While we make no claim that the acceptance of germ theory precipitated the emphasis on mothers' responsibility, the latter could easily incorporate the notion that many diseases were the result of invisible microorganisms. Previously, the predominant theory of disease causation had stressed the role of atmospheric miasmata, produced by environmental filth, as agents of disease (Rosenberg 1987). Sources of filth included sewers, cesspools, swamps, slaughterhouses, and decaying vegetation (Richmond 1954). Exposure to miasmata disrupted the body's balance, and physicians often attempted to restore balance through purgatives, diuretics, and emetics.

Szreter (1988) argues that some of the early popularity of miasmata theories in England resulted from convenient implication that it was the public environment of streets and courts, rather than domestic space, that required regulation and control. Libertarian respect for domestic privacy and a resistance to centralizing government authority had made it easier for officials to meliorate public space than private space. However, the splendid isolation of the Englishman's home was no longer tenable after the publicity given to the microscopic findings of bacteriologic science in the 1880s and 1890s (Szreter 1988:32).

Tomes (1990) suggests a less critical role for the germ theory in the United States, where much attention was being paid to domestic hygiene and the healthful configuration of homes even before the general acceptance of the germ theory. The recognition that germs caused disease focused attention, however, on the transmission of germs from person to person, including transmission within the household. Writing a fifty-year retrospective on the American public health movement, Chapin (1921) noted that during that period, *people,* rather than *things,* came to be seen as the source of infection. Certainly the idea of contagion was widely accepted for the most visible and episodic diseases such as cholera and yellow fever and had led to successful campaigns of quarantine (Kunitz 1983, 1986). But the endemic infectious diseases of childhood, such as diarrhea and pneumonia, were so constant a condition of life that they called less attention to their infectivity. Tomes does note that the germ theory led to a "pathologizing of life" in the United States, with bacteria becoming invisible foes against which constant vigilance was required.

Change in the understanding of disease, particularly the notions that were developing about the role of microorganisms in their etiology, can be illustrated by discussions of infant diarrhea found in successive editions of the leading pediatric textbooks in the United States. L. Emmett Holt's *Diseases of Infancy and Childhood* went through eight editions between 1897 and 1923. Holt died in 1924 and the revisions on two subsequent editions in 1928 and 1933 were made by others. Within two years of first publication, sales had surpassed those of any other text. Abraham Jacobi produced three editions of *Therapeutics of Infancy and Childhood* in 1895, 1898, and 1903. He had earlier published the specialized text, *The Intestinal Diseases of Infancy and Childhood* in 1887, and an article on cholera infantum in *The Medical Times* in 1897. The general pediatric textbooks of Holt and Jacobi followed the voluminous *Encyclopedia of the Diseases of Children* edited by William J. Keating in 1890. Keating's *Encyclopedia* contained contributions by both Jacobi and Holt, the latter's chapter entitled "The Diarrheal Diseases, Acute and Chronic."

Although their careers overlapped in the early period, Jacobi's work represents a distinctly earlier view and Holt's the future of thinking about diarrheal diseases in young children. As late as 1887, Jacobi's discussion of the etiology of "acute intestinal catarrh," a category that included most forms of "cholera infantum," displayed a noticeable lack of emphasis on the role of microorganisms.

> The causes are food, given in improper quantity or quality; improper artificial food mostly. But even mother's milk may cause it. Mothers who are sick, or convalescing, or the subjects of strong emotions, who suffer from tuberculosis or syphilis, who are pregnant, some who are menstruating, and all anemic persons, secrete improper milk. (Jacobi 1887:194)

Jacobi listed the heat of summer, the diminution or increases of atmospheric moisture, and the settling of ground water as factors in the etiology of diarrhea. Drugs, exposure to cold, typhoid, dysentery and severe forms of malaria, and finally disturbances of circulation, lungs, liver, and heart could explain diarrhea in the infant or young child. In only one sentence suggesting that the infant's mucous membrane, compared to the adult's, was more "irritated by the results of fermentation such as phenol, indol, scatol, bacteria and bacilli" does Jacobi (1887:194) refer to bacterial involvement when discussing the causes of diarrhea, and even here the source of the bacteria was fermentation of improper food in the infant's stomach. Jacobi's view embraced ideas of disease causality that had prevailed but would soon be overtaken by an emphasis on microorganisms as the source of the disease.

Jacobi, the first President of the American Pediatric Society, never saw germs as the chief causal agent in the etiology of diarrhea. In all three general pediatrics texts, he repeated his 1887 list of the causes of diarrheal diseases in young children, adding only some further considerations of overfeeding and an acknowledgement that bacteria had some minor role in the etiology of the disease. He noted the "obvious contagiousness" of diarrheal diseases as the major reason to think bacteria important (Jacobi 1903:347). In the 1898 article, "Cholera Infantum," he stated his position quite clearly. The theories explaining cholera infantum had changed with the more general theories of disease.

> Fifty years ago almost all the diseases of the infant and some of the mother were traced back by Thomas Ballard to "fruitless sucking." Infant cholera was by some considered identical with Asiatic cholera. Some unknown atmospheric influence, sewer emanations of undescribed nature, evaporations of the upper strata of the earth, malaria, moisture, the oscillations of the barometer, or of the subsoil water were charged with being the causes of cholera infantum, with equal and positive fervor.

When etiology incorporated bacteriology, microbes were accused, for instance those of the genus ascophora by Bouchut; others looked for poisons, as Sonnenberger, for the presence in the food of plant alkaloids (Jacobi 1898:261). However, he argued, "the temptation to attribute cholera infantum to the direct influence of microbes was combatted" by the fact that it was impossible to identify a single one as the cause of cholera infantum.

Jacobi noted the prevalence of the disease among children under two in hot weather, but for Jacobi, heat had both a direct and indirect effect in causing cholera infantum.

> By fermenting and spoiling the baby's food, mainly cow's milk, it produces deleterious ptomains. By paralyzing its nervous system it causes the characteristic gastric and intestinal disturbances, oversecretions and non-absorption. (Jacobi 1898:264)

Even the greater susceptibility of breastfed babies did not convince him that the major link between hot weather and mortality was food and the microorganisms that it contained when it was improperly maintained in the summer. Breastfed babies, he argued, were less likely to swelter in their beds, because they were occasionally picked up and moved around; bottles, however, could be fed to babies without changing their positions in their cribs. In addition, mothers drank more water in hot weather and passed the fluid via diluted breast milk to their babies.

Writing in 1890, Holt, on the other hand, argued that the understanding of the pathology of diarrheal diseases was in a state of transition and summarized the state of knowledge as follows:

> The predisposition to diarrheal diseases is furnished by age (under two years), enfeebled constitution, bad hygienic surroundings, and a chronic disorder of digestion depending upon improper methods of feeding or nursing and the habitual use of improper food.
>
> Their chief exciting cause is something to the development of which two things have a fixed and constant relation — viz, a certain degree of atmospheric heat and the practice of artificial feeding. Both these conditions are necessary. We believe the chief causative factor to be bacteria, and that these act in most cases by inducing changes in the food. (Keating 1890:70)

The idea that the chief precipitating agents in diarrheal diseases were bacteria was obviously new. Holt admitted that with regard to diarrhea:

> Many ancient fallacies have been exposed and dropped, but the building up of newer views upon surer foundations than those upon which the old rested is slow, and can scarcely be said to be much more than begun. We know enough to know that micro-organisms play an important part of these diseases, but which ones, and how, are still to a large degree unsolved problems. (Keating 1890:61)

Other factors, previously thought to be important, were either rejected entirely or labelled, as in the example above, "predisposing" rather than "exciting" causes of the disease.

Holt's major focus was on the relationship between feeding practices and diarrheal diseases, and here the connecting link seemed to him to be bacteria, although he by no means excluded other links — overfeeding, giving food unsuitable for a child's age, irregular feeding, or too frequent feeding. However, impure cow's milk resulting from diseased cows, from adulteration or pollution of milk in the process of transportation or delivery, or from its improper use at home was an important source of diarrheal disorders in young children. Almost all the changes in milk, he argued, were due to bacteria.

Holt's views about the importance of microorganisms in the etiology of diarrheal diseases had strengthened by 1897 when the first edition of his own pediatric textbook was published. Points made tentatively in 1890 about the role of bacteria in the disease were reasserted more strongly in 1897 and repeated in subsequent editions of Holt's text. Each edition furnished more references to new studies of milk, infant feeding practices, and their influence on diarrhea.

By 1916, however, Holt was worried that the bacterial contamination of cow's milk and the bacteria link itself had been overemphasized as a source of diarrheal diseases. Although he readily credited milk inspection and the general use of sterilized milk in summer for the decline in diarrheal diseases that had occurred, remaining high rates of diarrhea were hard to explain. Indeed by 1916, Holt found it "irresistible that heat itself has a direct, injurious effect upon the infant" (Holt 1916). Disillusionment with the focus on microorganisms resulted not only from the failure of the disease to disappear with the efforts to clean up the milk supply but also from the failure to isolate the bacterium causing the disease. Many different bacteria were present in the stool and intestines of infants having diarrhea or dying from it, but many of them were likewise present in healthy children. No single pathological agent was found to be present in all sick children and absent in all who were well.

Holt's concern that he and others had overemphasized bacteria, especially those found in contaminated milk, was repeated in later editions of his text. By 1928 death rates from diarrheal diseases under age two had declined substantially, but diarrhea deaths among infants and one-year-olds in New York City still equalled deaths at all ages from measles, scarlet fever, pertussis, typhoid, and diphtheria. In that year, Holt lamented:

> This leads us to question whether the bacterial contamination of milk is the great cause of diarrheal diseases, and whether the lowered mortality in summer has not been brought about quite as much by other conditions, such as better hygiene and care and a better understanding of infant feeding, as by the exclusion of germs from milk or their destruction by heat. (Holt and Howland 1927).

By 1928 Holt believed the role of bacteria was surely secondary, and the explanation for most cases of diarrhea lay elsewhere. Atmospheric heat, especially the stagnant heat inside houses and apartments, regained a primary position in the causal chain.

In summary then, an important change in the view of this major disease began at the end of the nineteenth century and continued throughout the first three decades of the twentieth century. Both Holt and Jacobi acknowledged the role of bacteria, but Jacobi, throughout his writings on the topic, considered bacteria relatively minor. Holt was in the forefront of a new way of thinking about this important cause of death among young children; bacteria were the immediate determinants of diarrheal diseases, and other conditions that had formerly been in the etiologic foreground were classified as background predisposing conditions. By 1890, Holt argued that the link between diarrheal diseases and contaminated food was strong, and he reaffirmed that view in subsequent editions of his text. Although by 1916 he had become somewhat disillusioned with the bacteriologic theories of the disease, he always acknowledged that bacteria were an important cause of it.

Diarrheal diseases were not alone; ideas about the etiology of many diseases were changing and with them some of the efforts to combat disease. The changing emphasis of health concerns is vividly revealed by a comparison of questionnaires prepared by the American Public Health Association. Among the 18 items on the questionnaire used for studying the sanitary conditions in each city, a number were changed between 1875 and 1921, including the following replacements (Chapin 1921):

1875 schedule	*1921 schedule*
Gas and lighting	Infant hygiene
Topography and geology	Laboratory, vaccination
Location, population, climate	Contagious diseases
Cemeteries and burial	Milk
Quarantine	Education, publicity

Methods Used for Educating Mothers

The changes in the broader concepts of disease exhibited in the pediatric textbooks may have influenced children's care and hence mortality through their direct contact with pediatricians and through books and pamphlets addressed to their mothers on the care and feeding of children that proliferated between 1890 and 1930. These efforts were certainly not entirely new; Buchan's *Domestic Medicine and Advice to Mothers* had gone through thirty-seven American editions before 1820, and the extraction of ideas from the most widely read English medical writers compiled in editions of the *Maternal Physician* in 1811 and 1818 provided mothers in the new world with sources to consult (Rosenberg 1972). However, in 1894, publication of Holt's *The Care and Feeding of Children*, marked the start of a new era of wide circulation of advice manuals.

During the first decades of this century, increased interest in ways to enhance child health was also reflected in increased coverage of these topics in the mass media. Fisher (1909:81) notes that popular magazines had taken up the fight against disease. Apple (1981) documents many exchanges on the relative merits of alternative infant feeding regimes in the popular press in the period from 1890 to 1920. Julia Lathrop, Director of the Children's Bureau, noted in 1912 that columns on baby care appeared in virtually every major newspaper, whereas a few years earlier there had been no interest in such a column when it had been proposed (Meckel 1990:122). Dwork (1987) cites comparable attention to issues of feeding and child survival in London newspapers. But at the Conference on the Prevention of Infant Mortality, it was noted that publication of child care advice in newspapers did not reach the class of people that it was most important to reach (Neff 1909).

In order to get the word out to mothers, health authorities had to take matters into their own hands. An immense number and variety of educational activities aimed at mothers were undertaken by public health officials. By 1910, 16 states had issued child care pamphlets, with more than 100,000 copies distributed. In Wisconsin, a state bulletin on the care of children was advertised on birth certificate cards (Sherbon and Moore 1919). North Carolina distributed a motion picture on hygiene for mothers (Bradley and Williamson 1918). *Infant Care*, published by the Children's Bureau, became the most widely distributed publication of the Government Printing Office, with over 12 million copies distributed by 1940 (Apple 1981).

Instructions were also delivered in verbal or written form at clinics, dispensaries, infant feeding stations, milk depots, and hospitals. In the United States, these were organized by municipalities and took a wide variety of forms. In Philadelphia, for example, a Child Hygiene Bureau was organized in 1910 to educate mothers regarding the preparation of food and the care of infants and children. The Bureau started clinics providing milk, ice, and education to mothers of infants. In addition, nurses in selected wards of the city visited the homes of expectant mothers and newborn babies. Between 1910 and 1914, clinics were set up in eight wards, and between 1915 and 1918 in nineteen others. Condran and Cheney (1982) report evidence that these clinics produced some desired results. Death rates from diarrheal diseases for children under age two had been higher in the wards where clinics were established but declined more rapidly in these than in other city wards. Acceleration in the rate of decline coincided with the establishment of clinics.

Milk depots were instituted in many American cities in the first two decades of the century with the ostensible purpose of distributing purified milk at subsidized prices to poorer families, especially during the hotter months when conventional milk supplies were known to be badly contaminated. But Ira Wile (1909), an administrator at a New York City depot, argued that the delivery of milk was the least important service supplied by the depots. Their main function was to be education, preferably delivered verbally both at the depot and in homes. Mothers were to be instructed in the value of breastfeeding, the dangers of flies and of the dirt that breeds them, the value of isolating family members with contagious disease, and how to purchase and prepare nutritious foods economically. A 1911 survey found that educational efforts were being made by 42 of the 43 agencies sponsoring milk stations in U.S. cities (Meckel 1990:125). The Children's Bureau found that virtually all of the over 500 infant welfare stations in cities over 10,000 in population that responded to a 1915 survey included some form of mothers' education among their activities. Most of the stations reported more than one of the following: conferences with doctors and/or nurses, formal classes for mothers' education, visitation of nurses to homes, and distribution of pamphlets on child care (Children's Bureau 1916).

Home visitation in connection with a clinic or as an independent program (which was most common in smaller cities) was another important effort to reach mothers. A program of home visitation was mounted in New York City in 1908 by Josephine Baker and proved so successful statistically that it was rapidly adopted by many other communities. Its main component was home visitation during summers by school nurses who instructed mothers in the basics of hygiene (e.g., sterilizing nipples and diapers) and of feeding, and directed mothers with sick infants to clinics (Meckel 1990:144-48).

Rochester (1923) provides some evidence on the numbers of babies reached by these programs in Baltimore. Of 10,397 babies born in 1915 and surviving at least two weeks, the care of 2935 (28.2 percent) had been supervised in some way by infant welfare agencies. Approximately one half of the 6624 babies whose fathers had low income received such supervision. The organizations were most successful in reaching black and foreign-born Jewish families; the proportions reached were 60.5 percent and 45.1 percent respectively. Among Poles and Italians, the agencies were more likely to reach mothers who spoke English, but the reverse was true for Jewish families (Rochester 1923:220).

Educational efforts were aimed at school girls as well as mothers, partly because they were the mothers of the future and partly because many already had child care responsibilities for younger siblings. In New York, a "Little Mother's League" was formed to provide instruction and support for girls with responsibility for child care, and 20,000 girls were attending the weekly meetings in 1912 (Apple 1981). In 1915, 45 cities with populations over 10,000 reported Little Mother's Leagues conducted by municipal agencies, and close to 50,000 girls attended classes during that year (Children's Bureau 1916). Another 500 leagues were sponsored by private agencies in these cities.

A final mode of disseminating information about child care was the celebration of "Baby Weeks." The initiative for sponsoring such weeks typically came from women's clubs or mothers' clubs, received endorsements and possibly financed support from municipalities and, after 1912, backing from the Children's Bureau. During 1912, 2000 Baby Weeks were sponsored in the United States. These celebrations, in addition to focusing on means of enhancing child survival, sometimes had a political angle, with pressure placed on localities to fund visiting nurses or milk depots. The Children's Bureau itself directly sponsored local "conferences" about child care. After one such conference in a remote area of Montana, it was reported, "Our post office is like a different place now on mail days. The mothers who come in, and even the fathers, ask one another what they are feeding their babies and whether they took the doctor's advice" (Paradise 1919). In 1919, Baby Weeks were supplemented by a Children's Year. Seventeen thousand committees were formed to organize its activities locally, on which some eleven million women served. More than 16,000 municipalities weighed and measured children during Children's Year (Abbott 1923).

All of these activities found a willing and eager audience. There is almost no mention by commentators of the need to stimulate interest in child survival. Children's Bureau statistical inquiries in rural North Carolina found mothers "enthusiastic", in rural Kansas "keenly interested", and in Montana "interested and enthusiastic" to learn more about ways of improving child health. By the 1920s, the Children's Bureau was receiving over 100,000 letters a year from mothers seeking child care advice (Meckel 1990:156). Furthermore, there was an increased assumption of responsibility not only for one's own offspring but also for those of the community. By 1915 in the United States, according to Dye and Smith (1986), "every dead child accused the community". Without this sense of community responsibility — partly fueled by declining birth rates and the prospect of "race suicide" — the public health activities undertaken would doubtless have been less vigorous.

The Message

The health information that mothers were to receive in the period 1900-1930, when the major dissemination efforts were undertaken, was primarily about the proper methods of feeding infants. Major emphasis was placed on breastfeeding and on providing clean food to a child who was not breastfed. The advice to breastfeed was, without a doubt, sound and important at a time when refrigeration was often inadequate and alternative food sources easily contaminated. From casual empiricism, the health advantages of breastfeeding had been known for centuries. As early as 1755, a Royal edict in Finland prescribed a fine of ten dollars for mothers who, by neglecting to suckle their babies for at least half a year, had "caused" the death of a child (Newman 1906:233). More systematic statistical studies in the nineteenth century supported the link, and it received its most striking confirmation in Woodbury's (1925) study commissioned by the Children's Bureau. Woodbury showed that in eight U.S. cities death rates among infants not breastfed were three or four times higher than among those who were.

Advice about the importance of breastfeeding was not new at the end of the nineteenth century. It was common among American physicians in the 1840s (Dye and Smith 1986), and both Buchan (1811) and *The Maternal Physician* devote major portions of their discussion of infant feeding to the joys and importance of nursing. In the last quarter of the nineteenth century this theme was taken up by health officials in large cities, who frequently advertised the advantages of breastfeeding. For example, copies of a pamphlet extolling breastfeeding and warning against weaning in the summer were distributed by public health authorities in Philadelphia in the 1870s and 1880s (Condran et al. 1984). A study of the history of infant feeding in the United States concludes that at the turn of the century, physicians generally advocated that mothers breastfeed their babies (Apple 1981). Undoubtedly, a large majority of women were taking this advice for the early months of an infant's life; however, the first quantitative data on the extent of breastfeeding in the United States are from the Children's Bureau studies carried out in the second decade of the twentieth century.

Efforts by public health authorities and self-help efforts by women's clubs to encourage breastfeeding expanded sharply in the first two decades of the twentieth century. These included instructional material and direct instruction through health clinics and home visits. For example, a Boston health officer in 1909 claimed credit for getting eighty mothers who were practicing mixed feeding to return to exclusive breastfeeding (Connolly 1909). In addition, Meckel (1990:179) argues that the belief among physicians that large fractions of women were incapable of breastfeeding began to wane in the first decade of the twentieth century.

Despite all these efforts, however, the trends in breastfeeding were almost certainly in the wrong direction to explain the decline in infant and childhood mortality. At the turn of the century, most mothers were probably already breastfeeding through six months, and the long-run trend was one of decline rather than increase. Indeed, it seems likely that the proliferation of advice to breastfeed was at least in part a response to the waning of the practice. Perhaps the efforts served to avert or slow down some of the decline that would otherwise have occurred, but breastfeeding was certainly not a key behavioral change accounting for the decline in mortality.

Changes in another aspect of infant and child feeding were more likely to have contributed to the decline in mortality, namely changes in feeding practices for babies and children who were not nursed. Cow's milk was a principal source of nutrients for children during the period, making up between seven and eight percent of the total calories consumed in the nation from 1890 to 1930 (Bennett and Pierce 1961). As late as 1900 the nation's milk supply was seriously contaminated with tuberculosis, typhoid, scarlet fever, diphtheria, and strep germs. Samples of milk supplies intended for consumption from around the country in 1905-10 showed that 8.3 percent contained tubercle bacilli (North 1921).

The germ theory unquestionably refocused attention that previously had been directed primarily towards adulteration or watering of milk to the bacterial contamination of the milk supply. North (1921) reports that only four articles about milk appeared in scientific journals in 1880, while ten appeared in 1890, and forty in 1900. But health authorities were slower to take steps to improve the cleanliness of milk than of water, partly because of the sheer difficulty of monitoring the quality of milk in the many stages between the birth of a calf and the consumption of the final product by customers, and partly because regulating private enterprise presented problems not encountered in regulating munici- pally owned water works. Moreover, at the turn of the century the public seemed largely indifferent to the quality of milk (Coit 1893; Chapin 1901). In 1911, only fifteen percent of the milk supply in New York City, one of the most progressive cities in public health, was pasteurized, even though the process had been known since the 1860s (Lentzner 1987).

But families had means at their disposal to sterilize the impure milk arriving at their doorstep. Heating of milk in the home was developed in Germany in 1886, and there is no evidence of its having been employed in the United States before 1888 (North 1921), although some physicians claim to have been recommending the procedure earlier. Apple (1981) suggests that the impetus for boiling or sterilizing milk was derived from the bacteriologic discoveries of the 1880s. Lentzner (1987) finds a recommendation for heating milk in a New York City newspaper in 1897. However, there was much disagreement about the process, with many physicians and lay people incorrectly believing that the process removed much of the nutritive value from milk. A widely cited empirical study in 1903 showed the merits of the process convincingly. Heating milk was shown to dramatically reduce bacterial counts, and infants fed with heated milk clearly had better outcomes in terms of diarrheal disease incidence and overall death rates (Park and Holt 1903).

Irving Fisher (1909:98) suggests that the practice caught on quickly, at least among the families with whom he was acquainted. He reports, "The times of a baby's meals, the quantity of feeding, the sterilization of milk, and the ventilation of rooms are now attended to with scrupulous care." Contemporaries believed, however, that boiling and sterilization were not practiced as widely among the poor as among the upper classes. Woodbury (1925:163) suggests that more safeguards on infant feeding existed in the upper income groups: more use of pure milk and more attention to proper sterilization of bottles. Presumably, upper income groups were also more likely to have refrigerators that protected the quality of milk.

While the feeding of infants and young children was the major focus of instruction, other personal health care practices could have affected infant and child mortality levels. A fifty-year retrospective of the American Public Health Association claimed that, even though homes were more crowded, they were much cleaner in 1920 than they had been in 1870 (Veiller 1921). This change probably affected urban homes more than rural ones. Contemporary observers often commented on the lack of hygiene typically found among farm families (Abbott 1900:71; Fox [1919] 1974:187). A Children's Bureau inquiry in northern Wisconsin in 1916 blamed the exceptionally high infant mortality among Polish farm families, despite their very long breastfeeding, on very unhygienic conditions of their homes and feeding practices (Sherbon and Moore 1919). Another Children's Bureau study of rural North Carolina commented that in this population "the intimate relation between good sanitation and good health is little understood" (Bradley and Williamson 1918:66).

Protection of household members from one another's germs also may have increased during the period 1900-1930. *Infant Care*, a 1914 publication of the newly-formed Children's Bureau, cautioned, "The rule that parents should not play with the baby may seem hard, but it is without doubt a safe one...The mother should not kiss the baby directly on the mouth, nor permit others to do so, as infections of various kinds are spread in this way" (Children's Bureau 1914:37). Tomes (1990) cites a baby's bib from the 1920s with the legend "Don't kiss me. I don't want to get sick."

In 1906, children in homes containing a person with tuberculosis, formerly considered a constitutional disease with a strong hereditary basis, were to be removed if at all possible. If not, "In order to avoid direct contagion the patient and children should be kept apart as much as possible... The patient must not cough, talk loudly or sneeze nearer than three feet from the children" (Morse 1906:891). In 1929, Richard Smith, Professor of Child Hygiene at Harvard, published a major review paper on the causes of infant mortality. He noted that respiratory disease could only be averted by "direct[ing] our efforts towards a protection of the infant from exposure to infection and bring[ing] his resistive powers to the point where he will be able to build up his own antibodies to combat the disease." To prevent infant deaths from tuberculosis, "contact must be prevented, and yet adults with open tuberculosis are allowed to remain in the home in close contact with the highly susceptible infant." Likewise, for whooping cough, "Our chief reliance rests upon the early isolation of suspected individuals and upon special efforts at avoiding the exposure of infants to positive sources of infection" (Smith 1929:982-83). It is likely that these efforts were more successful among prosperous families.

An additional carrier of disease became recognized in the 1890s: the domestic fly. Meckel (1990) traces a campaign against the "fly menace" in the U.S. to a convincing 1907 epidemiologic investigation by the New York City Water Pollution Committee, a campaign that included lectures, circulars, newspaper and magazine articles, and even a motion picture, *The Fly Pest*. Detailed advice about domestic hygiene after 1900 often included information about the importance of keeping flies away from milk and other food.

Handwashing also became an important ally in the fight against disease. Chapin (1917), in a short popular book *How to Avoid Infection*, urged parents to "Wash the hands well before eating and always after the use of the toilet. Teach this to children by precept and especially by example. Modern sanitary science enables the individual to protect himself even if his health department is inefficient" (cited in Starr 1982:190). He went on to comment that purification of the municipal water supply may require millions of dollars but washing the hands costs nothing.

The period 1900-1930 also saw major advances in nutritional sciences. There was no recognition of the role of vitamins in food until experiments conducted in 1906. At that point there was hypothesized to be one growth-enhancing substance contained in butter fat and cod liver oil. By 1921, two additional vitamins were recognized (North 1921). If they were to be effective, these advances in nutritional sciences had to be applied in daily doses in millions of homes. That they were being applied is suggested by an ironic comment by the Chairman of the 1931 White House Conference on Child Health and Protection, who refers to "The modern parent with his or her ideas regarding vitamins, cod-liver oil, and conduct, [who] is at times an undesirable associate in the views of many of our children" (Wilbur 1931:1079).

Finally, another component of behavioral change may have been an increase in the use of the medical professionals. Advice to that effect became increasingly prominent as the period advanced. Mothers needed to consult physicians, especially when disease symptoms were apparent (Starr 1982: Chapter 5).

Advice for Mothers in Two Prominent Manuals

We have attempted to evaluate more systematically some of these notions about behavioral change by examining the advice given to mothers in manuals prepared for their education. L. Emmett Holt published the first edition of *The Care and Feeding of Children* in 1894. The book was a huge success; it went through numerous editions, seventy-five printings, and was translated into many languages. Many other books had been written on the topic but none seemed "to hit the nail on the head as did this one" (Duffus and Holt 1940). The format of the book was to present a simple and straightforward series of questions that mothers presumably needed to have answered by a physician. It originated as a manual for the Practical Training School for Nursery Maids connected to the Babies' Hospital of New York, and was published so that it could serve its purpose in other institutions and schools and similarly "be of value to many mothers in the care of their own children, or a book they may safely put into the hands of the ordinary (untrained) child's nurse" (Holt 1894:5).

The first edition in 1894 was a slender volume; three years later, its size had nearly doubled, as a result, said the author, of "three years of daily use of the catechism" (Holt 1897). In the 1897 edition, the chapter on feeding introduced new material on the preparation and use of cow's milk for infant feeding, and the preface to the third edition claimed that both mothers and nursery maids expressed the need for still more information about infant feeding, especially regarding the modification of cow's milk. Subsequent editions contained expanded sections on illness, and in 1926, L. Emmett Holt, Jr. revised his father's manual, citing the increase in medical knowledge as the reason for revision.

While Holt's *Care and Feeding* was clearly directed toward middle class mothers, the Children's Bureau was attempting to reach the less affluent with its pamphlets on infant care. Three editions of *Infant Care* published in 1914, 1921, and 1929 allow us to trace advice directed to a somewhat different audience than that of Holt's manual.

We have focused on advice given to mothers in areas that were suggested by the above discussion to have been associated with important behavioral changes influencing infant and childhood mortality. These are: (1) the advice on feeding infants, especially the promotion of hygienic practices among those who were not nursing their infants, (2) advice about contagion and the isolation of children from sick household members, (3) the advice about handwashing and more general hygiene, and finally (4) advice about when to consult a physician.

Advice About Feeding

Throughout all editions of Holt's *Care and Feeding* from 1894 through 1926 and in the Children's Bureau pamphlets as well, breastfeeding was extolled as the most appropriate method of feeding infants. Neither the length of breastfeeding nor the reasons for nursing changed significantly over the time period. Mothers were told to nurse their infants for most of the first year because breast milk was the perfect food for infants and there was no equivalent substitute.

Holt argued, however, that breastfeeding did not have to be used exclusively. In all the editions of *Care and Feeding* that we have examined, mothers were advised that there were no objections to mixed feeding, i.e., to a baby's being partly nursed and partly bottle fed. In fact, mixed feeding was considered desirable in order that the mother's sleep not be disturbed at night. This advice on mixed feeding suggests that the major motivation for breastfeeding was something other than the avoidance of artificial, potentially contaminated foods. For both Holt and the Children's Bureau, breastfeeding was better because it was natural; cleanliness of breast milk was always a secondary consideration.

Weaning early or artificially feeding from the start could be necessary if a breastfed baby failed to thrive. Over time, Holt expanded the list of symptoms of unsuccessful nursing, and in later editions he advised mothers who had tuberculosis or a serious chronic disease against nursing at all.

The Children's Bureau made a stronger case for breastfeeding than did Holt, as evidenced by both the content of its message and the relative lack of attention to alternatives. The Children's Bureau was always very optimistic about the ability of mothers to breastfeed their babies. Most of the reasons for or symptoms of failure, elaborated by Holt, were not mentioned in the Children's Bureau pamphlets. Early weaning might be necessary but the Children's Bureau expressed grave concerns about what they perceived to be insufficient reasons for discontinuing nursing. Only another pregnancy was viewed as sufficient cause for early weaning in the two early editions of the pamphlet. In 1929, a mother with active tuberculosis, a chronic illness or epilepsy was warned against nursing.

As noted earlier, the trends in breastfeeding were almost certainly in the wrong direction to explain the mortality decline. We found little in the way of change in the content of the advice on breastfeeding to explain the defection from the practice. Mothers were always urged to breastfeed their infants. The impact of the message to breastfeed may have changed over time, however, as a result of the expansion of the advice on how to feed the infant who could not be nursed.

For Holt, the problems in breastfeeding were great enough that a carefully elaborated alternative was necessary. Therefore, instructions on artificially feeding the child who could not be nursed dominated *The Care and Feeding* and increased with every edition of his manual through 1926. Scheduling of feedings, applied as well to nursing infants, was very important. Quantities to be given were crucial for artificially fed infants whose quantity would not be limited by nature. Composition of cow's milk and efforts to make it approximate breast milk filled pages of Holt's advice manual. However, of more interest to us is Holt's advice on the care of milk, bottles, and nipples in the home. Was the increasing recognition of germs as a causal agent in disease accompanied by additional advice on the hygiene of feeding infants?

In 1894 and 1897 the focus was clearly on the composition of cow's milk. Although Holt advised mothers to obtain clean fresh milk from a healthy herd of cows, most of his advice concerned the modifications that could be made to cow's milk to make it closer in composition to breast milk. In 1903 Holt added that cleanliness was as important a consideration as the composition of cow's compared to mother's milk (Holt 1903:51-52).

The 1903 edition significantly added a number of questions and their answers regarding how milk should be handled; the 1903 advice was given with little or no change in subsequent editions. To the question, "What are the two essentials in milk handling?", the answer was first, "that it be kept clean and free from contamination," and second, "that it be cooled immediately after leaving the cows, and kept at as low a temperature as possible; to be efficient this should not be above 50 F"

(Holt 1903:47). None of the previous editions contained as much emphasis on cleanliness of milk and hygienic rules for milk handling as did the 1903 and subsequent editions.

Holt argued that milk fed to babies should be sterilized and/or pasteurized, especially in the city in the summer. In 1894, he noted that milk should be sterilized to kill germs in it, some of which could cause the milk to sour and some of which could cause disease. In 1897, Holt was more specific about the circumstances in which sterilization was essential. It always had to be sterilized in warm weather when not obtained fresh, i.e., always in cities in the summer. It was to be sterilized if there was any uncertainty about the health of the cows or the handling of the milk. Finally, it had to be sterilized if the milk was to be kept for more than twenty-four hours, especially without ice. In 1903, he added another condition requiring sterilization of the milk, namely the presence of epidemics of typhoid or scarlet fever, diphtheria, or diarrheal diseases. The advice remained the same until 1926 when Holt argued that all milk needed to be sterilized. In the 1917 edition, Holt issued another warning: mothers could not rely on milk pasteurized before delivery. Milk pasteurized at a dairy needed to be sterilized at home.

The distinction between pasteurizing and sterilizing milk at home was an important one. The processes were different and the effects on the quality of the milk were also believed to be different. In 1894, pasteurization involved heating milk to 170 degrees Fahrenheit for thirty minutes; sterilization required 212 degrees Fahrenheit. Pasteurization was not believed to alter the taste or digestibility of the milk, but pasteurized milk would keep for only three or four days. Sterilized milk would taste like boiled milk and be less digestible, but would keep much longer. Pasteurization required special equipment that could be ordered from a New York store; sterilizing required only ordinary pots or pans. The latter process, however, changed over time. In 1897, sterilizing required one and a half hours of heating at a temperature of 212 degrees Fahrenheit. In 1920, Holt acknowledged that milk was usually effectively sterilized by boiling for 15 minutes. In 1926, he argued milk could be sterilized by boiling for a minute or two.

The advice to sterilize or pasteurize milk was given with a cautionary note, however. The question of whether pasteurization and/or sterilization harmed the milk was raised throughout the period. The nutritive properties of milk were thought to be adversely affected by sterilization as were its taste and digestibility. This was a particular problem if the milk were the infant's sole food, and was thought important enough a problem that sterilization was not recommended for general use in the early editions of the manual. Pasteurization was widely recommended, and in 1897, Holt argued that it had not been shown to produce any unfavorable effects. By 1903, Holt was quite specific that the use of sterilized milk would cause scurvy and also was less certain that the lower temperature for a shorter time required to pasteurize milk had no ill effects. The effects of the latter, however, if they existed at all, were so slight as to be no deterrent to its general use. In 1917, Holt changed his view and argued that sterilized milk could be more digestible than raw milk for some children. Throughout, however, the dangers of scurvy and the need to supplement the milk with other food were emphasized. This advice was extended to the use of pasteurized milk in 1920. In that year, he continued his warning against reliance on dairy pasteurized milk. By 1926, Holt no longer recommended home pasteurization. Most milk purchased was already pasteurized, and mothers were advised to sterilize dairy-pasteurized milk by boiling it for one or two minutes. Until the 1926 edition, it is important to note, however, that Holt advocated the purchase of clean fresh milk so that heating of any sort would be unnecessary.

Finally, the notion that bacteria were the source of disease for babies, especially bottle-fed babies, extended to the care of bottles and nipples. In the 1894 edition of *Care and Feeding*, mothers were advised to wash bottles with a brush and hot soapy water and place them for twenty minutes in boiling water before filling with milk. The entire quantity for the day was to be prepared at once, the bottles stoppered with cotton and placed on ice. Black rubber nipples that fit straight over the bottle were to be kept in a borax solution and carefully washed three or four times a day. After use, bottles were to be rinsed in cold water and soaked in borax water. Before feeding, milk was to be heated in the bottle, not poured into a saucepan. Holt could not recommend boiling nipples regularly until 1926, when new transparent nipples that could be boiled everyday became available. In 1909, he emphasized the need to turn nipples inside out for thorough cleaning. With the minor changes noted above, the advice about the care of bottles remained the same from 1894 through 1926.

In its first pamphlet on infant care published in 1914, and in all subsequent editions, the Children's Bureau was quite explicitly concerned with the cleanliness of milk and the equipment used in storing it or feeding it to infants. They eschewed any long discussion of the appropriate "formula" to be fed to babies, a topic that dominated much of the discussion in Holt's *Care and Feeding*. According to the Children's Bureau, authorities differed so much on the question of how milk should be modified for feeding infants that they could make no recommendation except that a mother seek the advice of a good doctor. The emphasis was rather on how to choose and care for the milk that was to be fed to infants. Mothers were advised to choose certified milk for their infants, even though the cost at 16 cents a quart in 1914 was quite high. If certified milk could not be obtained, then the milk had to be heated to kill the germs in it. It also had to be kept cold to retard the growth of germs, and it had to be protected from dust and flies. The Children's Bureau pamphlet gave instructions for the building of a homemade icebox for homes that had no regular refrigeration.

Cleanliness of all equipment was also important according to the Children's Bureau pamphlets. Following advice contained in a New Zealand pamphlet on the subject, the Children's Bureau recommended boiling for 15 minutes everything that would come in contact with the baby's food. Bottles were to be washed in hot soapy water and then boiled. Nipples would be ruined by soaking and therefore they simply were to be rinsed and boiled for five minutes after each use, and then rinsed in boiled water just before using. Less explicit instructions were given in the subsequent editions of the pamphlet, but the general advice to boil everything prevailed.

The 1914 edition explained home pasteurization and gave instructions on how to do it without purchasing a pasteurizer. Milk could also be boiled for three quarters of an hour in bottles or three minutes directly in a saucepan before being fed to babies, or it could be scalded to free it from germs. However, unlike Holt, the Children's Bureau expressed no concerns about the effects of heating on the quality of the milk; therefore, mothers were free to choose among heating methods that would destroy the germs in milk.

The 1921 edition of the pamphlet listed several other kinds of milk — condensed milk, canned milk and proprietary foods — that a mother might choose for her infant; however, it strongly proscribed proprietary infant foods. This edition also contained no recommendation favoring one method of heating over another. By the end of the 1920s, mothers were being advised to use only dairy pasteurized milk; but they were warned, "Pasteurization does not take the place of boiling milk before giving it to a baby; all milk given to a baby must be boiled" (Children's

Bureau 1929). Scalded milk was no longer mentioned as an alternative to boiling.

In summary, both Holt and the Children's Bureau were recommending cleanliness of milk and all equipment used in food preparation, and for Holt the emphasis on cleanliness clearly increased after the turn of the century. The Children's Bureau was more dogmatic about the importance of breastfeeding than Holt, no doubt at least in part because they had less interest in the alternatives and the enhancement of pediatric medicine that these alternatives suggested. The class difference in the audiences to which the Children's Bureau and Holt were directing their respective messages also affected the content of the messages. The Children's Bureau was concerned with the costs of its recommendations and with suggesting low cost ways to achieve the desired ends. The pamphlets paid little attention to the composition of formulas to be fed to infants or to the complicated feeding procedures, emphases apparent in Holt. Leaving this message out had the effect of highlighting the cleanliness issues in their pamphlets. With hindsight, we could argue that the lower class audience targeted by the Children's Bureau was being provided with a more effective and precisely targeted message with regard to infants' health than were the middle and upper class readers of Holt.

Advice on Contagion and the Isolation of Sick Children

As more and more diseases were considered to be transmitted directly from one person to another, advice that mothers could protect their children's health by isolating them from household members who were ill became more important in infant care manuals. In the 1894 edition of Holt's *Care and Feeding*, three childhood diseases — measles, scarlet fever and diphtheria — were listed as contagious diseases requiring isolation of the patient from other children. As shown in Table 8-3, the list of the contagious diseases expanded over time; however, the length of isolation required for each disease changed very little except for a shortening of the length of isolation for diphtheria.

The Children's Bureau list of contagious diseases was quite different from Holt's. In 1914, the following were considered contagious and required quarantining the patient: measles, whooping cough, tuberculosis, vulvovaginitis, and trachoma. Although these diseases were spread from person to person, isolation periods were not specified. The 1914 pamphlet rather emphasized disinfecting the rooms of patients after the

Table 8-3 Advice on Isolation of Sick Children

1894	1897	1903, 1909	1917, 1920, 1926
Measles	Measles	Measles	Measles
Diphtheria	Diphtheria	Diphtheria	Diphtheria
Scarlet Fever	Scarlet Fever	Scarlet Fever	Scarlet Fever
	Whooping Cough	Whooping Cough	Whooping Cough
		German Measles	German Measles
		Chicken Pox	Chicken Pox
			Mumps

illness was over and the careful washing and disposing of towels, cloths, napkins and handkerchiefs used by patients suffering from these diseases. Tuberculosis was an important part of the list; mothers with tuberculosis were advised that they and their babies must "live constantly out of doors" (Children's Bureau 1914:73). Hookworm and syphilis were also listed as contagious diseases, but their prevention involved neither isolation nor hygienic care of things with which the patient had contact.

Like Holt, the Children's Bureau expanded the list of contagious diseases, and by 1921 the following diseases were considered communicable, and isolation was recommended as shown below:

Whooping cough	Six weeks from the time of infection
Measles	One week or longer if there is a discharge from the nose or ears
German measles	Two weeks
Scarlet fever	Four weeks or longer if discharges exist
Chicken pox	As long as the crusts are present
Smallpox	None given
Diphtheria	Until all symptoms have disappeared and a negative throat culture is obtained
Infantile paralysis	Four weeks
Tuberculosis	As long as the case is active, the baby should not live in the same house as the infected person.
Gonorrhea and syphilis	None given

While the discussion of contagious diseases expanded a great deal between 1914 and 1921 in the Children's Bureau pamphlets, in the 1929 editions, detailed quarantine advice was no longer given and the list of communicable diseases was shortened by dropping German measles, scarlet fever, chicken pox, smallpox, and infantile paralysis.

Concern about the transmission of disease from one person to another was also manifest in the advice about kissing young children and babies. In 1894, the issue was not raised by Holt, but in 1897 he wrote that there were many serious objections to kissing infants. The proscription against kissing infants remained in the manuals throughout the three decades of the twentieth century that we have examined. In 1917, syphilis was added to the list of diseases that could be transmitted to infants by kissing them. The Children's Bureau gave similar advice about kissing babies throughout all editions. Kissing was especially important in the spread of tuberculosis and therefore persons with a cough should never be allowed to kiss the baby. However, even healthy mothers were advised against the practice.

The isolation of children from ill family members was no doubt good advice. The new theories of disease, while not responsible for initiating the idea, probably increased the emphasis on contagion and the isolation practices that this emphasis implied. The isolation of children from other children with diphtheria and the separation of infants and young children from tubercular adults were the most likely avenues by which this practice could have influenced mortality.

Advice on General Hygiene

While cleanliness of homes and general hygiene practices have been suggested as important behavioral changes during the time period, these topics were not a major concern in the manuals examined here. That literature was located in several specialized magazines and has been analyzed by Tomes (1990). Holt paid no attention to general housekeeping and made only oblique references to handwashing. In the 1920s, Holt urged mothers to encourage older children to wash their hands after toileting and before eating. In 1903, in describing the preparation of infant formula, Holt noted, "The nurse's hands, bottles, tables, and all utensils should be scrupulously clean." This advice was, however, embedded in a long description of how to prepare the additions to milk for the infant, a topic that clearly had more importance than handwashing in Holt's mind. In addition, Holt argued that diapers were to be cleaned regularly and carefully. In general, however, mothers surely did not leave Holt's volume with a sense of the importance of cleanliness in the home or specific hygiene practices such as handwashing.

The Children's Bureau pamphlets were somewhat more explicit about general hygiene than Holt, a fact that may reflect the belief that poor hygiene was a problem particular to lower class families. In 1914 mothers were given advice on selecting a home:

> In every case the house and its surroundings should be carefully inspected. The cellar or basement should be clean and dry; if there is a well it should be so located as to prevent the water from being poisoned by the foul drainage from stable or outhouses. Pools of stagnant water, manure heaps, piles of garbage, refuse or rubbish of any sort, or open privies are all dangerous to health and furnish breeding places for disease-carrying insects, such as flies and mosquitoes. (Children's Bureau 1914:10)

It further advised that the health of the baby was so dependent on sanitary surroundings that mothers should consult an appendix to the pamphlet that provided a list of government publications related to hygiene of the home. The appendix listed publications under the following topics: milk, other foods, insects, the house, privies, sewage disposal, disease, drugs, disinfectants, hygiene of children, and birth registration. The discussion on selecting a home was the same in 1921 as in 1914, but the appendix was dropped. In 1929, the reference to the inappropriateness of an apartment for raising children, stated in 1914 and 1921, was deleted, and the discussion focused on the cleanliness of the water supplied to the house and the control of insects by screening all windows. A new appendix in 1929 contained only pamphlets on child care.

The 1914 edition contained a section on general health conditions including discussions of germs and flies. The section on germs simply stated that infectious diseases were caused by germs and that disease germs could be removed by disinfection, "which means simply cleanliness" (Children's Bureau 1914:75). A long discussion of flies as carriers of disease was followed by advice that infants could be protected by destroying flies' breeding grounds and by installing sanitary privies to prevent flies' contact with human excrement. The sections on germs and flies were omitted from the two later editions of the manual.

Changes in general hygiene practices seem a less likely source of mortality decline than either specific hygienic feeding practices or the isolation of children from sick family members. General hygiene appeared to be more strongly emphasized in the earliest edition of the Children's Bureau pamphlets than in later editions. Holt largely ignored the issue throughout the time period in question.

Advice on Consulting a Physician

Nowhere did the Children's Bureau and Holt differ more than on the explicit recommendations about when to consult a physician. Holt was much less likely than the Children's Bureau to encourage a mother to seek a physician's advice. The lack of explicit statements may reflect Holt's feeling that the manual was as good as consulting one's own physician or that his audience was already tied to physicians and did not need to be reminded to call the doctor. For whatever reason, the need to call a physician appeared much less frequently in Holt than in the Children's Bureau pamphlets. For Holt, writing in 1894, the following conditions required a physician's attention:

> eyelids sticky (not controllable with Vaseline)
> convulsions
> foreign body in the ear or nose
> croup if breathing becomes difficult
> first symptoms of a serious illness (none specified)
> prolonged constipation
> presence of bad habits (sucking, bed wetting, nail biting, masturbation)

Additions were made to the list as follows:

> 1897 advice regarding bathing for an infant with eczema
> 1903 none added
> general bad habits deleted and replaced by specific reference to bed wetting after age 3 or 4 and masturbation
> 1917 enlarged tonsils or adenoids
> smallpox vaccination
> tight foreskin
> 1920 rupture
> anemia
> 1926 toxin-antitoxin immunization against diphtheria following Shick test
> premature birth (required hospitalization if possible)

The changes in the list reflected some changes in medical technology, but noticeably absent are recommendations for well baby care by a physician even as late as 1926.

The Children's Bureau urged the use of a physician more strongly than Holt and the conditions requiring a physician were more numerous. Before birth the mother needed advice from a physician about the care of her breasts. After nursing was begun, she needed a physician if her breasts were cracked or sore or to apply a binder if nursing were to be discontinued. A physician was needed to advise the mother on artifical feeding, whether temporary because of the mother's acute illness or permanent. At the first signs of indigestion in either the nursing or the bottle fed infant, a physician was to be consulted. A lack of teeth by the end of the first year had to be brought to the attention of the doctor, as did red swollen gums in the teething infant. For the latter condition a physician was needed to lance the gums. In addition, almost all illness or symptoms of illness required a physician's advice or treatment.

By 1921 the list was greatly expanded and a physician was said to be required as well in the following circumstances:

    physical examination of any nursemaid
    physical examination of wet nurses
    care of city babies (well baby care at health centers)
    lack of proper development
    masturbation
    teaching a mother to read a thermometer
    swallowing pills or poison

Problems associated with teething were removed from the list; lancing of swollen gums appears to have disappeared as a treatment and with it the need to call a physician.

By 1929 the entire tone of the Children's Bureau pamphlets had changed. Even a baby with no observable problems needed the regular attention of a doctor. A well baby was to be seen by a physician weekly for weighing, monthly for advice, and quarterly for health examinations. Regular visits did not mean that a mother could let down her guard about specific conditions requiring a physician's attention, and the list of these conditions expanded even further.

Over the time period the advice to consult a physician on the part of the Children's Bureau was greatly extended. Again as with Holt some of the changes reflected changing medical technology. The largest change, the introduction of the notion that a baby had to be regularly examined regardless of the baby's health status, occurred only at the end of the time period examined. Advice to see a physician was, however, only one part of the medical picture. The treatment or care that a physician was giving was also changing so that consulting a physician might have different implications at different times.

Changes in Medicine and Medical Practice

During the period under discussion, several tools were developed that enhanced the powers of the physician. The most important of these were diphtheria antitoxin and tetanus antitoxin, both developed in 1894, and salvarsan, an anti-syphilitic drug discovered by Paul Ehrlich in 1907 (Pellegrino 1979; Ackernecht 1973). Diphtheria antitoxin had the most dramatic impact on the status of physicians, who were for the first time clearly able to arrest the progress of a killing disease. Its use spread quickly in major cities, sometimes aided by free distribution of the antitoxin by public health agencies, and death rates from the cause often registered major declines (Vogel 1980; Preston and Haines, 1990). The practice of vaccination against smallpox had also spread to a majority of urban children during the period, and the use of immunization against diphtheria was becoming widespread by 1923 (Research Division, American Child Health Association 1925).

Obstetrics also improved. Midwives delivered about half of the nation's births in 1900 and 20 percent in 1930, although the evidence of this is imprecise (Kobrin 1966; van Blarcom 1930). A variety of attempts were made to improve the practices of these "traditional health workers", beginning around the turn of the century. These included, in various localities, licensing, the institution of formal training requirements, free provision of silver nitrate to prevent eye disease, and inspection of bags. Where these reforms were successfully carried out, as in Providence by 1917, the mortality of babies delivered by midwives could even fall below average (Chapin 1919). The proportion of births occurring in hospitals increased after the turn of the century. Only 5 percent of births in New York City were delivered in hospitals in 1900, compared to 50 percent in 1939 (Apple 1981). Devitt (1977) estimates that 36.9 percent of births in the entire country took place in a hospital in 1935. Hospitals were becoming much safer places to give birth over the time period, largely as a result of antiseptic practices that improved greatly beginning in the 1870s, but whether they became safer than home births is not clear. The lack of improvement in maternal mortality before 1930 suggests that hospital delivery may have had little to do with the improved life chances of infants (Wertz and Wertz 1989; Leavitt 1986).

Each of Holt's pediatric textbooks contained a section on general therapeutics that outlined the measures available to physicians treating children. Holt claimed that sick children needed treatments that were different from those rendered to adults. The changes over time in his list of general therapeutics suggest both the increasing differentiation of the treatment of children and the changes in technology that were occurring. The 1897 edition of Holt's pediatric text shows the limits of treatment available at the time. The doctor's therapeutic repertoire included such antipyretic measures as ice caps, cold packs and baths, and a small number of drugs that would reduce fever. A physican could prescribe a number of drugs: stimulants, primarily alcohol; tonics such as cod liver oil, iron preparations, arsenic and bitter tonics; opiates, including morphine, codeine and paragoric; and anodynes, namely belladonna and chloral for the treatment of convulsions and nerve disorders. Holt believed that all these were well tolerated by infants and young children; opium and cocaine, however, were to be used only with great care. Doctors could also use a list of treatments labelled counterirritants, including mustard packs and paste, turpentine, stimulating liniments, local bloodletting with leeches and dry cups. Poultices and hot fomentations, cold and hot packs, and a number of baths could be recommended as treatments, but the preferred treatment for pulmonary inflammation was an oiled silk jacket that would maintain a constant temperature when worn by the child. Nasal spray, nasal syringing, and inhalations were recommended for infants whose illness involved congestion. An infant could be force fed through a tube, a technique called gavage. Stomach washing and irrigation of the colon were recommended as noted previously in the treatment of diarrhea. The hypodermic needle was available but not often used. Finally, massage could be used to treat a number of ailments, but especially anemia and malnutrition.

The list was remarkably slow to change. In 1906, Holt added anesthetics to the list. In 1911, a section on vaccines was added. He argued at that time that "their application in pediatrics is confined to therapeutics, as a prophylactic measure they are seldom called for except for prevention of typhoid fever" (Holt 1911:54). Noticeably absent was any reference to smallpox vaccination. Even as a therapeutic, vaccines were a disappointment according to Holt. For most conditions, he argued, "experience thus far does not warrant one forming a sanguine opinion of their value" (Holt 1911:54). In 1911, Holt also added hypodermoclysis, i.e., the subcutaneous injection of fluids, as a treatment for diarrhea, and sedatives to the drugs available. Only the oiled silk jacket was deleted from the original list at this time. From time to time, minor changes were made in the drugs listed for use. In 1916, digitalis, caffeine, strychnine and camphor were added to alcohol as stimulants. In that edition, blood transfusions were also described. In 1923, interperitoneal and intrasinus injections as a means of introducing fluids into the system were added. The prophylactic use of vaccines was extended to pertussis, but the negative view of vaccines in treatment persisted. The recommended uses for counterirritants diminished during the late 1910s and early 1920s and the use of leeches disappeared. In addition a change in the method of blood transfusion differentiates the 1927 from the 1923 edition.

Significant changes in the list were deferred until 1933, when the format of the list changed and the contents were pared down. Counterirritants, poultices, and hot fomentations no longer appeared. A number of drug treatments were removed, e.g., the use of strychnine as a stimulant. The use of tonics was also labelled unnecessary for the well-fed child. The new therapies included oxygen administration and serum treatment. The latter probably represents the most significant change in treatment and was discussed in each disease where applicable.

In general, advances in therapeutics, as outlined by Holt, were not impressive during the first three decades of the twentieth century. We have, however, examined the recommendations for the treatment of diarrheal diseases in infants and young children as a case study of the changes in therapeutics over that time period.

Changes in Recommended Treatment: An Illustration

All of Holt's pediatric textbooks contained lengthy discussions of the treatment of diarrheal diseases in children. Most of the recommendations for treatment changed very little until the 1923 edition of the text. However, modifications in two aspects of the treatment are especially interesting to follow over time. One, the use of cathartics and purgation, was a treatment that no doubt added to the problem and reflected a holdover from earlier theories of disease. The second, rehydration therapy, is currently recognized as the key factor in treating severe diarrhea, but required a knowledge of physiology and technical advances only beginning to evolve at the turn of the twentieth century.

Between 1897 and 1923 the emphasis on cathartics in the treatment of diarrhea grew stronger. Germ theory probably enhanced the rationale for cathartics; contaminated food could not be digested, fermented in the stomach and intestines of the infant, and required removal. It was not until the ninth edition of his pediatrics text, in 1928, that Holt began to retreat from the extensive use of cathartics. In that year, he wrote that cathartics might be needed in some circumstances, but "if the diarrhea has been profuse, cathartics should not be employed" (Holt and Howland 1927:293).

Finally in 1933, Holt's textbook, as revised by L. Emmett Holt, Jr. and Rustin McIntosh, contained the recognition that dehydration was a major problem and the use of cathartics entirely inappropriate.

> The practice of purging, once universal, has largely been discontinued. It adds to the discomfort of the patient and to the severity of dehydration. It is seldom that indications for cathartics arise....If the diarrhea is profuse, cathartics should not be employed; the intestine requires no aid in expelling its contents. (Holt and McIntosh 1933:189)

While Holt recognized throughout this period that water loss was a problem, understanding the seriousness of the problem depended on developments in physiology and particularly observation of the changes in blood chemistry that accompanied diarrhea.

In addition, the technological changes required for safe administration of fluids were slow in coming and certainly postdated most of the decline in diarrheal deaths. In 1911, the general therapeutics section of Holt's textbook contained a section on hypodermoclysis and recommended subcutaneous injections of saline solutions as a therapeutic technique in the treatment of acute diarrhea. In 1916, the directions for subcutaneous injection were expanded; in 1923, a section on intraperitoneal injections was added; and finally in 1933, intravenous introduction of fluids was described. However, Holt noted that because of the "technical difficulties in giving prolonged intravenous infusion in infants, this route is seldom used in the treatment of dehydration" (Holt 1933).

However, by 1933, although the practice of intravenous administration of fluids was still not well developed, the knowledge about infant physiology had greatly expanded. The 1933 edition contained long sections on dehydration, electrolytes and mineral loss, and noted that "the maintenance of life depends upon a series of physiochemical processes controlled by balanced equilibrium" (Holt and Mcintosh 1933). There was no doubt that the implied treatment was dangerous, but the use of cathartics was totally discredited by the recognition of dehydration as a serious problem.

How did these changes in the view of the treatment of diarrhea get transmitted to mothers, who needed to treat the sick child, at least until the doctor arrived? Beginning with the 1897 edition of *Care and Feeding*, Holt provided mothers with advice on how to treat children with diarrheal diseases. His advice to mothers followed closely the changes in treatment recommended in his pediatric text. He recommended that all solid food be stopped and milk greatly diluted when an infant had diarrhea. If there was vomiting, all milk was to be stopped and the infant fed broth or boiled water only. A cathartic, usually castor oil, was to be given. The feeding recommendations changed slightly; mothers were advised to reduce the fat content of milk, reduce the amount of milk in the infant's formula and to stop food for even longer periods in later editions. The recommendation for using a cathartic remained the same until the 1926 edition. Holt asked and answered the obvious question, "Why is a cathartic necessary if the movements are already frequent?" Diarrhea was nature's way to get rid of an irritant in the bowels resulting from undigested food; mothers could help nature by administering a cathartic. In 1920, the rationale for using a cathartic added that the irritation of the intestines was caused by fermenting food that had not been digested. In 1926, a reversal of opinion was couched in terms of a typology of diarrhea; there were two forms, one due to lack of digestion of food, the other, dysentery, due to the dysentery germ, which caused an inflammation of the bowels. The latter was more serious and required careful prophylaxis. Treatment was secondary to prevention but required only changes in food. "A cathartic is not required, and particularly in infants may produce much harm" (Holt 1926:232). Mothers could prevent dysentery in infants and young children by isolating them from people who had the disease, by using mosquito netting because dysentery could be spread by flies, and by washing hands after contact with anyone with diarrhea and whenever handling the baby's food. These precautions were especially important in the summer.

The Children's Bureau emphasized prevention more than treatment in all three editions of its manual (1914, 1921, 1929). Diarrhea, especially in the summer, could be prevented by keeping the baby cool, by reducing the amount of food, and by increasing the quantities of water given. For nursing babies, the interval between feedings had to be extended and the length of the feeding shortened in as much as diarrhea was most often caused by too frequent nursing. If the diarrhea continued, nursing should cease altogether for several hours. For bottle fed babies, if the diarrhea was mild, the volume of feedings should be reduced by half, milk should be skimmed, and all sugar omitted. For more severe diarrhea, mothers were advised to stop all milk, give only boiled water, and consult a physician.

By 1921, breastfeeding, pure milk, hygienic surroundings, and proper methods of artificial feeding were seen as the means of preventing diarrhea in infants. Once it occurred, all food was to be stopped, boiled water given to replace lost fluids, and the physician called. If no physician was available, then castor oil would be given and all milk stopped for 24 hours. The Children's Bureau was always more moderate than Holt in its recommendations for purgatives; a single dose would suffice and was really only required if spoiled food was the cause of the diarrhea. Diarrhea stemming from overfeeding would be checked by simply withholding food. In the 1929 edition, the administration of castor oil was no longer recommended. Milk was to be withdrawn from the child with diarrhea for 24 hours and feeding would then resume with diluted skim milk that had been boiled for five minutes. For mothers using the Children's Bureau manuals, the fatal error before the late 1920s would have been to call a physician who would likely prescribe the excessive use of cathartics in the treatment of the illness.

Conclusions

Child mortality differences by ethnicity were clearly visible in the United States at the turn of the century. In particular, French-Canadians had extraordinarily high mortality and Jews exceptionally low mortality. These differences were not related to the educational levels of mothers, which was a minor factor in mortality at the time and which favored French-Canadians. The mortality differences were almost certainly a reflection of specific child raising practices relating to infant feeding and standards of hygiene. We have suggested, consistent with Caldwell's proposals, that these differences were in turn a reflection of a different degree of child-centeredness of French-Canadian and Jewish families.

Partly influenced by such observations, great emphasis was placed by health authorities on improving maternal practices during the period 1900-1930, and they used a wide variety of means to influence these practices. We have questioned whether this advice about domestic health practices, if followed by sufficient numbers of mothers, could have accounted for some of the decline in the mortality of children from 1900 to 1930. Cause-of-death data linking the decline in childhood mortality to a list of causes headed by diarrheal diseases lend credence to the notion that private health and child care practices may have been important.

In a number of areas, notably that of infant feeding, which dominated the advice literature, the advice given to mothers was largely sound by current standards. As they were in the nineteenth century, mothers were being urged to breastfeed their children. The weight of evidence, however, is that breastfeeding diminished during the period of rapid mortality decline. When breastfeeding was not practical because of problems encountered or because of the age of the child, mothers were encouraged to supply clean, bacteria-free food to children. An increase in the emphasis on the importance of sterilizing milk and and bottles was an important change in the first decades of the twentieth century and might well have had a positive effect on the life chances of bottle fed babies. In addition, increased emphasis was placed on isolating house-hold members with an infectious disease. For both artificial feeding practices and isolation, a shift in the message was certainly in line with improvements of the health of children. Furthermore, the number receiving these messages was vastly expanded by organized efforts to improve maternal practices and an outpouring of interest in child health on the part of mothers themselves.

On the other hand, we found little evidence in the advice literature that we examined of an increased concern with general hygiene practices, such as handwashing or fly control. Acceptance of germ theories of disease causality certainly focused some attention on these issues, but they never held a prominent position in the child care literature. Finally, we find little in the extension of the use of physicians to suggest that it played a prominent role in the mortality decline. Physicians had several new and effective drugs at their disposal and an increased appreciation of hygienic practices themselves, but therapeutics changed very slowly during this period. Indeed, our analysis of diarrheal diseases shows that the treatment of these diseases changed remarkably slowly, given the radical shifts in the etiologic framework that occurred at the end of the nineteenth century. Improved personal health care practices undoubtedly contributed to the decline in infant mortality during the first three decades of the twentieth century, but the successes were principally in the domain of prevention rather than treatment.

Acknowledgement

We are grateful to our collaborators on work related to this topic for their many contributions to this paper: Michael Haines, Douglas Ewbank, Mark Hereward, and Ellen Kramarow.

Note

1 This section and the two following draw heavily on Ewbank and Preston (1990).

References

Abbott, S.W. 1900. *The Past and Present Condition of Public Hygiene and State Medicine in the United States.* Boston: Wright & Potter Printing Company.

Abbott, G. 1923. "Ten years' work for children." *North American Review.* 189–200.

Ackernecht, E.H. 1973. *Therapeutics From the Primitive to the 20th Century.* New York: Hafner Press.

Ashby, H.T. 1922. *Infant Mortality.* Second edition. Cambridge: Cambridge University Press.

Aykroyd, W.R. 1971. "Nutrition and mortality in infancy and early childhood: Past and present relationships." *American Journal of Clinical Nutrition,* 24: 480–87.

Apple, R. 1981. "How Shall I Feed My Baby? Infant Feeding in the United States, 1870–1940." Ph.D. dissertation, History of Science. Ann Arbor: University of Michigan. University Microfilms.

Bennett, M.K., and R.H. Pierce. 1961. "Change in the American national diet, 1879–1959." *Food Research Institute Studies,* 2(2): 97–118.

Bradley, F.S., and M.A. Williamson. 1918. *Rural Children in Selected Countries of North Carolina.* U.S. Department of Labor Children's Bureau Rural Child Welfare Series, 2. Washington, DC: Government Printing Office.

Buchan, W. 1811. *Advice to Mothers, on the Subject of Their Own Health and the Means of Promoting the Health, Strength, and Beauty of Their Offspring.* Boston: Joseph Bumstead.

Caldwell, J.C. 1988. "Family change and demographic change: The reversal of the veneration flow." In K. Srinivasan and S. Mukerji, eds. *Dynamics of Population and Family Welfare 1987.* Bombay: Humalaya.

Caldwell, J.C., P.H. Reddy, and P. Caldwell. 1988. *The Causes of Demographic Change: Experimental Research in South India.* Madison: University of Wisconsin Press.

Chapin, C.V. 1901. *Municipal Sanitation in the United States.* Providence, RI: Snow and Furnhum.

Chapin, C.V. 1919. "The control of midwifery." In W.L. Chenery and E.A. Merritt, eds. *Standards of Child Welfare.* New York: Arno Press. 1974. Reprint of U.S. Department of Labor Children's Bureau, *Standards of Child Welfare.* Report of the Children's Bureau Conferences, May and June, 1919. Bureau Publications No. 60. Washington, DC: Department of Labor.

Chapin, C.V. 1921. "History of state and municipal control of disease." In M.P. Ravenel, ed. *A Half Century of Public Health.* New York: American Public Health Association.

Cheney, R. 1984. "Seasonal aspects of infant and childhood mortality: Philadelphia, 1865–1920." *Journal of Interdisciplinary History,* 14: 561–85.

Children's Bureau. 1914. *Infant Care.* By Mrs. Max West. Care of Children Series No. 2. Children's Bureau Publication No. 8. Washington, DC: Government Printing Office.

Children's Bureau. 1916. *A Tabular Statement of Infant-Welfare Work by Public and Private Agencies in the United States.* The Children's Bureau, Infant Mortality Series No. 5. Washington, DC: Government Printing Office.

Children's Bureau. 1917. *Baby Week Campaigns.* Miscellaneous Series No. 5. Bureau Publication No. 15. Washington, DC: Government Printing Office.

Children's Bureau. 1921. *Infant Care.* Care of Children Series No. 2. Bureau Publication No. 8. (Revised).

Children's Bureau. 1929. *Infant Care.* Bureau Publication No. 8. Washington, DC: Government Printing Office.

Clelland, J.G., and J.K. van Ginneken. 1988. "Maternal education and child survival in developing countries: The search for pathways of influence." *Social Science and Medicine,* 27(12):1357–68.

Coit, H.L. 1893. *A Plan to Procure Cow's Milk Designed for Clinical Purposes.* Newark, NJ. Reprinted in part in R.H. Bremner, *Children and Youth in America.* Vol II. 1866–1932. Cambridge, MA: Harvard University Press, 1971: 867–69.

Condran, G.A., and R.A. Cheney. 1982. "Mortality trends in Philadelphia: Age and cause–specific death rates, 1870–1930." *Demography,* 19(1): 97–123.

Condran, G.A., H. Williams, and R.A. Cheney. 1984. "The decline in mortality in Philadelphia from 1870 to 1930: The role of municipal services." *The Pennsylvania Magazine of History and Biography*, 108: 153–77.

Condran, G.A., and E.A. Kramarow. 1990. "Child mortality among Jewish immigrants to the United States." *Journal of Interdisciplinary History*, 22: 223–25.

Connolly, J.M. 1909. "Discussion." In Conference on the Prevention of Infant Mortality. *Prevention of Infant Mortality*. New Haven, CT: American Academy of Medicine.

Davis, M.M. 1921. *Immigrant Health and the Community*. New York: Harper and Row.

Devitt, N. 1977. "The transition from home to hospital birth in the United States, 1930–1960." *Birth and the Family Journal*, 4 (Summer): 47–56.

Duffus, R.L., and L.E. Holt, Jr. 1940. *L. Emmett Holt*. New York: D. Appleton and Company.

Dwork, D. 1987. *War is Good for Babies and Other Young Children: A History of the Infant and Child Welfare Movement in England, 1898-1918*. London: Tavistock Publications.

Dye, N.S., and D.B. Smith. 1986. "Mother love and infant death, 1750–1920." *Journal of American History*, 73(2): 329–53.

Ewbank, D., and S.H. Preston. 1990. "Personal health behavior and the decline in infant and child mortality: The United States, 1900–30." In J.C. Caldwell, S. Findley, P. Caldwell, G. Santow, W. Cosford, J. Braid, and D. Broers-Freeman. 1990. *What We Know About the Health Transition: The Cultural, Social and Behavioural Determinants of Health, Health Transition Series*, No. 2, Vol. 1 Canberra: Health Transition Centre, Australian National University.

Fishberg, M. 1911. *The Jews: A Study of Race and Environment*. New York: Charles Scribner's Sons.

Fisher, I. 1909. *Report on National Vitality, Its Wastes and Conservation*. Bulletin of the Committee of One Hundred on National Health. Prepared for the National Conservation Commission. Washington, DC: Government Printing Office.

Fox, E.G. [1919] 1974. "Rural problems." In W.L. Chenery and E.A. Merritt, eds. *Standards of Child Welfare*. New York: Arno Press. Reprint of U.S. Department of Labor Children's Bureau, *Standards of Child Welfare*. Report of the Children's Bureau of Conferences, May and June, 1919. Bureau Publication No. 60. Washington, DC: Department of Labor.

Gauvreau, D. 1990. Personal communication. Centre interuniversitaire de recherches sur les populations. Université du Quebec à Chicoutimi, Canada.

Glover, J.W. 1921. *United States Life Tables, 1890, 1901, 1910, and 1901–1910*. Washington, DC: Goverment Printing Office.

Hareven, T., and R. Langenbach. 1978. *Amoskeag: Life and Work in an American Factory-City*. New York: Pantheon.

Hareven, T. 1982. *Family Time and Indstrial Time: The Relationship Between Family and Work in a New England Industrial Community*. Cambridge: Cambridge University Press.

Hedger, C. 1909. "The relation of infant mortality to the occupation and long hours of work for women." In Conference on the Prevention of Infant Mortality. *Prevention of Infant Mortality*. New Haven, CT: American Academy of Medicine.

Holt, L.E. 1894. *The Care and Feeding of Children*. New York: D. Appleton and Company.

Holt, L.E. 1897. *The Care and Feeding of Children*. Second Edition. New York: D. Appleton and Company.

Holt, L.E. 1897. *The Diseases of Infancy and Childhood*. New York: D. Appleton and Company.

Holt, L.E. 1903. *The Care and Feeding of Children*. Third Edition. New York: D. Appleton and Company.

Holt, L.E. 1906. *The Diseases of Infancy and Childhood*. Third edition. New York: D. Appleton and Company.

Holt, L.E. 1909. *The Diseases of Infancy and Childhood*. Fifth edition. New York: D. Appleton and Company.

Holt, L.E. 1909. *The Care and Feeding of Children*. New York: D. Appleton and Company.

Holt, L.E. 1911. *The Diseases of Infancy and Childhood*. Sixth edition. New York: D. Appleton and Company.

Holt, L.E. 1916. *The Diseases of Infancy and Childhood*. Seventh edition. New York: D. Appleton and Company.

Holt, L.E. 1917. *The Care and Feeding of Children*. Eighth edition. New York: D. Appleton and Company.

Holt, L.E. 1920. *The Care and Feeding of Children*. Tenth edition. Revised and Enlarged. New York: D. Appleton and Company.

Holt, L.E. 1923. *The Care and Feeding of Children*. Twelfth edition. Revised and Enlarged. New York: D. Appleton and Company.

Holt, L.E. 1926. *The Care and Feeding of Children*. Thirteenth edition. New York: D. Appleton and Company.

Holt, L.E., and J. Howland 1923. *The Diseases of Infancy and Childhood*. Eighth edition. New York: D. Appleton and Company.

Holt, L.E., and J. Howland. 1927. *The Diseases of Infancy and Childhood.* Ninth edition. New York: D. Appleton and Company.

Holt L.E., and R. McIntosh. 1933. *Holt's Diseases of Infancy and Childhood.* Tenth edition. New York: D. Appleton and Company.

Jacobi, A. 1887. *The Intestinal Diseases of Infancy and Childhood.* Detroit: George S. Davis.

Jacobi, A. 1895. *Therapeutics of Infancy and Childhood.* Philadelphia: J.B. Lippincott Company.

Jacobi, A. 1898. *Therapeutics of Infancy and Childhood.* Second edition. Philadelphia: J.B. Lippincott Company.

Jacobi, A. 1903. *Therapeutics of Infancy and Childhood.* Third edition. Philadelphia: J.B. Lippincott Company.

Jacobs, J., and M. Greene. 1990. "Race and ethnicity, social class and schooling 1910." Presented to Workshop on the Social Demography of the United States in 1910. Philadelphia: University of Pennsylvania. February 8–10.

Keating, W.J. 1890. *Cyclopedia of the Diseases of Children.* Vol. III. Philadelphia: J.B. Lippincott Company.

Kobrin, F.E. 1966. "The American midwife controversy: A crisis of professionalization." *Bulletin of the History of Medicine*, 40: 350–63. Reprinted in J.W. Leavitt and R.L. Numbers, eds. *Sickness and Health in America: Readings in the History of Medicine and Public Health.* Madison, WI: University of Wisconsin Press.

Kunitz, S.J. 1983. "Speculations on the European mortality decline." *Economic History Review*, 36:349–64.

Kunitz, S.J. 1986. "Mortality since Malthus." In D. Coleman and R. Schofield, eds. *The State of Population Theory.* Oxford: Basil Blackwell.

Leavitt, J.W. 1986. *Brought to Bed: Childbearing in America, 1750 to 1950.* New York: Oxford University Press.

Lentzner, H.R. 1987. "Seasonal Patterns of Infant and Child Mortality in New York, Chicago and New Orleans: 1870–1919." Dissertation in demography. University of Pennsylvania.

Lentzner, H., and G.A. Condran. 1985. "Seasonal patterns of infant and childhood mortality in New York, Chicago, and New Orleans: 1870–1920." Paper presented at the meetings of the Population Association of America, Boston.

McKeown, T. 1976. *The Modern Rise of Population.* New York: Academic Press.

McKinlay, J.B., and S.M. McKinlay. 1977. "The questionable contribution of medical measures to the decline of mortality in the United States." *Health and Society*, 55(Summer): 405–28.

Meckel, R.A. 1990. *Save the Babies: American Public Health Reform and the Prevention of Infant Mortality, 1850–1929.* Baltimore, MD: Johns Hopkins University Press.

Morse, J.L. 1906. "The protection of infants and young children from tuberculosis infection." Transactions of the National Association for the Study and Prevention of Tuberculosis: 624–26. Reprinted in R.H. Bremner, *Children and Youth in America.* Vol. II. 1866–1932. Cambridge, MA: Harvard University Press. 1971: 890–92.

Nagnur, D. 1986. *Longevity and Historical Life Tables, 1921–81, Canada and the Provences.* Ottawa, Canada: Minister of Supplies and Services.

National Center for Health Statistics. 1984. *Vital Statistics of the United States, 1980.* Life Tables. Vol. II, Section 6. Hyattsville, MD: National Center for Health Statistics.

Neff, J.S. 1909. "Discussion." In conference on the Prevention of Infant Mortality. *Prevention of Infant Mortality.* New Haven, CT: American Academy of Medicine.

Newman, G. 1906. *Infant Mortality: A Social Problem.* London: Methuen and Company.

North, C.E. 1921. "Milk and its relation to public health." In M.P. Ravenel, ed. *A Half Century of Public Health.* New York: American Public Health Association.

Paradise, V.I. 1919. *Maternity Care and the Welfare of Young Children in a Homesteading County in Montana.* U.S. Department of Labor Children's Bureau Rural Child Welfare Series, 3. Washington, DC: Government Printing Office.

Park, W.H., and E. Holt. 1903. "Report upon the results with different kinds of pure and impure milk in infant feeding in tenement houses and institutions of New York City: A cultural and bacteriological study." *Archives of Pediatrics,* 20(12): 881–909.

Pellegrino, E.D. 1979. "The sociocultural impact of twentieth-century therapeutics." In M.J. Vogel and C.E. Rosenberg, eds. *The Therapeutic Revolution.* Philadelphia: University of Pennsylvania Press.

Preston, S.H. 1975. "The changing relation between mortality and level of economic development." *Population Studies,* 29(2): 231–48.

Preston, S.H. 1980. "Causes and consequences of mortality declines in less developed countries during the twentieth century." In R.A. Easterlin, ed., *Population and Economic change in Developing Countries.* Conference Report No. 30. Universities-National Bureau Committee for Economic Research. Chicago: University of Chicago Press.

Preston, S.H. 1985. "Resources, knowledge and child mortality: A comparison of the U.S. in the late nineteenth century and developing countries today." Paper presented at the International Population Conference. Florence, Italy: International Union for the Scientific Study of Population.

Preston, S.H., and M. Haines. 1991. *Fatal Years: Child Mortality in Late Nineteenth Century America*. Princeton, NJ: Princeton University Press.

Preston, S.H., D. Ewbank, and M. Hereward. 1990. "Ethnic differences in American child mortality." Paper presented at a workshop on the 1910 Conference. Philadelphia: University of Pennsylvania.

Research Division, American Child Health Association. 1925. *A Health Survey of 86 Cities*. New York. Reprinted in part in R.H. Bremner, *Children and Youth in America*. Vol. II. 1866–1932. Cambridge, MA: Harvard University Press. 1971: 924–28.

Richmond, P.A. 1954. "American attitudes towards the germ theory of disease (1860–1880)." *Journal of the History of Medicine*, 9: 428–54.

Rochester, A. 1923. *Infant Mortality*. Results of a Field Study in Baltimore, MD. Washington, DC: Government Printing Office.

Rosenberg, C.E., ed. 1972. Reprint of 1818 edition of *The Maternal Physician*. New York: Arno Press & The New York Times.

Rosenberg, C.E. 1987. *The Care of Strangers*. New York: Basic Books.

Schmelz, U.O. 1971. *Infant and Early Childhood Mortality Among Jews of the Diaspora*. Jerusalem: Institute of Contemporary Jewry, The Hebrew University.

Schaftel, N. 1978. " A history of the population of milk in New York, or 'How, now, brown cow?'" In J.W. Leavitt and R.L. Numberg, eds. *Sickness and Health in America: Readings in the History of Medicine and Public Health*. Madison, WI: University of Wisconsin Press.

Sherbon, F.B., and E. Moore. 1919. *Maternity and Infant Care in two Rural Counties in Wisconsin*. U.S. Department of Labor Children's Bureau Rural Child Welfare Series, 4. Washington, DC: Government Printing Office.

Smith, R.M. 1929. "The important causes of infant mortality." *Child Health Bulletin*, 5: 97–109. Reprinted in part in R.H. Bremner, *Children and Youth in America*. Vol II. 1866–1932. Cambridge, MA: Harvard University Press. 1971:976–83.

Starr, P. 1982. *The Social Transformation of American Medicine*. New York: Basic Books.

Strong, M.A., S.H. Preston, A.R. Miller, and M. Hereward. 1989. *User's Guide, Public Use Sample, 1910 United States Census of Population*. Philadelphia: Population Studies Center, University of Pennsylvania.

Sydenstricker, E. 1933. *Health and Environment*. New York: McGraw Hill.

Szreter, S. 1988. "The importance of social intervention in Britain's mortality decline c.1850–1914: A reinterpretation of the role of public health." *Social History of Medicine*, 1: 1–37.

Tesh, S.N. 1988. *Hidden Arguments: Political Ideology and Disease Prevention Policy.* New Brunswick: Rutgers University Press.

Thornton, P., and S. Olson. 1990. "Infant mortality and fertility: Cause or effect? Some evidence from 19th century Montreal." Paper presented at the Annual Meetings of the Population Association of America. Toronto.

Tomes, N. 1990. "The private side of public health: Sanitary science, domestic hygiene and the germ theory, 1870–1900." *Bulletin of the History of Medicine,* 64(4): 509–39.

United Nations. 1985. *Socioeconomic Differentials in Child Mortality in Developing Countries.* Population Study No. 97. New York: United Nations.

U.S. Bureau of the Census. 1933. *Fifteenth Census of the United States: 1930.* Population Volume II. Washington, DC: Government Printing Office.

U.S. Bureau of the Census. 1934. *Mortality Statistics 1930.* Washington, DC: Government Printing Office.

van Blarcom, C.C. 1930. "Rat pie among the black midwives of the south." *Harper's Monthly Magazine,* CLX:322–32. Reprinted in part in R.H. Bremner, *Children and Youth in America.* Vol. II. 1866–1932. Cambridge, MA: Harvard University Press. 1971: 989–94.

Veiller, L. 1921. "Housing as a factor in health progress in the past fifty years." In M.P. Ravenal, ed. *A Half Century of Public Health.* New York: American Public Health Association.

Vogel, M. 1980. *The Invention of the Modern Hospital: Boston, 1870–1930.* Chicago: University of Chicago Press.

Wertz, R.W., and D.C. Wertz. 1989. *Lying In: A History of Childbirth in America.* New Haven: Yale University Press.

Wilbur, R.L. 1931. "We want our future men and women to be self-starters." White House Conference on Child Health and Protection, 1930. Address and Abstracts. New York. In R.H. Bremner, ed. *Children and Youth in America.* Vol. II. 1866–1932. Cambridge, MA.: Harvard University Press. 1971:1077–80.

Wile, I.S. 1909. "Educational responsibilities of a milk depot." In Conference on the Prevention of Infant Mortality. *Prevention of Infant Mortality.* New Haven, CT: American Academy of Medicine.

Winslow, C.E.A. 1909. "The educational session, introductory remarks by the chairman." In Conference on the Prevention of Infant Mortality. *Prevention of Infant Mortality.* New Haven, CT: American Academy of Medicine.

Woodbury, R.M. 1925. *Causal Factors in Infant Mortality: A Statistical Study Based on Investigations in Eight Cities.* Washington, DC: Government Printing Office.

9

The Value of Particularism in the Study of the Cultural, Social, and Behavioral Determinants of Mortality

Stephen J. Kunitz

Introduction

Whether from savagism through barbarism to civilization; from slavery through feudalism and capitalism to communism; from gemeinschaft to gesellschaft; from traditional to legal-rational authority; from mechanical to organic solidarity; from traditional to modern and even post-modern; from pre-transition through transitional to post-transition demographic and epidemiologic regimes, it is a habit of western thought to view history in stages. Often these stages have implied progress and improvement, sometimes decline and decay.

The generalizations implied in these typologies are of course useful. It is possible to commit the historicist fallacy (Hill 1986), however, and assume that developmental stages are everywhere the same and follow one another in some inevitable progression. The result may be that diverse phenomena are forced into a procrustean bed where they are shaped to conform to pre-existing theories. In the case of changing patterns of morbidity and mortality, it is generally assumed that pre-transition rates characteristic of "traditional" societies are high and the result of infectious diseases. As a result of economic development and technical interventions, mortality declines. And in the post-transition phase, noninfectious diseases cause low rates of mortality.

There is a great deal of truth to this broad outline, but as I hope to show in this chapter, it masks astonishing diversity and fails to include many explanatory variables that are of significance if we are to adequately understand the distribution and change of health and diseases in populations, particularly their cultural, social, and behavioral determinants. While it is true that stages of development may be usefully regarded as ideal types — that is to say, as models or heuristic devices — such constructs may be misleading because they may cause us to generalize inappropriately and to reify what began simply as an abstraction based upon one or a few cases.

These attempts to create taxonomies of developmental stages are examples of the necessity we often feel to generalize about the sociocultural determinants of health status. This entirely understandable wish to enunciate law-like explanations of social phenomena has, I think, often diverted attention from unique historical or social features that are of great explanatory value. Therefore in this chapter I shall attempt to redress the balance by providing a series of examples of the gains to be had by distinguishing between societies, cultures, historical periods, and diseases when attempting to explain the sociocultural determinants of mortality.

Differentiating among Cultures

Most of the time when mortality differences among societies are analyzed, the variables that we depend upon are those that can be readily and perhaps even accurately measured: per capita gross national product, physicians per 1,000 population, average number of calories consumed per person per day, proportion of the population residing in urban areas, life expectancy at birth. Many come from estimates provided by national governments. Others derive from survey data of national or subnational populations. The general rubric under which they are subsumed is "the level of economic development." Useful insights have certainly resulted from such analyses.

But the label of economic development obscures many of the processes that are directly associated with mortality and which ought to be disaggregated to be made more visible. Consider for example the differences in mortality between Eastern and Western Europe in the 18th and 19th centuries. It would be easy enough to say — and many do — that the core countries of Western Europe were economically developed, and the peripheral countries of the East were not, and that accounts for the differences in mortality between regions. Such a generalization, however broadly true, prevents one from discovering a variety of particular social, cultural, and agricultural patterns that bear directly on mortality.

While the causal relationships among these factors are impossible to establish, one can certainly describe their collective impact on mortality.

I shall do so by first describing the two different social and economic universes of Western and Eastern Europe, and then discussing their associations with patterns of death.

In Western Europe, agriculture consisted of a mixture of dairy and arable farming practiced on individually held lands of 20 to 50 hectares, a high proportion of which were operated by neolocally organized families, often with the help of servants. Marriage was late for both men and women, childbearing began relatively late, and thus fertility was considerably less than the biological maximum. Marriage was not universal, and usually a new household was formed at marriage. By the 18th century, breastfeeding was medically recognized as important for the health of the infant and seems to have been widely although not universally practiced.

By contrast, in Eastern Europe agriculture tended to be practiced on large estates often owned by noblemen, which were devoted to single grain crops grown for export. The labor was performed by an impoverished peasantry, either as serfs or as agricultural wage laborers. Their household organization tended to be extended and patrilocal (sons brought their wives to live in their natal household rather than forming a new household at marriage), marriage was virtually universal, and childbearing began early and continued late. The need for female labor in the fields generally meant that breastfeeding did not extend very far into an infant's first year of life, and weaning to adult foods occurred early.

The very enumeration of these factors suggests their implications for the populations' health. For example, early marriage associated with early childbearing increased the risk of both maternal and infant death. Crowded households increased the risk of contracting both airborne infections in especially heavy doses as well as diseases spread by body lice. Indeed, typhus continued to be endemic in Eastern Europe and the Balkans into the 20th century. While infants would have been at especially high risk, adults experienced high morbidity and mortality as well from such chronic infectious diseases as tuberculosis and typhus. Households tended to be clustered in villages rather than isolated, and thus the risk was enhanced of microepidemics from contaminated common wells as well as from close personal contact. And the need to exploit female labor in the fields led to increased physiological stress on mothers and to diminished breastfeeding of their newborns. The transfer of infants to watered down versions of adult table foods rather than to more suitable diets increased malnutrition and the lethality of weanling diarrhea (Kunitz 1983: 357). (Similar patterns were found in Italy, particularly southern Italy, and the Iberian peninsula, although households tended to be stem rather than extended in organization.)

In summary, the areas of Europe that were characterized by monocropping on large estates worked by an impoverished peasantry tended to be characterized not simply by rural poverty but by a form of agricultural and domestic organization that contributed to the risk of early death.

By way of contrast, rural household organization in Western and Northern Europe was conducive to lower mortality at all ages. Childbearing began later, thereby reducing the risk of both maternal and infant death. Since dairying was more common, the availability of milk for the weanling was increased (though it was not without risks itself). A more varied diet reduced the risk of nutritional deficiencies such as pellagra. In addition, although data are not available, it is plausible that other factors also reduced risk. Though average household size may have been about the same density of people per room, and thus crowding may have been somewhat less in the West than in the East, so the risks of respiratory infections and the spread of typhus by body lice may have been somewhat diminished as well. Residence on relatively more isolated farms than existed in Eastern Europe would have more likely confined microepidemics to households rather than villages. It is clear from this that rich versus poor, though obviously important, is inadequate as an explanatory concept. One must finely analyze the particularistic features of nations, cultures, regions and localities. If one does not, one inevitably slips into decontextualization.

Yet another distinction of importance is that between urban and rural. Until the late 19th century it was rural mortality that accounted for the differences across Europe. Urban mortality in Western Europe was as high as mortality in Eastern Europe. It declined only in the second half of the 19th century. The causes of this decline have stimulated debate between those who attribute it to increased living standards and those who attribute it to improvements in public health (e.g., McKeown 1976a, 1976b; Szreter 1988). The debate has drawn attention away from the crucial fact that from the mid-18th to the late 19th century it was the agricultural and domestic patterns of life in rural areas that determined the mortality differences among regions of Europe. Once again this illustrates the need to particularize.

Even within smaller geographic units disaggregation is sometimes necessary. If we look at groups with different cultures within the same cities and countries in Europe which are exposed to roughly the same epidemiologic regimes, we make a discovery we otherwise would not make. In neighboring, equally poor Jewish and Gentile populations, infant mortality rates were consistently lower among the former than the latter from the late 18th century to the early 20th century (Schmelz 1971; Sawchuck et al. 1985; Herring and Sawchuck 1986; Ashby 1922; Woodbury 1926). It has never been entirely clear what accounts for the lower risk of death among Jews — observation of dietary prohibitions, the devoted attention of Jewish mothers, or the bacteriostatic qualities of chicken soup. Whatever the cause, Jewish cultural practices were clearly associated with increased chances of survival, even holding environmental conditions roughly constant.

It would not be possible to make this sort of observation if one relied exclusively upon extremely broad analytic generalizations such as economic development. Taken alone, that generalization obscures many critical social and cultural variables that are essential in explanations of historical, regional, and even community differences in mortality across Europe.

Differentiating among Colonial Cultures

The same kind of particularistic disaggregation is also critical in the analysis of mortality in colonial cultures. Commonly analysts use measures of GNP per capita, mean educational achievement of mother, and other such variables in multiple regressions in which the units of analysis are entire nations. More can be learned by examining sociocultural factors — both the culture of the colonizers as well as of the colonized.

In respect to the differences between colonizers, in the Americas, for example, it is obvious that the difference between the demographic patterns in Anglo and Latin America are traceable to the differences between England on the one hand and Spain and Portugal on the other. The settlement of North America by the British was a commercial venture, with numerous settlements reflecting the economic and religious diversity of the English reformation and the growing economic complexity of Britain itself. By contrast, Spain imposed its own authoritarian culture on the New World. As Lang put it, "In Spanish America, the diverse conditions of an entire continent had to find expression in the same set of standard institutions" (Lang 1975: 221-2).

Socioeconomic conditions differed strikingly in the two Americas. In Anglo America, when the British, intent on expanding their neolocally organized households and individually held farms, encountered native cultures, they were unable to incorporate or use them in their own institutions. Thus they forced westward or killed the natives. In Latin America, when the Spanish and Portuguese encountered indigenous populations, they were able to replicate the semifeudal relations with which they were familiar. Thus they subjugated the natives and exploited their labor. Elsewhere, primarily in Caribbean islands and in what became Brazil, both the Iberians and the British (who included both slave owners and slavery haters) imported captive blacks to work their plantations. Inevitably they created the New World in the image of the Old.

To this very day we see the impact on mortality of these different patterns of colonization. One can still state, as Stein and Stein put it, speaking of the 19th century: "In Latin America the colonial heritages reinforced by external and internal factors produced economic growth without appreciable sociopolitical change" (Stein and Stein 1970: 173). Even now beneath the turbulent and changing surface, the ancient colonial heritages shape mortality patterns. In Latin America, as in Southern and Eastern Europe, rural poverty, early and universal marriage, crowded households, inadequate sewerage, and malnutrition increased the risks of early death and, right up to the present, have kept rural mortality higher than urban mortality.

By contrast, the traditions established in English America led to very different mortality patterns. The settlers in English America came from a society "which generally treated literacy, toleration, individual rights, economic liberty, savings and investment as inseparable elements of the process of change and growth" (Stein and Stein 1970: 127). In Anglo America the availability of land for farming resulted in early marriage and high fertility, but, as in Northern Europe, it also resulted in very good nutrition, low density of population, and good health, which resulted in rural mortality being lower than urban mortality until the second decade of the present century.

Once again, we see that it is not sufficient to rely exclusively on a few measures of economic development. The cultures of both colonizers and colonized play a critical role in explaining mortality patterns.

Further important distinctions must be made within these two broad colonial categories. I start with Latin America. The mortality patterns I have just described are actually characteristic of the majority of colonies, those where there were indigenous agricultural populations — e.g., parts of Mexico, Guatemala, Ecuador, Peru, and Bolivia. A strikingly different mortality pattern can be found in those few regions which lacked an indigenous agricultural population — the lowland areas of Argentina, Uruguay, Chile, and Southern Brazil, as well as Costa Rica. Such areas did not lend themselves to semi-feudal agriculture and mining, and were not of early interest to the Iberians. All except Costa Rica attracted extensive European immigration in the late 19th century, and all developed commerce and industry earlier and more extensively than the other regions of Latin America. The impact of these conditions on mortality patterns in the first decades of this century occasions no surprise. In contrast to other countries for which data are available, Uruguay and Argentina had far lower crude mortality rates (Sanchez-Albornoz 1974, Kunitz 1986: 293).

This sharp differentiation between the two types of Latin American societies began to fade in the 1920s and 1930s when the rates of improvement of life expectancy increased in all of Latin America, most impressively in the poorest, high mortality countries (Arriaga and Davis 1969). This was the result primarily of the success of imported public health technologies, particularly the prevention of malaria and yellow fever. After World War II, rates of improvement in, and convergence of, life expectancy accelerated even more. Nonetheless, old colonial institutions cast long shadows into the present. Infectious and parasitic causes of death in the most agricultural countries are still more significant than in the least agricultural countries (Kunitz 1986), where cerebro-vascular and ischemic heart disease have become more common (see Table 9-1).

These differences within Latin America suggest that the legacy of the past is likely to be observable even after several centuries, that it is embedded in social institutions and in the culture that one generation transmits to the next, and that it continues to be reflected not only in ways of life but in ways of death. Yet again, these critical differentiations are obscured by almost symbolic economic concepts such as the number of physicians per 1,000 population.

In Anglo America, too, important cultural and political distinctions ultimately produced differing mortality patterns. Though both the United

Table 9-1 Age Adjusted Mortality from Selected Causes, The Americas, early 1980s

Age-Adjusted Rate per 100,000

Country	Total age-adj. rate per 1,000	Infectious & parasit.		Cervical cancer		Hypertensive disease		C.V.D.		I.H.D.		Accident & viol.	
		rate	%	rate	%	rate	%	rate	%	rate	%	rate	%
Argentina	5.2	26.6	5.1	3.3	0.6	7.3	1.4	38.6	7.4	43	8.3	49	9.3
Chile	4.9	20.7	4.2	8.4	1.7	5.5	1.1	39.5	8.0	42	9	70	14.3
Costa Rica	3.9	17.7	4.5	6.8	1.7	3.6	0.9	27.9	7.1	54	14	35	8.9
Ecuador	7.6	126.1	16.6	4.2	0.5	5.6	0.7	27.2	3.5	17	2	74	10
Guatemala	10.0	242.7	24.2	3.7	0.3	5.9	0.6	14.1	1.4	8	0.8	199	20
Honduras	5.2	72.6	13.9	0.3	.05	2.6	0.5	16.2	3.1	4	0.8	61	12
Mexico	5.7	68.3	11.9	8.7	1.5	5.1	0.9	22.5	3.9	24	4.2	95	17
Panama	3.6	23.3	6.4	7.1	1.9	5.1	1.4	26.5	7.3	39	11	49	14
Paraguay	5.8	69.3	11.9	4.9	0.8	7.1	1.2	41.0	7.0	29	4.9	40	6.8
Peru	4.4	81.8	18.5	4.5	1.0	2.9	0.6	15.4	3.5	15	3.4	29	6.6
Uruguay	4.9	21.0	4.2	3.1	0.6	5.4	1.1	46.0	9.3	51	10.3	40	8.2
Venezuela	4.9	48.9	9.9	6.7	1.3	10.5	2.1	32.6	6.6	57	11.6	70	14.2
Canada	3.2	2.3	0.7	1.8	0.5	1.9	0.5	20.0	6.2	73	22.7	43	13.2
U.S.A.	3.7	4.6	1.2	1.9	0.5	4.7	1.2	21.1	5.7	79	21.4	49	13.6

Source: PAHO 1986: Table 111-5b.

States and Canada were settled by the English, the United States was settled largely by middle class religious dissenters who broke decisively with the mother country in the late 18th century. Canada was settled by loyalists and remained firmly in the English orbit. Pierre Berton has written of the Canadian response to the War of 1812: "This attitude — that the British way of life is preferable to the American; that certain sensitive positions are better filled by appointments than by election; that order imposed from above has advantages over grass-roots democracy (for which read 'license' or 'anarchy'); that a ruling elite often knows better than the body politic — flourished as a result of an invasion repelled. Out of it, shaped by an emerging nationalism and tempered by rebellion, grew that special form of state paternalism that makes the Canadian way of life significantly different from the more individualistic American way" (Berton 1980: 313-4).

The "state paternalism" that Berton says characterizes Canadian political and civic culture has been, and continues to be, manifested in numerous ways. As Canadians themselves point out, their frontier was pacified by the Royal Canadian Mounted Police, who represented the authority of the state. Individualistic frontiersmen and Indian fighters played a far less significant role than they did in America. Canadian political life is collectivist and has included a socialist party that has controlled several provincial governments and even knocked at the doors of national political office. In America, similar political movements have found representation only as one among many interest groups in the Democratic Party. And the Canadians, with their paternalist-collectivist orientation, have developed universal health insurance which, at the national level, Conservatives as well as Liberals have supported. In contrast, the Americans have not created universal health insurance but have assumed that the individual can care for himself or herself, and have created programs for exceptional categories of beneficiaries: veterans, Indians, the elderly, and the very poor.

A further distinction between the two countries that is crucial, but of a different nature, is that Canadians did not import black slaves to work on plantations. Americans did.

Many of the effects on mortality of these differences in political and civic culture and institutions are subtle, as the data in Table 9-1 indicate. Age-adjusted total mortality rates are nearly identical in the two countries; the Canadian rate is 86 percent of the American. Similarly, age-adjusted death rates from cervical cancer, cerebro-vascular disease, and ischemic heart disease are only very slightly lower among Canadians (92-95 percent of the American rate). Death rates from accidents and violence among Canadians are 88 percent of the American rate. But if one examines the broad category of violence more closely, one sees that some of the mortality patterns are dramatically different. Canadians have less than a third of the American rate of homicide (2.3 versus 7.3 per 100,000). Also death rates from infectious diseases among Canadians are 50 percent of the American rate, and from hypertension, 40 percent.

While it is possible that diagnostic fashions explain some of the dramatic differences, it is even more plausible that they may be explained by the social and cultural differences described above. Infectious diseases and hypertension are widely regarded as conditions amenable to preventive and therapeutic interventions by the health care system. To the degree that universal health insurance makes services more accessible in Canada than the United States, such treatable conditions may well be dealt with more effectively in the former than the latter country. In respect to homicide, it seems likely that the Americans' jealously defended right to bear arms, combined with a glamorized frontier and gunslinger tradition, as well as an explosive and violent underclass, all conspire to elevate the American rate well beyond the Canadian.

The moral of this tale is similar to the one that emerged from the discussion of Latin American mortality. Even in countries that seem — and are in fact — similar in many important ways, the legacy of past differences continues to be reflected not simply in ways of life but in ways of death as well. Clearly such issues are submerged by a reliance on analytical categories (such as mean household size) that offer not the substance but an illusion of understanding.

Differentiating between the Effects of Economic Development and Public Health

One of the liveliest debates about death is what has been called the standard of living debate. In origin it is concerned primarily with the impact of industrial development in England in the late 18th century and first half of the 19th century. On one side are the pessimists who argue that industrialization and urbanization were paid for by the lower classes, whose situation deteriorated as a result of these developments. On the other side are the optimists, who argue that as a result of these developments, average incomes increased, income inequalities decreased, and both the quantity and quality of life improved for everyone, including the lower classes.

Among writers concerned with the history of mortality, Thomas McKeown (1976a, 1976b) would be considered an optimist, for he argued that public health interventions were unimportant until the end of the 19th century; curative measures only became significant in the present century; and thus, improved nutrition — a manifestation of improved living conditions — must have been the primary cause of the historic decline of European mortality. Simon Szreter (1988) is an example of the "pessimistic" school inasmuch as he argues that living standards cannot be given credit for the decline of mortality and that human agency — improvements in public health — deserve credit for the decline.

It is significant that the debate has been primarily about England, the first industrial nation, where the ideas of the free market and of economic individualism were born. It is this debate about England that has largely determined our understanding of the past, and that has set the terms for debates about contemporary changes in mortality in less developed countries as well. That is to say, whether one believes in the efficacy of the free market or centrally planned economies, economic development is often posed as the alternative to preventive and curative health services. The latter are considered either technical aid or technological fixes, again depending on the persuasion of the commentator.

But England was not the only nation whose mortality rates declined in the second half of the 19th century and early decades of this century. It is illuminating to consider some of those other historical experiences, for they illustrate the point that there was more than one way that mortality declined in the past, and they thus may contribute to the enlargement of the terms of contemporary debate as well.

Several authors have shown, for example, that life expectancy was approximately the same in 19th century Japan as it was in England and Western Europe at the same time. Yet Japanese cities were as large as or larger than European cities, per capita income was substantially lower in Japan, and industrialization, economic development and increased living standards had not occurred as they had in the West. These authors all argue that several factors were involved in explaining the equally low mortality of Japan in the face of economic backwardness. There was a high degree of governmental control over social life in Japan, which made possible the planning and construction of sophisticated water supplies beginning in the 17th century. Human feces and urine were regarded as an economic good to be sold as fertilizer, not as waste to be disposed of in unsanitary cesspits or in rivers that also provided drinking water. Due to concern about damage from earthquakes, houses could not be more than one story tall, so multistory tenements such as existed in western cities were unknown in Japan. Moreover, habits of personal cleanliness deriving from traditional religious values made bathing, handwashing and laundering common. The custom of drinking tea meant that much of the water consumed had been boiled. Virtually all food was eaten cooked, so contamination from the nightsoil used as fertilizer was reduced. Each member of the household had his or her own eating utensils. And so on. The point is that a different sociocultural system created both the environment and personal behavior which led to rather low mortality in the absence of economic development (Mosk and Johansson 1986; Johansson and Mosk 1987; Hanley 1987; Jannetta 1987).

Turning to a European example, John C. Brown (1988, 1989) has suggested that the very rapid improvement in mortality in German cities in the late 19th and early 20th centuries was the result of improvement in public health initiated by local elites who controlled town councils. He observes that by 1900, Germany, with a per capita income three-fifths of England's and perhaps half of America's, had slightly higher male life expectancy than either, both at birth and at age 10. Typhoid fever deaths, typically used as a measure of the quality of urban water supplies, were considerably lower in Germany than in the United States, and slightly lower than in England as well.

The motives of the elites were undoubtedly mixed. They themselves benefited by having a healthy workforce. High mortality and slowing urban migration from the countryside were thought to threaten labor shortages in some places. Furthermore, like Bismarck's reforms in the 1880s, improvements in the quality of urban life may have been aimed at reducing the power of the Social Democrats. Whatever the reasons for their implementation, the evidence suggests that public health measures did have a measurable and significant impact on improvements in life expectancy, even in the face of low per capita income.

The point of these two examples is that economic expansion, as it occurred in England and the United States in the 19th century, may well have been the engine that propelled improvements in life expectancy. One must be careful, however, not to generalize from those historical cases to every other case. As the German and Japanese data indicate, other societies with different political and civic cultures had attained similar levels of mortality by other means.

Differentiating among Historical Variables

Variables that are of value in explaining mortality in one period are often thought to be of value in another. This can be true, of course, but extrapolation from one period to another can also be misleading. We know, for example, that population density as a measure of crowding was a useful explanatory variable of mortality in 19th century cities, but Hong Kong and the Netherlands, two of the most densely settled areas in the world, now have among the lowest rates of mortality. A startling example of such an extrapolation from past to present is one that will probably bear in perpetuity the name of Thomas McKeown, though it has by now been widely shared. I am not going to discuss all of McKeown's work nor the standard of living debate to which it has been such an important contribution. I will isolate only this unusual example of the belief that the insignificance of an explanatory variable in one country may be extrapolated to another.

In both of his books, McKeown published a series of graphs which showed for England and Wales the decline since the early 19th century in age-adjusted mortality rates due to specific diseases, with an arrow at the year at which an effective or definitive preventive measure or therapy first became available. The results were impressive because they showed clearly that the vast majority of decline in mortality from virtually all infectious diseases had occurred well before the definitive technology had become available. McKeown's point — one among many — was clear; the personal physician system had no impact on mortality in the 18th and 19th centuries.

McKeown had been saying something similar since the 1950s, largely in response to the status revolution that had occurred in medicine with the development of antibiotics and pesticides. Suddenly therapeutic medicine, the care of the individual patient, was in the ascendant, and social medicine, the care of the community, was déclassé. McKeown's historical work served the purpose (embraced by many cost-conscious policy makers in the 1970s) of denigrating medicine's inflated claims to past accomplishments, and thus deflated the pretensions of high status in the present. For some, his work clearly provided a rationale for the cost containing activities on which they were embarking. For others, no doubt it was immediately persuasive and had an impact on their perceptions of the efficacy of the personal physician system of care.

This is a striking example of a misleading extrapolation from the past to the present. Most of what McKeown said about the ineffectiveness of doctors in the past was true, but this was actually irrelevant to the mortality patterns and modes of prevention and therapy that predominated in his own time. The world had changed; diseases were different and so were the preventive and therapeutic measures available to deal with them.

Indeed, in the very year that McKeown's two books were published, a Working Group on Preventable and Manageable Diseases (Rutstein et al. 1976) assessed the available literature to ascertain what diseases of contemporary significance in developed nations were amenable to prevention and treatment by the health care system. A number of studies were subsequently done in which the rates of decline of diseases amenable to prevention and treatment were compared with the rates of decline of diseases not thought to be amenable. The amenable diseases invariably declined more dramatically. What is more, they were sufficiently diverse that no common environmental, genetic, or behavioral change could account for a simultaneous decline in all of them. Table 9-2 displays the results from a study of mortality change in six countries. Similar results were observed in Finland (Poikolainen and Eskola 1986) and in the Netherlands (Mackenbach 1988). In every instance, the causes of death amenable to prevention and treatment had declined far more dramatically than the non-amenable conditions.

In addition, and particularly telling, studies in the United States indicated that: 1) deaths from amenable causes (hypertension and diabetes) increased when health care benefits for the poor were terminated (Lurie et al. 1984); and 2) deaths from amenable causes were higher among blacks than whites in Alameda County, California (Woolhandler et al. 1985). Both studies suggested that lack of access to health services had a measurable impact on mortality.

In all the above studies of death rates from diseases previously identified as amenable or not amenable to medical intervention, it was always the amenable causes that proved to be most responsive to the availability or lack of availability of medical services. Which is to say, while McKeown may have been right in his assertions about the past futility of medical care, they were not applicable to the present and were not a reliable guide for policy makers. Indeed, a more pressing concern,

Table 9-2 Proportionate decline in mortality from 1956 to 1978 in six nations; Causes of death amenable and not amenable to medical intervention

Causes of death	England & Wales	U.S.A.	France	Japan	Italy	Sweden
Infant Mortality	48	48	73	58	67	55
Tuberculosis	90	90	92	93	90	90
Cervical Cancer	20	63	34	6	61	15
Hodgkin's disease	40	38	40	59	34	77
Chronic rheumatic heart disease	84	83	54	68	79	80
Hypertensive dis.	71	90	10	60	49	90
Stroke	33	47	51	61	36	47
Appendicitis	84	79	72	91	86	75
Cholelithiasis & cholecystitis	66	77	20	83	46	83
Maternal deaths	81	75	72	86	85	82
All causes (ages 5-64)	12	18	26	53	25	12
Amenable causes (ages 5-64)*	51	55	64	72	57	61
All other causes (ages 5-64)	4	9	19	43	17	3

* Includes tuberculosis, cervical cancer, chronic rheumatic heart disease, hypertensive disease, stroke, and cholelithiasis and cholecystitis, ages 5-64.

Source: Charlton and Velez 1986: 296.

as the United States examples immediately above suggest, is the accessibility of health care in circumstances where its efficacy is demonstrable and its lack undeniably deleterious.

To recapitulate: the moral of the story is that extrapolations of variables critical in one era to another may often prove useful, but can on occasion be amazingly misleading. Policy makers in Great Britain, Canada, and the United States still use this invalid extrapolation as a justification for cost containment.

Differentiation in a Homogenized World

There is a tendency to believe that as infectious diseases recede with Westernization and economic development, we approach ever closer to the adamantine bedrock of death, that the structure of mortality becomes both more rigid and more resistant to change. The differentiation between diseases amenable and not amenable to prevention and treatment should help dispel some of that belief. Other differentiating data are even more compelling.

Cancer is a superlative refutation of the notion of a rigid structure of mortality. Indeed it reveals that mortality is astonishingly malleable. In low mortality populations cancer ranks among the most important of the non-infectious diseases and accounts for a high proportion of all deaths. And yet, "Whereas the total...incidence varies less than four-fold from one part of the world to another, the incidence of cancer at individual sites may vary a hundred times or more" (Doll and Armstrong 1981: 93). The incidence of colon cancer is 30 per 100,000 among men in Connecticut in the United States, 12.7 in Norway and 6.0 in Poland (Hutt and Burkitt 1986: 28). The incidence of cancer of the breast is about 50 per 100,000 among women in England and 75 in Canada (p. 116). The incidence of carcinoma of the endometrium is about 30 per 100,000 women in the United States and 10 in Poland (p. 111). In a span of 500 miles along the Caspian Sea in Iran and the Soviet Union the incidence of esophageal cancer varies between 2.3 and 195.3 per 100,000 women (p. 9). As these numbers indicate, death from cancer(s) is not a fixed, rigid phenomenon.

Ischemic heart disease is equally malleable. There are dramatic temporal and regional differences in mortality rates from this disease. Beginning in the early 1950s the previously rapid decline in mortality in the United States all but ceased. The common explanation at the time was that with the virtual elimination of the infectious diseases, the bedrock of mortality had been reached and henceforth heart disease, cancer, and stroke were to be the lot of modern man. At the end of the 1960s, however, it became evident that mortality was beginning to decline rapidly once again. The decline was due largely to the decline in ischemic heart disease, and it has persisted to the present.

Studies at the individual and ecological level have shown that the decline in ischemic heart disease is real, that it is a result first of declining incidence and second of declining case-fatality rates, and that it began first in metropolitan areas with the highest proportions of white collar workers. Communities with high proportions of white collar workers continue to have the lowest rates of death from this disease (Wing et al. 1986, 1987, 1988; Kaplan et al. 1988; Pell and Fayerweather 1985; Gomez-Martin et al. 1987). A similar class difference has occurred in England, where Marmot et al. (1978: 1111) have shown that "the failure of total mortality to continue to decline in classes IV and V, as it has in classes I and II, is substantially due to the rise in the prevalence of heart disease" in the two lower classes.

Changes in deaths due to ischemic heart disease are also reflected in widely different patterns of rates of change in life expectancy in Europe and North America, as Table 9-3 indicates. From the period between the 1950s and 1970s to that of the 1970s and 1980s, the rate of improvement in Eastern Europe and the U.S.S.R. all but ceased for both males and females. In Southern Europe the high rate of improvement slowed for both sexes. In Northern and Western Europe and the United States and Canada the rates for men increased, whereas for women they either remained constant or declined slightly. That these patterns are not the result of an asymptotic effect is suggested by the fact that life expectancy in Eastern Europe, where improvement has all but ceased, is lower than in Northwestern Europe and North America, where improvement has accelerated.

Table 9-3 Average Annual Rates of Change in Life Expectancy at Birth in Europe and North America (%).

Country	From c. 1950s to 1970s*		From c. 1970s to 1980s**	
	males	females	males	females
Eastern Europe	.56	.6	0	.15
U.S.S.R.	.3	.6	.11	0
Northern Europe	.22	.33	.37	.33
Western Europe	.28	.4	.47	.41
Southern Europe	.64	.67	.35	.39
Canada	.2	.4	.36	.31
United States	.2	.3	.33	.26

*UN 1982: 9.

**European rates calculated from UN 1982: 9 and World Bank, 1986: Table 27. North American rates calculated from UN 1982: 9 and PAHO 1986:22.

The investigation of differences within the patterns of noninfectious diseases reveals quite clearly that even after infectious diseases have diminished in significance, one finds no adamantine stratum of bedrock made up of an unchanging mix of noninfectious diseases. Richard Doll has observed: "Westernization is not...an indivisible package. There is no necessary set of cancer outcomes that must follow economic development. Depending on the presence or absence of individual components of Western lifestyle, the overall incidence of cancer may either rise (as in black Americans) or fall (as it is now doing in Japan)" (Doll and Armstrong 1981: 106). Clearly, the same is true for other diseases. Thus improper generalization is to be avoided; differentiation among diseases, even in low mortality populations, is crucial.

The End of an Era: Differentiation within the Third World
It is becoming part of the conventional wisdom that we are at the end of an era of spectacular declines in mortality in the "Third World". A good many reasons are given, which I shall list, not discuss: the world economy has made it less likely that the needed support will be forthcoming to achieve the World Health Organization's goal of health for all by the year 2000; the diminution of infectious diseases has meant that noninfectious diseases have become more important, and these are intrinsically more difficult to prevent or treat: "Third World" countries must now deal with a combination of infectious and noninfectious diseases that are most likely to be susceptible to changes in individual behavior and that require improvements in education that these countries must provide for themselves.

The countries in which the problems are greatest are in Africa and Asia. Even in Latin America, however, there is evidence of a diminution in the rate of improvement in some high mortality countries such as Guatemala and Honduras (see Table 9-4).

The "Third World," however, is a highly diverse world and differentiations must be made within it. It is therefore imperative to examine the countries that are lumped under the rubric "Third World". Indeed, having advocated the value of searching for anomalies, I have found a group of scientists who set out to do just that. Ironically, they wind up providing us an object lesson in what not to do when one has discovered an anomaly. This cautionary example is to be found in the publication *Good Health at Low Cost* (Halstead et al. 1985). In this study, the authors wisely recognized that "Third World" anomalies merited their close attention —

Table 9-4 Average annual rate of change in life expectancy (%) in Latin America.

Country	Average annual rate of change in life expectancy		
	1950-60	**1960-70**	**1970s – 1985**
Costa Rica	.88	1.12	.53
El Salvador	1.86	.23	1.06
Guatemala	1.44	1.33	.97
Honduras	—	2.01	1.49
Mexico	1.72	.48	.69
Nicaragua(f)	—	.40	.92
Panama	—	.48	.72
Argentina	.65	-.12	.46
Chile	.50	.74	.98
Uruguay	—	.06	.23
Bolivia	—	—	.51
Brazil	1.0	—	.39
Colombia	—	.04	.80
Peru	—	—	.61
Venezuela	—	.59	.29
Ecuador	—	—	.86
Paraguay	—	—	.21

Sources: Rates of change 1950-60, and 1960-70, UN 1982: 142. 1970s-1985, calculated from UN 1982: 174-6 and PAHO 1986: 22.

[1] Caldwell (1986) has made a similar point about the importance of the political and cultural backgrounds of these unusual countries in attempting to account for their low levels of mortality.

namely, those countries that contradicted the conventional observation that higher mortality rates would always be associated with lower per capita income. This was not the case in the anomalous countries, e.g., Costa Rica, Sri Lanka, Kerala State (India), and China, where low per capita income coexisted with low mortality.

The authors of the various studies therefore asked what it was about these countries that made them unique. Despite some lack of unanimity among the conferees, there was general agreement that certain common-alities existed among the anomalous countries that provided lessons that could be learned and were transferrable to equally poor countries with high mortality.

The conferees concluded that a "political and social commitment to equitable distribution" would account for the unexpected phenomena in the anomalous countries. Given such a commitment to equity, three additional factors were necessary to produce the same low mortality rates in other "Third World" countries:

A. Equitable distribution and access to public health and health care beginning at the primary level and reinforced by secondary and tertiary stystems.

B. A uniformly accessible educational system emphasizing the primary level and then moving to secondary and above [stressing *maternal* education — S.J.K.].

C. Assurance of adequate nutrition at all levels of society. (Halstead et al. 1985: 248).

These extraordinary conclusions implied that the other "Third World" countries could develop such attributes by choice. This prescription for the exercise of political and social will is similar to a physician's urging an addict to get a grip on himself, exercise will power, and simply say no to drugs. It does not suggest a very profound understanding of either individual psychology or the processes underlying addiction. Similarly, the recommendations made by Halstead et al. did not suggest a profound understanding of the social and political processes underlying the evolution of different nations, and were approximately as useful as the doctor's advice to the addict. In fact, the only likely result of these recommendations would be to justify limits on the generosity of donor institutions. Once "Third World" countries had revolutionized them-selves by an act of will, the donor institutions would need only to provide technical and training assistance. That in fact may be all that is possible in this era of "aid weariness" (Arndt 1987: 143), but First World exhaustion does not validate the scientific conclusions of Halstead et al.

> Their advocacy of primary health care and nutrition are standard. Their originality lies in their stress on maternal education. Unfor-tunately, maternal education — their one non-biological recom-mendation — is treated by Halstead et al. as though it were just another biomedical intervention. They prescibe it in yearly doses as one does DPT and other vaccines. But maternal education is not

a biomedical phenomenon, it is a cultural phenomenon and means something quite different in different cultural contexts. To fail to recognize this creates not understanding but the illusion of understanding. Does maternal education mean a change in the balance of power within the household? Does it represent an increase in instrumental knowledge about hygiene and nutrition? Does it signify a change in the way a woman thinks of herself quite apart from the content of the education? Finally, what difference does the social environment make in the effectiveness of education? Why do four years of maternal education reduce the risk of child mortality more in Cuba than Bolivia? To think of education as a vaccine that prevents infant mortality the way measles vaccine prevents measles is to ignore the cultural and socio-political context within which education occurs and which endows it with significance.[1]

Halstead et al. teach us that anomalous cultures call our attention to important exceptions to what we may have thought were universally true observations, and for this they deserve enormous credit. They also teach us, however, that anomalous cultures may be studied in vain if one extrapolates baselessly and fails to understand the history and institutions of each culture. This may be one of the most important lessons we can learn in considering mortality patterns in what is unfortunately packaged under the label of the "Third World."

Conclusions

I began by saying that my observations have both epistemological and policy implications. In respect of the former, we generally think of science as the establishment of elegantly simple, universal truths. In this sense scientific truths transcend the particularity of time and place. It is irrelevant to the effectiveness of smallpox vaccine whether a society is organized neolocally or patrilocally. Once one can find and vaccinate all susceptible individuals, the spread of the disease will cease. It is in this sense that science may be said to transcend culture. That is indeed its great attraction. And on occasion the consequences of a science-based technological intervention are every bit as successful as we hope they will be. The impact of antibiotics on the transformation of infectious diseases in rich societies beginning in the late 1930s, the great success of the smallpox eradication campaign, and the possibility of preventing and treating iodine deficiency disorders are all examples.

Such interventions, based on the assumption that science is universal, overleap the barriers of national borders and cultural boundaries. Indeed what is so powerfully attractive about this vision of scientific knowledge is precisely its universality: its accessibility to all and its applicability to all. In this sense science is liberating and deeply democratic. Penicillin can cure pneumococcal pneumonia regardless of the moral or financial worth of the patient no matter what his or her skin color. It is the culture of the infecting organism, not the patient, that is relevant.

This vision is so seductive because its elegance, its simplicity, and its universality allow us to forget the many ways in which diseases are expressions of particular cultures in particular social and ecological settings. So seductive is it, indeed, that it becomes synonymous with science itself. This is a problem, for not all disease conditions are susceptible to explanations based upon the idea of a necessary cause, the absence of which always assures the absence of the particular condition. Many health problems in both rich and poor countries are still best explained by multiple weakly sufficient causes, or risk factors, and understanding their incidence, prevalence, and distribution, as well as their prevention and treatment, may require intimate understanding of particular people and settings. This demands a different kind of science, one based on local knowledge of social organization, cultural beliefs and values, and patterns of behavior, rather than simply universal knowledge of the behavior of viruses and GNP per capita.

There are a number of policy implications that flow from this. One has to do with the politics of science itself. It is clear that these different ways of understanding the causal attribution of diseases in populations characterize different professional disciplines. Physicians tend to accept a universalistic notion of attribution. Many demographers, sociologists, and economists tend to take a similar approach, using social or economic measures rather than tubercle bacilli or vitamins as explanatory variables. Anthropologists and historians tend to be more particularistic. These different ways of understanding causation (e.g., "the biomedical model," "the anthropological approach") may — and ideally should — cross-fertilize one another in mutually beneficial ways. Because they are attached to concrete professional interests, however, they are even more likely to become ideological weapons with which different groups may attack one another. This will remain a contentious issue for which no general solution exists. Nonetheless, as we become increasingly concerned about the social, cultural, and behavioral determinants of health, it would be prudent not to be prematurely attracted to easy generalizations based on inferences from historical or contemporary cases but to study in fine-grained detail the settings in which interventions are planned.

Such an approach has broader implications, for it suggests that one ought not assure "policy makers" that, for example, all they need to do to improve health is provide a modicum of primary education and a minimum amount of food to even the poorest members of their societies. To offer such assurances would be to assume that which must be demonstrated. Minimal education and food are important, even necessary; whether they are sufficient is far from certain. Moreover, while it may be good tactics to package educational reform as a technological fix, most government officials will understand that it is likely to be far more than that; that increasing the literacy of mothers may have profound consequences not only for child survival but for the structure of families and for the fate of political leaders themselves.

The point I wish to make, finally, is not that generalizations are impossible and to be avoided. It is rather that generalizations based on either national statistics or extrapolations from case studies must be treated with caution because the sociocultural determinants of health and of mortality and morbidity are far too complex to be captured by formulaic abstractions. They can best be understood by immersion in the lives of the people whose deaths we are seeking to explain.

Acknowledgments

I am grateful to George Alter, Theodore Brown, Anthony Carter, Edith Efron, and Stanley Engerman for helpful comments. This article originally appeared in J.C. Caldwell, et al., eds. 1990. *What We Know About the Health Transition: The Cultural, Social and Behavioural Determinants of Health, Health Transition Series,* No. 2, Vol. 1: 92–109. Canberra: Health Transition Centre, Australian National University.

References

Arndt, H.W. 1987. *Economic Development: The History of an Idea.* Chicago: University of Chicago Press.

Arriaga, E.E., and K. Davis. 1969. "The pattern of mortality change in Latin America." *Demography,* 6: 223–42.

Ashby, H.T. 1922. *Infant Mortality.* Cambridge: Cambridge University Press.

Berton, P. 1980. *The Invasion of Canada, 1812–1813*. Toronto: McClelland and Stewart.

Brown, J.C. 1988. "Public reform for private gain? Public health and sanitary infrastructure in German cities 1877–1910." Paper presented at the Annual Meeting of the Social Science History Association, Chicago, November.

Brown, J.C. 1989. "Public health reform and the decline of urban mortality: The case of Germany, 1876–1912." Paper presented at the Annual Meeting of the Population Association of America, Baltimore, MD., March.

Caldwell, J.C. 1986. "Routes to low mortality in poor countries." *Population and Development Review*, 12: 171–220.

Charlton, J.R.H., and R. Velez. 1986. "Some international comparisons of mortality amenable to medical intervention." *British Medical Journal*, 292: 295–301.

Doll, R., and B. Armstrong. 1981. "Cancer." In H. Trowell and D. Burkitt, eds. *Western Diseases*. Cambridge, MA: Harvard University Press.

Gomez-Martin, O., A.R. Folsom, R.E. Kottke, S.C.H. Chen, D.R. Jacobs, R.F. Gillum, S. A. Edlavitch, and H. Balackburn. 1987. "Improvement in long-term survival among patients hospitalized with acute myocardial infarction, 1970 to 1980." *New England Journal of Medicine*, 316: 1353–9.

Halstead, S.B., J.A. Walsh, and K.S. Warren. 1985. *Good Health at Low Cost*. New York: The Rockefeller Foundation.

Hanley, S.B. 1987. "Urban sanitation in preindustrial Japan." *Journal of Interdisciplinary History*, 18: 1–26.

Herring, D.A., and L.A. Sawchuck. 1986. "The emergence of class differentials in infant mortality in the Jewish community of Gibraltar, 1840 to 1929." *Collegium Antropologicum*, 10: 29–35.

Hill, P. 1986. *Development Economics on Trial: The Anthropological Case for a Prosecution*. Cambridge: Cambridge University Press.

Hutt, M.S.R., and D.P. Burkitt. 1986. *The Geography of Non-Infectious Diseases*. Oxford: Oxford University Press.

Jannetta, A.B. 1987. *Epidemics and Mortality in Early Modern Japan*. Princeton, NJ: Princeton University Press.

Johansson, S.R., and C. Mosk. 1987. "Exposure, resistance and life expectancy: Disease and death during the economic development of Japan, 1900–1960." *Population Studies*, 41: 207–235.

Kaplan, G.A., B.A. Cohen, and J. Guralnik. 1988. "The decline in ischemic heart disease mortality: Prospective evidence from the Alameda County Study." *American Journal of Epidemiology*, 127: 1131–42.

Kunitz, S.J. 1983. "Speculations on the European mortality decline." *The Economic History Review*, 36: 349–64.

Kunitz, S.J. 1986. "Mortality since Malthus." *The State of Population Theory.* Oxford: B.H. Blackwell.

Lang, J. 1975. *Conquest and Commerce: Spain and England in the Americas.* New York: Academic Press.

Lurie, N., N.B. Ward, M.F. Shapiro, and R.H. Brook. 1984. "Termination from Medi-Cal: Does it affect health?" *New England Journal of Medicine,* 311: 480–4.

McKeown, T. 1976a. *The Modern Rise of Population.* New York: Academic Press.

McKeown, T. 1976b. *The Role of Medicine.* London: Nuffield Provincial Hospitals Trust.

Mackenbach, J.P. 1988. "Mortality and Medical Care." Unpublished Ph.D. thesis, Erasmus University, Rotterdam, The Netherlands.

Marmot, M.G., A.M. Adelstein, N. Robinson, and G.A. Rose. 1978. "Changing social class distribution of heart disease." *British Medical Journal,* 2: 1109–12.

Mosk, C., and S.R. Johansson. 1986. "Income and mortality: Evidence from modern Japan." *Population and Development Review,* 12: 415–440.

Pan American Health Organization. 1986. *Health Conditions in the Americas, 1981–1984:* Vol. 1. Scientific Publications No. 500. Washington, DC: PAHO.

Pell, S., and W.E. Fayerweather. 1985. "Trends in the incidence of myocardial infarction and associated mortality and morbidity in a large employed population, 1957–1983." *New England Journal of Medicine,* 312: 1005–11.

Poikolainen, K., and J. Eskola. 1986. "The effect of health services on mortality: Decline in death rates from amenable and non–amenable causes in Finland, 1969–1981." *The Lancet,* 1: 199–202.

Rutstein, D.D., W. Berenberg, T.C. Chalmers, C.G. Child 3rd, A.P. Fishman, and E.B. Perrin. 1976. "Measuring the quality of medical care: A clinical method." *New England Journal of Medicine,* 294: 582–8.

Sanchez-Albornoz, N. 1974. *The Population of Latin America: A History.* Berkeley: University of California Press.

Sawchuck, L.A., D.A. Herring, and L.R. Waks. 1985. "Evidence of a Jewish advantage: A study of infant mortality in Gibraltar, 1870–1959." *American Anthropologist,* 87: 616–25.

Schmelz, U.O. 1971. *Infant and Early Childhood Mortality among the Jews of the Diaspora.* Jerusalem: The Institute of Contemporary Jewry, The Hebrew University.

Stein, S.J., and B.H. Stein. 1970. *The Colonial Heritage of Latin America.* New York: Oxford University Press.

Szreter, S. 1988. "The importance of social intervention in Britain's mortality decline 1850–1914: A re-interpretation of the role of public health." *Social History of Medicine,* 1: 1–37.

United Nations. 1982. *Levels and Trends of Mortality since 1950.* New York: UN.

Wing, S., C. Hayes, G. Heiss, E. John, M. Knowles, W. Riggan, and H.A. Tyroler. 1986. "Geographic variation in the onset of decline of ischemic heart disease mortality in the United States." *American Journal of Public Health,* 76: 1404–8.

Wing S., M. Casper, C.G. Hayes, P. Dargent-Molina, W. Riggan, and H.A. Tyroler. 1987. "Changing association between community occupational structure and ischemic heart disease mortality in the United States." *The Lancet,* November 7: 1067–70.

Wing, S., M. Casper, W. Riggan, C. Hayes, and H.A. Tyroler. 1988. "Socio-environmental characteristics associated with the onset of decline of ischemic heart disease mortality in the United States." *American Journal of Public Health,* 78: 923–6.

Woodbury, R.M. 1926. *Infant Mortality and its Causes.* Baltimore: The Williams and Wilkins Company.

Woolhandler, S., D.U. Himmelstein, R. Silber, M. Bader, M. Harnly, and A.A. Jones. 1985. "Medical care and mortality: Racial differences in preventable deaths." *International Journal of Health Services,* 15: 1–22.

10

Parallels between the Mortality Transition and the Fertility Transition

Joseph E. Potter

Starting with the earliest formulations of demographic transition theory, demographers have attached considerable importance to the causal relations that might exist between levels of fertility and mortality. Yet they, along with other social scientists, have tended to view and approach the two phenomena in quite different ways. Fertility has always been considered "social" or "behavioral" in nature, while mortality has been considered a direct result of living standards, hygiene, and medical technology. At a time when we are considering new ways in which social scientists might approach the study of health, it is useful to review the relations between fertility and mortality and to compare and contrast these two areas of research. By juxtaposing the different sets of issues and methods, we may identify opportunities for each field to benefit from the experience of the other. Beyond that practical endeavor lies the strategic question of how to organize and approach research on mortality, fertility, and their interrelations.

After offering a brief characterization of recent social science research on fertility, I will outline what appear to be the reasons social scientists have subjected mortality and fertility to quite different sorts of inquiries. The discussion then proceeds to the numerous similarities between the two fields of research. The thrust of the argument is that, at least among demographers, the "social" and "behavioral" nature of health and mortality has heretofore been severely underestimated, that considerable overlap and complementarity exists between research on fertility and mortality, and that most of the customary reasons for thinking that mortality research is inherently less social and behavioral than fertility research are not valid.

Social Science Research on Fertility

A very large part of recent work on the determinants of fertility, particularly with reference to contemporary developing societies, is focused on the demand for children (Caldwell 1983; Bulatao and Lee 1983; Miró and Potter 1980). Researchers commonly assume that fertility decisions respond to the balance of benefits and costs that childbearing entails, and that shifts in this calculus underlie the transition from high to low fertility. The costs of children are thought to be both direct (e.g., expenditures on food, clothing, and education) and indirect (e.g., expenditures of time), while their benefits have been construed as the money the children may eventually remit to their parental household as well as the labor they contribute toward household maintenance and domestic production. A variety of historical, development-induced changes, such as urbanization, industrialization, proletarianization of the labor force, the appearance of consumer goods, increases in the opportunities for and the returns to education, and the establishment of social security institutions that provide support for the elderly, are thought to affect this economic calculus, leading either to increases in the costs of children or to reductions in their relative benefits.

Development or modernization is also seen as leading to changes in norms, beliefs, and attitudes that adversely affect the demand for children. Such change is held to be especially important with respect to consumption and to relations within the family. Increasing aspirations for newly available consumer goods provided by improved transportation and communication networks are seen as displacing aspirations for large families (Freedman 1978). Much is also made of changes in intra-familial relationships. Of particular importance are the collapse of patriarchy, strengthening of the conjugal bond, and the advent of shared decision-making between spouses (Caldwell 1976). The hypothesis is that the emergence of the nuclear family and of sentiment lead to greater expression of a mother's maternal feelings, and, eventually, to a broadening of the range of issues perceived as requiring active decision-making. Prominent among the "new issues" that spouses may address is fertility control.

Another substantial segment of the fertility literature deals directly with the use of contraception. The basic issue is, given motivation to space pregnancies or limit their number, what determines whether a woman will practice contraception, and, if she does so, what sort of method she will use (Lapham and Simmons 1987). Much of the debate regarding fertility determinants has hinged on the relative importance of efforts to increase the availability of contraceptive technology, and changes — programmatic or otherwise — that may have led to increased motivation of couples or mothers to restrict fertility. Controversy also surrounds the influence of tastes, norms and ideas regarding birth control on the disposition to use contraception (Cleland and Wilson 1987; Bogue 1983), as compared with the influence of either the "objective supply environment" (Hermalin and Entwistle 1985) or the underlying demand for children.

While fertility research has undoubtedly reached a certain maturity in the sense that a substantial literature has been amassed along with a considerable methodological apparatus, there is no consensus on the major issues toward which attention has been directed (McNicoll 1978). Debate continues concerning the factors underlying the rapid fertility change that has occurred in many parts of the third world, and there is uncertainty as to the trajectory that fertility will follow in Sub-Saharan Africa and other subregions where no appreciable downward change has been seen to date. Perhaps the most important and indisputable result of the study of fertility determinants is that people no longer believe there are easy generalizations to be drawn about the relationship of fertility to development, nor do they harbor the illusion of an easy "technological fix" for the problem of high fertility.

Social Science Research on Mortality

Although there is an obvious correspondence between the "living standards versus technical change" debate regarding the determinants of secular change in mortality and the "development versus family planning program" debate with respect to fertility decline, the research issues surrounding the transition in mortality have long been thought of as different from, and distinctly less behavioral than, those pertaining to the fertility transition. One difference between the two areas of inquiry that may account for this perception is the absence in mortality research of an analog to the demand for children. The demand for survival is taken for granted. In Stolnitz's words, "Greater longevity is probably the most universally and readily accepted of major human values" (1953, p.45). This idea was clearly spelled out in a once-popular introduction to demography, as follows:

"The tendency of mortality to decline earlier and initially more rapidly than fertility results in large measure from the difference in human attitudes toward death and procreation. Death is usually an altogether involuntary, though, inevitable event, whereas procreation is the outcome of a motivated act and often represents the fulfillment of a cherished individual and social goal." (Wrong 1956, p. 31)

The author later notes:

"...the vigor with which men have sought to postpone the inevitable coming of death has been amply attested throughout history. The intensity of their desire to procreate, however, is a far less certain quantity as the rapid decline of the birth rate in the past century indicates. The motivations and cultural norms underlying and governing fertility are much more elaborate and variable than in the case of mortality." (p. 49)

The implication is that demographers, in their search to understand the determinants of mortality, need not concern themselves with the behavior and motivation of individuals.

Similar contrasts are often drawn with respect to societal goals and social programs. A program or policy to reduce fertility can only be justified in terms of the effect this will have on economic growth, or on some other widely accepted goal. On the other hand, since longevity is a universal value, reduced mortality is clearly an objective for society to pursue in its own right. Indeed, the same premium placed by all members of the society on health and longevity leads one to expect "there is apt to be less resistance to reforms that will lower mortality than to the adoption of practices that will reduce fertility" (Wrong 1956, p. 32).

One of the most intriguing aspects of fertility policy for social scientists is the possibility, perhaps even the likelihood, of a discrepancy between the goals and objectives of individuals and those of society (Demeny 1971). The problem arises when some of the costs of high fertility, e.g., higher unemployment sometime in the future, are not borne by those making the reproductive decisions. A solution is to change the incentive structure so that the private costs of children are brought into line with their social costs. How this might be done so as to bring reproductive behavior around to some socially desirable level has been the subject of much theorizing as well a sizable amount of post hoc analysis of both successful and unsuccessful policies (Berelson 1969; McNicoll 1980).

While there are no analogous externalities involving differences between individual ambitions for a long life and the general welfare of society, arguments related to the difference between private and public evaluations of the consequences of particular actions or measures are one of the primary justifications for government intervention in the health sector. Indeed, for such reasons virtually all "public health" activities such as malaria spraying, immunization campaigns, and collective improvements in sewage disposal and water supply are viewed as being the responsibility of the community rather than the individual. The contrast with fertility is not so much in the nature of the policy problem, as in the scope for mandating action without engaging in what might be viewed as the coercion of individuals.

The distinction is an important one, in part because much of the improvement in life expectancy that has taken place in different parts of the world is often attributed to public health measures (Stolnitz 1953). The idea, simply put, is that individuals can be ordered to have their children immunized, their houses sprayed, or their garbage disposed of in certain ways without infringing on their civil liberty. The presumption is not only that improved health is an important social objective that warrants such interference in private life, but that there will be little resistance to such measures since they are consonant with individual goals. Moreover, changing people's ideas, values, and ambitions has not usually been seen to be as necessary to the success of an immunization campaign, for example, as it is to the success of a family planning program. The institutional change and behavioral modification that are viewed as central to policies to alter fertility figure much less prominently in the design and implementation of public health policies.

If the social and behavioral determinants of fertility have often been seen as more complex and variable than those of mortality, the contrary is clearly true with respect to the complexity and variability of the underlying biological processes (Mosley 1984). Indeed, it is easily argued that the dominance of the biomedical model of causation in the health field has been so great as to leave little room for attention to social and behavioral influences on health outcomes (Starr 1982). Moreover, this biomedical dominance creates substantial barriers to entry for social scientists. Two disparate examples serve to make the point. First, those who would research illness behavior and health seeking using an anthropological perspective are often encouraged to get both an M.D. and a Ph.D if they wish to be taken seriously. Second, for a sociologist to argue that a phenomenon such as social relationships affects survival, he or she must have a plausible hypothesis concerning the underlying biological mechanisms to be credible (House et al. 1988).

At least by comparison, the biological processes underlying fertility are less imposing. And while debates about certain biological issues related to fertility, such as the influence of malnutrition on fecundity, have sometimes been heated (Bongaarts 1980; Frisch 1978; Trussell 1978), they have commanded relatively little attention. The main biological or biomedical challenge confronting the field of human reproduction is, of course, the development and testing of new contraceptives. Efforts on this front have absorbed a considerable fraction of the resources devoted to fertility research, but have not dominated attention (and budgets) as completely as have laboratory and clinical research related to disease processes. Indeed, on numerous occasions it has been argued that contraceptive development is severely under funded relative to other areas of biomedical research (Greep 1976; Commission on Health Research for Development 1990).

Some of the difference in the priority accorded social science research on mortality and fertility, and a certain amount of the separation between the two enterprises, may be construed as resulting from disparate diagnoses of the state of knowledge, the nature of the respective policy problems, and of the interrelations that exist between poverty, poor health, and high fertility. For much of the last three decades, a marked contrast has colored perceptions of what social science or applied programmatic or clinical research might contribute to solving the problems of high fertility and high mortality in poor countries. With respect to high fertility, there was the question of what needed to be done. Would simply providing family planning services induce a change in behavior? A good case was made for more potent measures, and social scientists were asked to estimate the impacts of incentive schemes, efforts at social engineering, or even of attempts to "restructure development" (Cassen 1976; Berelson 1977). In contrast to this perceived need for innovative interventions to reduce fertility, there were few if any questions regarding what remedial policy measures were necessary to lessen mortality differentials and accelerate improvement in life expectancy. The reigning view in the mid to late 1970s was that a reallocation of resources from metropolitan hospitals to primary health care and preventive medicine would be sufficient (World Bank 1975). The issue was not what needed to be done, but how to get it done. The missing ingredient was "political will" (see Reich, chapter 15, this volume), and there was no perceived need for complex social interventions of the sort that might alter the incentive structure for reproductive behavior.

Further, in some quarters, the notion was commonplace that the two research enterprises were working at cross purposes. In attempting to explain why health interests received such a low priority in development planning in less developed countries, Knowles (1980) noted that public health programs were often blamed for the population explosion. Efforts to improve health were viewed as counterproductive, and there was "silent resistance" to spending more money on them. Such reasoning was never prevalent among the demographers and social scientists involved in population research. That it held sway among those responsible for funding research and development assistance is, however, attested to by the recent effort of the independent Commission on Health Research for Development to argue strenuously that the negative consequences of rapid population growth and high fertility were *not* reasons "to delay or constrain health advances" (1990: 8). Whether differences of opinion on this issue have been responsible for the bureaucratic divisions between health and population funding that evolved in the U.S. Congress, in the United Nations system, and in agencies such as the Rockefeller Foundation is, at this point, an open question.

The Striking Similarities Between the Two Endeavors

Social scientists tended to view mortality and fertility differently, and donors and policy makers sometimes failed to see the complementarity between health and population programs in spite of numerous parallels and considerable overlap between the two behavioral and programmatic domains. The similarities between family planning programs and programs to promote child survival are particularly striking. As Bhatia et al. (1989) have noted:

> Both have demographic objectives; family planning is concerned with altering the levels of fertility while child survival is concerned with reducing the levels of infant and child mortality. In both cases, the primary actors in producing these demographic changes are families, especially mothers, who are concerned with reproduction and the household production of health. Programs designed to assist families and mothers in this process are essentially social interventions facilitated by technologies (p. 2).

The new technology in both cases is medical technology, and more often than not it is promoted and delivered by the same individuals. Typically, these are medical personnel, broadly defined, in the employ of private or public health institutions. Doctors are critical actors on both fronts, along with nurses, pharmacists, and community health workers. Both family planning and child survival, despite some wishful thinking to the contrary, are highly medicalized endeavors in the contemporary third world.

There is, of course, a marked contrast between this level of medicalization and the level that probably existed in the now-industrialized countries as they passed through their fertility and mortality transitions 100 years ago. As has been repeatedly pointed out by students of both transitions, very little in the way of effective technology was available either to control fertility or to deal with disease (McKeown 1976; Knodel and Van de Walle 1979). The declines in demographic rates were obtained by quite different means, and presumably without the friction between traditional and modern medical systems observed today (Shedlin and Hollerbach 1981; Muecke 1976; Young 1981).

Turning to the determinants of the two transitions, further similarities and points of contact can be found. To a considerable extent, and at varying distances, the determinants seem to be the same. One of the enviable successes of population research is the development of a parsimonious and relatively well-documented account of the proximate determinants of fertility decline (Bongaarts and Potter 1980). A strong case has been made that only four such variables determine the level of fertility: age at first marriage, breastfeeding, contraceptive use, and abortion. Each, of course, has important health consequences. Contraceptive practice may enhance the health of both mothers and their children, by lengthening intervals between births and by providing a means of avoiding high-risk pregnancies (Hobcraft et al. 1985; National Research Council 1989). Early age at first marriage is responsible for considerable maternal mortality and morbidity in Africa (Harrison and Rossiter 1985), as is unhygienic abortion in many parts of the world. Breastfeeding is essential to child survival, both for the protection and nutrition it affords the child and for its influence on birth spacing. One immediate example of the importance of these proximate determinants of fertility for mortality is provided by Kunitz (chapter 9, this volume), who attributes much of the difference in life expectancy between Eastern and Western Europe in the 18th and 19th centuries to differences in age at first marriage and breastfeeding.

The dominance of the biomedical model, with its emphasis on diseases as the immediate causes of death, has been held responsible for the absence of a similar framework for mortality. But efforts in this direction (Schultz 1980, 1984; Mosley and Chen 1984) have included maternal factors and nutrient deficiency as important parts of the proposed schema. Clearly there is more to child survival and good health than late marriage, breastfeeding, and contraception; but these practices are viewed as central factors, particularly where maternal and child health problems loom large.

At one remove from the proximate determinants are factors that, in addition to being "socioeconomic" and "institutional" in nature, are themselves determined by the larger structural changes taking place in a society. Faria (1989) calls these the proximate structural determinants. One of these, education, has received close scrutiny as a factor underlying changes in both fertility and child survival. Indeed, the realization that infant and child mortality are closely related to the educational attainment of mothers, together with an appreciation that the association exists at higher ecological levels, has probably been of paramount importance in convincing health experts that mortality is socially as well as biologically determined (Mosley 1983; Caldwell 1979).

The statistical evidence showing an association between women's schooling on the one hand, and reduced fertility and reduced child mortality on the other, as well as the causal relationships that might account for the association are carefully reviewed by LeVine et al. (chapter 12, this volume). On causality, they suggest first that schooling permits the acquisition of skills that influence a woman's later interactions with the health bureaucracy. Second, education is a route to and symptomatic of advantages in the emerging "occupational prestige hierarchy and thus in the social strata emerging from economic development." Finally, schooling leads to a revised concept of the parent-child relationship, ultimately producing a healthier and more demanding child.

This schema is useful for conceptualizing how other proximate structural determinants such as coverage by social security, exposure to the mass media, and incorporation in the modern health care system could affect fertility and mortality. These too can be expected to confer skills, change aspirations, affect conceptions of parenting, and increase access to health and family planning services. As variables, factors such as social security and exposure to the mass media and the modern medical system are harder to measure than education; yet all three have expanded dramatically in most parts of the developing world that have experienced major demographic change in recent decades. And, in each case, there is ample reason to hypothesize that the change has exerted a major influence on both mortality and fertility.

Social security varies widely in the third world, but in many cases the programs associated with formal, salaried employment offer such benefits as insurance for disability and employment-related accidents, maternity leave, a retirement pension, and coverage for a variety of medical expenses (Mesa-Lago 1981). Enrollment in such programs may reduce motivation for children as a source of old age security or risk insurance, and it directly increases access to the health care system. More broadly, the expansion of social security programs may consecrate retirement with a pension as a strategic dimension of citizenship (Faria 1989), and alter the nature of the intergenerational contract between parents and children. The rapid expansion in the reach of television may have even more pervasive effects. Messages conveyed by soap operas, advertising, and news shows boost consumerism and sexuality, and they may also influence ideas about family relationships and family size, transmit a considerable amount of health-related knowledge, and enhance the image of modern medicine.

The advent of specialized, clinic and hospital-based curative care and the increasing medicalization associated with such care, can be construed as having exerted a strong influence on behavior. Fertility, as well as health, has been affected. Hospitals, clinics and pharmacies have become the places where contraceptive supplies and services are obtained. Additionally, increased exposure to the medical subculture and the progressive inclusion of new aspects of social behavior under medical authority have undermined the legitimacy of such "traditional" authorities as priests, parents, brothers, and husbands to dictate behavior related to sexuality and reproduction. Clearly, it has also legitimized intervention in biological processes, imposed new standards of hygiene and body care, and lent credibility to the efficacy of surgical procedures and allopathic medicine (Faria 1989). As a final possibility, just as LeVine et al. suggest that girls identify with the role of teacher as they have experienced it in the classroom, so also may they identify with the role of doctor as they have experienced it in a hospital or clinic setting. In one case mothers tend to become "teachers" of their children; in the other, they tend to become "doctors" to their children (and perhaps to others in the household). The latter possibility is quite consistent with the growing literature on lay referral in a variety of settings (Angel and Thoits 1987).

There are two remaining types of determinants. One refers to the "less proximate" structural determinants, the other to the shifts in norms and ideas that may underlie changes in parenting and other health-related behaviors as well as contraceptive practice. The latter are of particular interest because their relevance in the health domain is not restricted to the health of mothers and children. The ideas that arguably matter to both reproductive behavior and health more generally are those pertaining to the family, the status and roles of women, beauty and sex, and the legitimacy of modern medicine.

A good example of the role of normative influences was recently set forth by Vallin (1988) in an effort to identify the factors underlying the enormous advantage in life expectancy enjoyed by females in most developed countries. He argues that, among other reasons, women live longer than men because they tend to be in closer touch with their bodies. There are two reasons for this rapport. The first is the influence of preventive gynecological and obstetric care in teaching the custom and the value of prevention and of watchfulness more generally. Men are not afforded this opportunity in their teens and early twenties. The second reason is the premium on beauty rather than on forcefulness that the society imposes on women. They are encouraged to stay young and healthy for as long as possible. Men have not been subject to the same norm, although Vallin notes that this now seems to be changing.

Vallin was writing about determinants of health and longevity, but the same normative pressures have clear relevance to ideas about childbearing and contraceptive practice. In many parts of the Third World, ideals regarding femininity are changing rapidly *pari passu* with an enormous increase in exposure to television. The ideal woman is no longer one who spends most of her reproductive years either pregnant or nursing, but someone who is physically attractive and well preserved. As a consequence, traditional forms of birth spacing and family limitation are viewed with increasing disfavor, and modern contraception becomes the only rational alternative.

What about the larger structural determinants? How are such phenomena as industrialization, urbanization, and changes in agrarian structure and family organization related to mortality and fertility? It has long been an article of faith that insertion in the economic mode of production had an important influence on people's incentives for reproduction (Notestein 1953). The kind of work an individual or family was engaged in presumably also influenced the environmental and occupational health risks, but in fact remarkably little attention has been given to the pathways through which changes in the mode of production may have influenced mortality. Indeed, Kunitz (chapter 9, this volume) provides one of the few available explorations of this set of relations. Arguing that "the label of economic development obscures many of the processes that are directly associated with mortality," (p 256) he highlights specific social, cultural, and agricultural patterns that account for the difference in mortality between Eastern and Western Europe in the 18th and 19th centuries, and between the various colonial regimes that were installed in the New World. For present purposes, the value of his chapter is to demonstrate how a number of structural factors that have long been credited with influencing fertility deserve an equally important place as determinants of mortality.

With respect to historical experience, Kunitz argues that many of the same features of economic and family organization in Western and Northern Europe that have been highlighted by Wrigley and Schofield (1983), Smith (1981), and Lesthaeghe (1980) as integral to a homeostatic system for regulating the level of fertility — in particular, the interlocking relations between farm ownership, agrarian service, and delayed marriage — had beneficial effects on life expectancy. In Eastern and Southern Europe, as in the Spanish colonies in the Americas, the institutions that led to high fertility — large estates devoted to single crops grown for export worked by an impoverished peasantry — also led to high levels of mortality. Kunitz tries to impart the lesson that debates about mortality which are centered on such general distinctions as rural versus urban, agricultural versus industrial, and low versus high living standards are bound to miss some of the most important aspects of the social and cultural determinants of mortality. A similar lesson was learned by fertility researchers some years ago (Demeny 1968; Knodel and Van de Walle 1979).

The parallels between fertility research and mortality research, underscore a variety of opportunities for profitable imitation. In next few years, those familiar with the fertility/family planning social scientific enterprise can be expected to come forward with sizeable agendas for increasing the pertinence and relevance of social science research on health. Indeed, Bhatia et al. (1989) have already prepared an impressive review of "family planning program strategies, operations, and research as a model for primary health care programs." The topics they cover extend from unmet need for contraception and client-provider relations to innovations in program evaluation. More generally, fertility research offers a host of approaches and methodologies that could be adapted to the realms of health, morbidity, and mortality. For example, lessons learned from studying the value of children, in carrying out retrospective surveys, and in studying the institutional determinants of fertility might have immediate implications for investigation of health related topics.

Clearly, there is much that fertility research has to offer, especially in Third World contexts. But it would be shortsighted to create or recommend a one-way line of communication. Fertility researchers studying the massive adoption of modern contraceptive technology also have much to learn from experienced students of illness perception, health-seeking behavior, and health care systems. Indeed, another implication of the parallels noted above is that, just as there has been an under-appreciation in some circles of mortality as a social phenomenon, so too has there been an under-appreciation of fertility as a medical phenomenon.

Transitions in Family Relationships, Medical Technology, Fertility and Mortality

Chenery and Srinivasan observed that it is useful to think of development as a spectrum of interrelated transitions (1988). It is plausible to argue that the links between the two transitions considered here, the mortality transition and the fertility transition, are particularly strong. It might be appropriate to think of them together as simply one transition, or at least as fields of inquiry that fit together naturally.

The argument for integration would seem to hinge on two essential hypotheses or postulates. The first is that a single behavioral shift underlies both transitions. The second is that the character and the source of the technology for both transitions is the same. The central behavioral shift is alluded to or described in many of the chapters in this volume. For example, Condran and Preston, in their analysis of the dramatic differential in child survival between French-Canadians and Jewish immigrants to the United States at the turn of the century (chapter 8, this volume), focus on the difference in the "child centeredness" of Jewish and French-Canadian families, as indicated by differences in the frequency with which mothers were employed away from home during pregnancy and during the infant's first year of life. And LeVine et al., as they explore the different ways that schooling may lead to increased child survival and reduced fertility, emphasize the changing nature of the mother-child relationship. The change they describe involves increased verbal and visual interaction, an increase in the demands the child places upon the mother, and a shift in the conception of the demands of parenting. Finally, the Caldwells, in their discussion of patriarchy and its pernicious effects on child survival, focus on shifts in relations between the sexes and generations within the family. They attach particular importance to the shift toward greater emotional nucleation.

Each of these chapters emphasizes a different dimension of a general shift in social and familial relationships that has clear and profound consequences for the health and welfare of children, and for the level of fertility. The first dimension refers to the place of children; the shift along this dimension involves the social invention of childhood as a protected period of maturation and education, and the *child* as someone to be loved and nurtured (Ariès 1962). The second dimension refers to patterns of communication and decision making within the family, with the shift consisting of an increase in interaction between mothers and children, and between husbands and spouses. The third and final dimension involves the pattern of authority and control, and the shift involves a breakdown in "traditional" patterns whereby the old control the young, and men control women.

What about the means of achieving reduced mortality and fertility? In the previous century and well into this century, medical technology and knowledge of disease processes were extremely primitive by modern standards (McKeown 1976). So too were the methods available to avoid pregnancy. Yet the shelf was by no means empty, as Condran and Preston (Chapter 8, this volume) have documented with respect to child care, and motivated parents or couples could take moderately effective steps toward attaining their reproductive and child health objectives. The contemporary situation is, of course, vastly improved. The means of reducing the incidence and fatality of the major infectious diseases of childhood and the means of avoiding or terminating pregnancy have advanced greatly as knowledge of the pertinent processes, and the technology for intervening in those processes has mushroomed since World War II. The means for disseminating this knowledge and technology have also grown. With this progress have come undreamed-of advances in the stature of the medical profession and in the size and influence of the health care and pharmaceutical industries (Starr 1982). It is this profession and these "industries" that have supplied the knowledge and technology underlying the post war transitions in both mortality and fertility, and that have exercised control over the vast majority of programs to accelerate these transitions.

Rather than argue for some over-arching process bringing all of these changes along as part of a universal pattern of development or modernization, I would contend that changes in family relationships and in the stature and reach of modern medicine are, in most Third World situations and places, over-determined. In short, so many possible vehicles and grounds for these changes exist that it is not necessary to believe that they are always brought about in the same way and for the same reasons. Nevertheless, the picture that emerges is one of interlocking and often simultaneous changes in fertility, mortality, parenting, and medicalization.

Several loose ends remain. One is the connection with adult health. What, if anything, does improved parenting and doctoring of children have to do with the health of others in the family? Some plausible connections hinge on the role of mothers in caring for and controlling others in the household. Women assume disproportionate responsibility for the elderly in settings where the elderly rarely live by themselves and where families rather than institutions are charged with providing for them. Needless to say, knowledge of disease processes, diagnostic skills, and familiarity with the health care system gained while caring for infants and small children have applications in this other realm. Moreover, if marriage and parenting provide external regulation and facilitate self-regulation of health behaviors (Umberson 1987), this medical knowledge may serve an important preventive function for all adult members of a household or family. There is room, though, for numerous negative outcomes. Even as the health of mothers and children improves, the health of adult males may deteriorate in response to increased consumption of harmful foods and substances, increased stress, increased exposure to risks of accidents or violence, and decreased social support (World Bank 1989).

The other open question concerns interrelations between mortality and fertility. Over the years, interest in the possible connections between one variable and the other has shifted from one type of link to another. Early on, there was interest in the timing of the two transitions. How soon after a sustained decline in mortality would fertility decline? In the original formulations of demographic transition theory, both transitions were thought to be caused by modernization, but modernization was seen as having a more immediate effect on mortality than on fertility (Notestein 1953). Consideration was also given to the societal and individual responses to the rapid population growth generated by a decline in mortality (Davis 1963). Later, the focus shifted to the ways in which mortality affected the demand for children. Do mothers substitute additional pregnancies for children who die early in life (Preston 1978)? Or, alternatively, does increased child survival lead parents to want fewer births so as to arrive at a certain (unchanged) number of surviving children (Easterlin 1975)? Most recently, interest has centered on the effects that a fertility decline may have on health (National Research Council 1989). At issue is whether the accompanying changes in birth spacing patterns and in the distribution of births by mother's age and parity lead, through both biological and behavioral mechanisms, to increased child survival.

If one shares the view that the two transitions — in mortality and in fertility — are closely tied to transitions in family relations and in medical technology and practice, such questions seem narrowly framed, even shortsighted. Contrast the arid calculus regarding mortality decline and the demand for children with a more complex picture in which greater emotional nucleation leads to increased expenditures of time and effort on childrearing. This shift, in turn, enhances the probability of child survival. It also reduces the number of (surviving) children that parents feel they can care for, yielding a twofold increase in the motivation to control fertility.

Similar mutually reinforcing influences result from the spread of the modern medical system. While medical technology increases child survival, medical advice urges mothers to adhere to new standards of hygiene and nutrition that make children more expensive. Again there is a twofold increase in the motivation to control fertility. Furthermore, the spread of the modern medical technology and practice tends to reduce the fear that women may have of modern methods of contraception, just as it increases their access to this new technology. The increase in the availability and acceptability of effective birth control, together with heightened motivation, leads to a smaller number of children who, in turn, will receive more intense care and have even higher survival prospects. Such an unfolding web of synergistic effects and tangled causality defies simple characterization or meaningful statistical estimation.

A closing caveat is in order. Passage through a transition involving shifts in family relationships, medical technology, fertility, and mortality may or may not imply a generalized increase in welfare. The challenge is not just to understand what is taking place, but to identify ways to guide the process so as to avoid excesses and to maximize the benefits of these transitions for all sectors of a population. How might this be done? Certainly one implication of the "one transition" hypothesis is that in addition to narrowly conceived programs to deliver family planning and primary health care, there is a need for enlightened social policy to guide the spread of modern medicine and to both accommodate and facilitate change in family relationships.

Acknowledgments

I am grateful for the opportunity to present earlier versions of this paper at the Australian National University, the University of Texas, and the University of Campinas. Comments from Elza Berquo, Monica Das Gupta, Vilmar Faria, Anibal Faundes, Omer Galle, Arthur Kleinman, Neide Patarra, and Debra Umberson were particularly helpful. An earlier version of the article appeared in J.C. Caldwell, et al., eds. 1990. *What We Know About the Health Transition: The Cultural, Social and Behavioural Determinants of Health, Health Transition Series*, No. 2, Vol. 1: 85–91. Canberra: Health Transition Centre, Australian National University.

References

Angel, R., and P. Thoits. 1987. "The impact of culture on the cognitive structure of illness." *Culture, Medicine and Psychiatry*, 11: 465–494.

Ariès, P. 1962. *Centuries of Childhood: A Social History of Family Life*. New York: Vintage Books.

Berelson, B. 1969. "Beyond family-planning." *Science*, 163: 533–543.

Berelson, B. 1977. "Paths to fertility reduction: The policy cube." *Family Planning Perspectives*, 9(5): 214–219.

Bhatia, S., F. Saadah, and W.H. Mosley. 1989. "Analytical review of the development of family planning program strategies, operations, and research as a model for primary health care programs." Paper prepared for the International Commission on Health Research for Development, January.

Bogue, D. 1983. "Normative and psychic costs of contraception." In R. Bulatao and R. Lee, eds. *Determinants of Fertility in Developing Countries*, Vol. 2. New York: Academic Press.

Bongaarts, J. 1980. "Does malnutrition affect fecundity? A summary of evidence." *Science*, 208: 564–569.

Bongaarts, J., and R. Potter. 1983. *Fertility, Biology, and Behavior.* New York: Academic Press.

Bulatao, R., and R. Lee, eds. 1983. *Determinants of Fertility in Developing Countries.* New York: Academic Press.

Caldwell, J.C. 1976. "Toward a restatement of demographic transition theory." *Population and Development Review*, 2: 321–366.

Caldwell, J.C. 1979. "Education as a factor in mortality decline: An examination of Nigerian data." *Population Studies,* 33:395–413.

Caldwell, J.C. 1983. "Direct economic costs and benefits of children." In R.A. Bulatao and R.D. Lee, eds. *Determinants of Fertility in Developing Countries*, Vol. 1. New York: Academic Press.

Cassen, R.H. 1976. "Population and development: A survey." *World Development*, 4: 785–830.

Chenery, H.B., and T.N. Srinivasan, eds. 1988. *Handbook of Development Economics*, Vol. 1. New York and Amsterdam: North Holland-Elsevier.

Cleland, J., and C. Wilson. 1987. "Demand theories of the fertility transition: An iconoclastic view." *Population Studies*, 41: 5–30.

Commission on Health Research for Development. 1990. *Health Research: Essential Link to Equity in Development.* New York: Oxford University Press.

Demeny, P. 1968. "Early fertility decline in Austria-Hungary: A lesson in demographic transition." *Daedelus*, 97: 502–522.

Demeny, P. 1971. "The economics of population control." In *Rapid Population Growth: Consequences and Policy Implications*, National Academy of Sciences. Baltimore: The Johns Hopkins Press.

Davis, K. 1963. "The theory of change and response in modern demographic history." *Population Index*, 29: 345–366.

Faria, V. 1989. "Politicas de governo e regulacao de fecundidade: Consecuencias nao anticipadas e efeitos perversos." *Ciencias Sociais Hoje, 1989.* Sao Paulo: Vertice, Editora Revista dos Tribunais, ANPOCS.

Freedman, R. 1978. "Theories of fertility decline: A reappraisal." *Social Forces*, 58: 1–17.

Frisch, R.E. 1978. "Population, food intake, and fertility." *Science*, 199: 22–30.

Greep, R. 1976. *Reproduction and Human Welfare: A Challenge to Research.* Cambridge, MA: MIT Press.

Harrison, K.A., and C.E. Rossiter. 1985. "Child-bearing, health, and social priorities: A survey of 22,774 hospital births in Zaria, Northern Nigeria." *British Journal of Obstetrics and Gynaecology*, 92 (Suppl. 5): 100–115.

Hermalin, A., and B. Entwistle. 1985. "Future directions in the analysis of contraceptive availability." In *International Population Conference, Florence, 1985,* International Union for the Scientific Study of Population, Volume III.

House, J.S., K.R. Landis, and D. Umberson. 1988. "Social relationships and health." *Science,* 241: 540–545.

Knodel, J., and E. Van de Walle. 1979. "Lessons from the past: Policy implications of historical fertility studies." *Population and Development Review*, 5: 217–246.

Knowles, J.H. 1980. "Health, population and development." *Social Science and Medicine*, 14C(2): 67–70.

Lapham, R., and G.B. Simmons, eds. 1987. *Organizing for Effective Family Planning Programs.* Washington, DC: National Academy Press.

Lesthaeghe, R. 1980. "On the social control of human reproduction." *Population and Development Review*, 6(4): 527–548.

McKeown, T. 1976. *The Modern Rise of Population.* New York: Academic Press.

McNicoll, G. 1978. "On fertility policy research." *Population and Development Review*, 4: 681–693.

McNicoll, G. 1980. "Institutional determinants of fertility change." *Population and Development Review*, 6(3): 441–462.

Mesa-Lago, C. 1978. *Social Security in Latin America: Pressure Groups, Stratification, and Inequality.* Pittsburgh: University of Pittsburgh Press.

Miró, C.A., and J.E. Potter. 1980. *Population Policy: Research Priorities in the Developing World.* London: Frances Pinter.

Mosley, W.H. 1983. "Will primary health care reduce infant and child mortality? A critique of some current strategies with special reference to Africa and Asia." Paper presented in International Union for the Scientific Study of Population Seminar on Social Policy, Health Policy, and Mortality Prospects, Paris. Paris: Institut National d'Études Démographiques.

Mosley, W.H. 1984. "Child survival research and policy." *Population and Development Review*, 10(Suppl): 3–24.

Mosley, W.H., and L.C. Chen. 1984. "An analytical framework for the study of child survival in developing countries." *Population and Development Review*, 10(Suppl): 25–48.

Muecke, M.A. 1976. "Health care systems as socializing agents: Childbearing the North Thai and Western ways." *Social Science and Medicine*, 10(7–8):377–384.

National Research Council. 1989. *Contraception and Reproduction: Health Consequences for Women and Children in the Developing World.* Washington, DC: National Academy Press.

Notestein, F.W. 1953. "Economic problems of population change." In *Proceedings of the Eighth International Conference of Agricultural Economists.* London: Oxford University Press.

Preston, S.H., ed. 1978. *The Effect of Infant and Child Mortality on Fertility.* New York: Academic Press.

Schultz, T.P. 1980. "Interpretation of relations among mortality, economics of the household, and the health environment." In *Proceedings of the Meeting on Socioeconomic Determinants and Consequences of Mortality.* New York and Geneva: United Nations and World Health Organization.

Schultz, T.P. 1984. "Studying the impact of household economic and community variables on child mortality." *Population and Development Review*, 10(Suppl): 215–235.

Shedlin, M., and P. Hollerbach. 1981. "Modern and traditional fertility regulation in a Mexican community: The process of decision making." *Studies in Family Planning*, 12: 278–296.

Smith, R.M. 1981. "Fertility, economy, and household formation in England over three centuries." *Population and Development Review*, 7(4): 595–622.

Starr, P. 1982. *The Social Transformation of American Medicine.* New York: Basic Books.

Stolnitz, G. 1955. "A century of international mortality trends: I." *Population Studies*, 9(1): 24–55.

Stolnitz, G. 1975. "International mortality trends: Some main facts and implications." In *The Population Debate: Dimensions and Perspectives* (Population Studies, No. 57). New York: United Nations.

Trussell, J. 1978. "Menarche and fatness: Re-examination of the critical body fat composition hypothesis." *Science*, 200(4349): 1506–1509.

Umberson, D. 1987. "Family status and health behaviors: Social control as a dimension of social integration." *Journal of Health and Social Behavior*, 28: 306–319.

Vallin, J. 1988. "Evolution sociale et baisse de la mortalité: conquête ou reconquête d'un avantage feminin." Conférence sur le statut de la femme et l'évolution démographique dans le cadre du développement, Asker (Norvege), 15–18 Juin.

World Bank. 1975. *Health Sector Policy Paper.* Washington, DC: World Bank.

World Bank. 1989. *Adult Health in Brazil: Adjusting to New Challenges.* Report No. 7807–BR. Washington, DC: World Bank.

Wrigley, E.A., and R.S. Schofield. 1983. "English population history from family reconstitution: Summary results." *Population Studies,* 37(2): 157–184.

Wrong, D.H. 1956. *Population.* New York: Random House.

Young, J.C. 1981. *Medical Choice in a Mexican Village.* New Brunswick, NJ: Rutgers University Press.

Section IV

Social, Behavioral, and Cultural Mediators

11

Illness Behavior and the Health Transition in the Developing World

Nicholas A. Christakis
Norma C. Ware
Arthur Kleinman

Introduction

The "health transition" refers to the ongoing, worldwide increase in life expectancy that has occurred since the beginning of the twentieth century, more especially since the 1960s. In the 25 years from 1960 to 1985, global life expectancy at birth increased from approximately 48 to 59 years. Since this increase occurred in all regions of the world, the mortality differential between the developed and developing world has persisted (United Nations 1985).

The health transition also encompasses the changing configuration of causes of death and the changing character of morbidity. Acute infectious disease now accounts for less of the morbidity burden in some countries (although it remains a serious problem in sub-Saharan Africa, India, and the Middle East), while chronic disease (e.g., heart disease, stroke, and cancer) and behavioral problems (e.g., substance abuse, child abuse, depression, anxiety disorders, and suicide) account for more. This has resulted in a so-called "triple burden" of acute illness, chronic illness, and behavioral pathology in the Third World. Medically speaking, then, the health transition has three essential aspects: a decline in mortality, a change in morbidity, and an increase in behavioral pathology.[1]

John Caldwell has cogently argued that the positive aspects of the health transition have resulted from the complex and synergistic interplay of modernizing social forces (e.g., urbanization, economic development, mass communication, and improved education) and direct biomedical interventions, such as childhood immunization, oral rehydration therapy, and village health systems (1986). This proposition is based on the premise that as a result of modernization, people in the developing world are somehow increasing their use of available biomedical health resources in ways that result in prolonged life and improved health. Generally, the argument is that in the developing world — under the pressures of modernization and socioeconomic change — people consider biomedicine to be more effective than traditional medicine, that they avail themselves of biomedicine whenever possible, that biomedicine is increasingly accessible, that biomedicine is indeed more effective than traditional medicine, and that, as a result of all of these, health improves.

Recognizing the value of this theoretical contribution to our understanding of the health transition, this chapter seeks to build upon Caldwell's formulation by probing some of the complexities it subsumes. The analysis is intended to show how these two types of factors — modernizing social forces and biomedical interventions — might result in the changes that characterize the health transition, and also how they are actually played out in local cultural settings in the developing world. A review of cross-cultural studies reveals that "biomedicine" assumes different forms in different contexts, and that it is not always either the preferred mode of healing or the most effective one.

By focusing on one aspect of modernizing socioeconomic change — maternal education — and by documenting cultural differences in the perception and use of biomedicine in situations of medical pluralism, we hope to demonstrate convincingly that any adequate explanation of the health transition must take local cultural variation into account. To organize and concretize the discussion of local differences, we will draw upon the notion of illness behavior — the constellation of meanings and activities exhibited by an individual and his or her social circle in response to bodily indications perceived as symptoms (Mechanic 1978).

Our primary aim here, then, is to advance the theoretical proposition that the effects of both modernizing social change and biomedical interventions upon health status in the developing world are mediated by local-level processes, in particular, illness behavior.

The available cross-cultural data suggest not only that illness behavior is a mediating variable in the health transition, but also that it is undergoing change. Worldwide transformations in health status are leading to rapid changes in illness behavior, at the same time that illness behavior — often motivated by large-scale socioeconomic changes —

is producing changes in health. In short, illness behavior is dynamic. Thus, our second aim is to argue that illness behavior should be considered part of the health transition.

Illness Behavior

In a given individual or social network, illness behavior involves monitoring the body, recognizing and interpreting symptoms, and taking remedial action (e.g., seeking lay or professional help) to rectify the perceived abnormality. Help may be sought from a number of sources in the patient's social network, including friends, family, folk healers, and professionals. To focus on illness behavior is to emphasize the response of human beings to morbidity — to sickness and suffering — rather than to mortality *per se*.

Illness behavior also encompasses the ongoing response of the sick individual and those around him or her to the course of the illness. Examples here include attention to symptoms, compliance with therapeutic advice, changes in treatment regimens, and evaluation of therapeutic efficacy and outcome.

The notion of illness behavior should be distinguished from that of health behavior. The latter includes advertent and inadvertent behaviors that maintain health, or, conversely, place persons and groups at risk for ill health. Thus, behavioral risk factors for acute infectious diseases (e.g., hygienic practices, sexual behaviors) and for chronic conditions (e.g., cigarette smoking, alcohol and drug abuse, dietary practices) can be thought of as health behaviors, as can practices that are health enhancing (e.g., exercise, proper diet).

Thus we see that illness behavior is one component of the larger category of health behavior. Although illness behavior is the primary focus of this discussion, we will also consider health enhancing behaviors (e.g., maintenance of adequate nutrition or use of vaccination services) that are initiated in the absence of illness. Health behavior and illness behavior are inextricably linked.

Included under the rubric of illness behavior is what is termed the health- or help-seeking process — a series of activities aimed at rectifying the perceived aberration in the individual's state of health (Chrisman 1977). Help-seeking begins with symptom definition or an evaluation of the bodily problem. A strategy for responding to the symptoms, the treatment action plan, is then devised. Treatment action may involve any combination of self care, family care, and care from folk and professional healers. The degree to which this plan is carried out by the ill person and his/her family is termed adherence (or compliance). Adherence is in turn strongly influenced by an ongoing evaluation of outcome. Both symptom definition and treatment action are affected by lay consultation and referral and by the social networks in which the individual participates.

Healer Choice in Medically Pluralistic Cultural Settings: A Preference for Biomedicine?

Cross-cultural data on illness behavior from situations of medical pluralism in the developing world indicate that both the perceived efficacy of biomedicine and the decision to use biomedical services are highly variable and subject to influence by a number of intervening factors.

Medical pluralism, or the existence of several distinct therapeutic systems in a single cultural setting, is an especially important feature of medical care in the developing world (Leslie 1978). Patients may feel uncertain as to what type of care provider can cure their illness, leading them to consult both traditional and biomedical practitioners. Or they may decide that treatment of certain illnesses requires more than one type of assistance. Generally, care is sought from several types of providers concurrently or sequentially, and the various types of care are often seen as complementary rather than conflicting.

Biomedicine is often highly regarded in the developing world — but not unequivocally so. Many studies, in fact, have shown that from the point of view of the patient, modern health services are often seen as no more effective than traditional medicine. For example, a study of illness behavior in Ethiopia found that traditional medicine was felt to be as effective as modern medicine in curing a variety of complaints (Kloos et al. 1987). Even in industrial East Asia, traditional medicine is often viewed as more effective than biomedicine for certain conditions, usually chronic disease (Locke 1980). Similarly, research in Singapore revealed that nearly 60 percent of patients visiting a traditional Chinese doctor reported effectiveness as their major reason for choosing such treatment (Ho, Lun and Ng 1984). Only a small minority gave "traditional beliefs" (7 percent) or cost (10 percent) as their major reasons for consulting a traditional practitioner. Indeed, patients in this setting had a well-articulated set of expectations regarding which type of healer — "Western" or "traditional Chinese" — was preferable for various conditions.[2] Finally, Sargent (1982) describes a setting in Benin where traditional birth attendants are perceived as more effective — and may actually be more effective — than biomedical services.[3] Indeed, perceived efficacy may accurately reflect actual efficacy. But the critical point is that it is perceived efficacy that guides healer choice.[4] In a study of the efficacy of traditional and modern healers in Taiwan, Kleinman and Gale (1982) compared matched sets of patients treated by shamans and physicians for similar illnesses. Overall, the two groups showed similar patterns of improvement across illness types. Efficacy was examined using both subjective measures (e.g., patient assessment of the effect of practitioner on outcome) and objective measures (evaluation of outcome by the research team).

Patient and community preferences for indigenous healing systems often reflect the realities of how biomedicine is practiced in much of the developing world. In fact, biomedical practice in third world settings is inadequate in a number of ways. A typical encounter between patient and health care provider may last less than two minutes (Reid 1984). Descriptions of symptoms may be limited to a single sentence. Physical or laboratory examinations may be cursory or even nonexistent. Potentially toxic medication may be prescribed without either a full course of treatment or follow-up to determine subsequent effects (Weisberg and Long 1984). Iatrogenesis, inappropriate and inadequate treatment, and failure to properly inform patients and families of potential toxicity or alternative treatment options are commonplace. Primary health care units are often staffed by practitioners who are absent while performing more lucrative private services or by medical students and junior nurses whose training is inadequate. Care may even be delivered by staff who lack the most basic medical knowledge, as has been reported in Nepal (Justice 1986).

The existence of biomedical services in the vicinity of ill people does not mean that these services will be utilized, even if they are perceived as efficacious. In an Ecuadorian Indian community, for example, the home is regarded as a refuge from illness, while the outside world is considered to be disease-promoting. Thus, one study of a Saraguro community demonstrated that Indian mothers chose to avoid therapeutic care, whether professional or traditional, that was delivered outside the home (Finerman 1987). In other research, Guatemalan peasants were shown to avoid government facilities that provided biomedical care because they lacked drugs and equipment (Annis 1981).

Young (1981a, 1981b) found that in one Mexican village the critical considerations in the decision not to use a physician were of three types: (1) preexisting preference for folk treatment, which was considered to offer a higher likelihood of cure (21 percent), (2) access problems, such as lack of money or transportation (58 percent), and (3) recent experience of failure in attempting to achieve a cure through consulting a physician (21 percent). Thus, while nearly half of the choices not to consult a physician in this Mexican village were based on perceived or proven lack of efficacy, slightly more than half were based on logistic concerns.

The results of an epidemiological study following a major outbreak of polio in Taiwan in 1982 further demonstrate that the availability of effective biomedical interventions does not *ipso facto* ensure that they will be used (Kim-Farley et al. 1984). Surveys in two counties, Yun Lin and Chia Yi, indicated that despite community-wide vaccination programs, the spread of the disease reached epidemic proportions. The most important risk factor for developing polio in this case was clearly the failure to vaccinate. An unvaccinated child was found to be 80 times more likely to contract polio than a child who had received three or more doses of vaccine. Less significant risk factors included, in decreasing order of importance, non-municipal water supply (making a child five times more likely to develop the disease), sharing of toilets by more than one family, fathers who were unemployed or in unskilled jobs, and fathers with little education. The investigators were unable to determine, however, whether these other factors contributed independently to polio incidence or simply correlated with failure to vaccinate (Morbidity and Mortality Weekly Report 1983). Clearly, an appropriate biomedical resource, namely polio vaccination, was available in this case. However, noncompliance with the recommendation to vaccinate prevented the biomedical intervention from averting the epidemic.

The distance that must often be traveled to reach a biomedical practitioner in contrast to various types of traditional healers also represents a significant constraint on the use of biomedicine.[5] A study of physician use in northern Nigeria found that per capita utilization of local government health dispensaries declined at a rate of 25% per kilometer (Stock 1983; Ayeni, Rushton and McNulty 1987). Distance has also been shown to reduce pharmacy use in Ethiopia (Kloos et al. 1986).

Research in Bangladesh has revealed a strong correlation between distance to a diarrhea clinic and visits to the clinic when an episode of diarrhea occurs. While about 95 percent of all episodes occurring in patients who lived within one mile resulted in visits to the clinic, only about 35 percent (for females) and 70 percent (for males) of episodes occurring to patients who lived between two and three miles from the clinic were treated there (Rahaman et al. 1982).

Annis (1981) provides further evidence of the limiting effect of distance on the use of biomedical services. Citing data from the highland provinces of Guatemala, Annis observed that while only 16 percent of the local population lived within one kilometer of the health post, more than 50 percent of patient visits were made by persons living within this immediate area. Conversely, patients living more than 3.5 kilometers from the health post accounted for only 15 percent of post visits, even though more than half the population of the area lived at this distance.

The difficulty in reaching biomedical practitioners may be contrasted with the availability of the more popular varieties of traditional healers. For example, in several rural and urban Brazilian communities studied by Nations and Rebhun (1988), the population ratio of traditional healers was 1:150 in the rural communities and about 1:75 in the urban shantytown. The corresponding ratio for biomedical physicians was 1:2,000. Data from Bangladesh yield ratios for traditional healers and allopathic practitioners of 1:240 and 1:400 respectively (Sarder and Chen 1981). Finally, Ahern's (1978) research in Taipei suggests that "symbolic distance" can influence the use of biomedical practitioners, who are perceived as symbolically "more distant" from the experiential world of patients than are traditional healers.

Other sociocultural differences may also work against the use of biomedicine. Welch (1980) explains that a health post set up for the Ningerum of Papua New Guinea was at one point not widely used because the clinic staff, being from another region, were regarded by the local population as a potential source of sorcery. In rural Nepal, Justice (1986) has shown that primary health care workers are perceived as unreceptive and inaccessible to local peasants, who have therefore turned to the health center's "peon" — an uneducated handyman and member of the local community— for assistance with health problems.

In his study of disease classification and health behavior in rural Ghana, Fosu (1981) concludes that the perceived cause of a disease determines the choice between traditional healers and local biomedical clinics. The inhabitants of Bereduso, Ghana, classify diseases as being caused by natural agents, supernatural agents, or both. Fosu found that for diseases considered to have a natural cause, 3 percent of patients consulted a traditional healer, while 53 percent sought help at a local clinic. However, for diseases considered to have a supernatural cause, 31 percent consulted a traditional healer while only 15 percent turned to the clinic. A mixed pattern of consultation emerged for diseases seen as having both kinds of causes. Significantly, diseases such as tuberculosis, insanity, epilepsy, pneumonia, asthma, and leprosy were all felt to have supernatural causes. In other words, those diseases perceived to be appropriately treated by biomedicine are sometimes not the ones for which effective therapy exists; alternatively, those diseases perceived to be appropriately treated by local healers are sometimes those for which biomedicine is effective.

A final set of variables that influence the choice of a healer are the patient's personal attributes, such as age, sex, education, residence, and occupation. Visits to a diarrhea clinic in rural Bangladesh, for example, were shown to be significantly associated with the patient's age and sex; older females and younger males tended to make fewer visits when ill (Rahaman et al. 1982).

The use of medical services for sick infants is profoundly influenced by the child's sex, with utilization rates often being considerably lower for females (McCormack 1988). Das Gupta (1989) demonstrates that in rural Punjab, the second and third female children, in particular, receive less expert attention for illness episodes. Citing research in South Indian villages, Caldwell (personal communication) has observed that when seeking treatment for sick children meant traveling outside the village to the nearest health center, boys were more likely to be brought to the clinic than girls. Since traveling to the health center meant taking time off from work, fathers brought children to the clinic on the weekly market day. They were more likely to bring sons than daughters because of concerns about leaving small girls in the marketplace all day.

The point here is that treatment decisions in the medically pluralistic settings typical of the developing world are complex. In reviewing selected cross-cultural research on illness behavior, we see that the choice of a healer is shaped by a wide range of factors, among them perceptions of efficacy, practical considerations (such as distance), symbolic considerations (such as the experiential distance between patient and practitioner), the perceived cause of the ailment and whether it is viewed as life threatening, and personal attributes of the patient. This body of research shows that the existence of biomedicine as a treatment option does not mean that it will be the preferred choice.

Socioeconomic Change Modifies Illness Behavior: The Case of Maternal Education

Maternal education provides a good tool with which to examine the issue of primary interest here: the relationship between the health transition, biomedical health interventions, and macrolevel socioeconomic change.

It has been repeatedly observed that societies with the highest levels of maternal education (which also tend to be those with the greatest female autonomy) are likely to show the highest rates of infant survival and to appear "healthier" according to other indexes. This is true of both developing and developed countries.[6] The reduction of illness and death among infants has a more profound impact on the overall health status of a country than do corresponding decreases in mortality and morbidity in adults. Indeed, some of the greatest gains of the health transition may have resulted from changes in the care of infants, that is, adult illness behavior directed toward the very young.

Analyzing data from the 1973 Nigerian segment of the Changing African Family Project, Caldwell (1979) points to maternal education as the single most significant determinant of observed differences in child mortality. His subsequent discussion of the possible explanations for this phenomenon posits two intervening factors in this relationship: increased use of Western biomedical services and changes in the "traditional balance of familial relationships." The latter is seen as acting through both a redistribution of family resources in the direction of child care (at the instigation of the mother) and an increase in maternal assertiveness. This, in turn, leads to increased use of medical care, particularly biomedical care, for children.

This is in some ways a valid argument. However, increased use of modern medical alternatives available to traditional women may not be the most important way in which maternal education works to improve health status. The significance of illness behavior as an intervening variable seems to be far greater.

The following is intended to broaden existing conceptualizations of the impact of educated mothers upon child health by reviewing the cross-cultural literature on illness behavior in relation to maternal education and the health status of children. Again, building on previous thinking in this area, we aim to document the complexity of this relationship by (1) reflecting on the nature of education for women in the developing world, (2) suggesting that maternal education works through a variety of mechanisms to affect child health, and (3) proposing that seeking biomedical care may be only part of a larger phenomenon that is influenced not only by maternal education, but by other key social changes as well. We emphasize that our theoretical model is one that is partially supported by the literature. In short, while illness behavior helps to explain some of the effect of maternal education, it cannot explain all of it.

In much of the developing world, education for women often means one-to-six years of primary education. Any putative effect of maternal education upon child health must therefore somehow be realized on the basis of as little as one or two years in school. This simple observation strongly suggests that it is not the content of what is taught in school that is important, since health education *per se* is unlikely to be part of such limited schooling.

Since education seems to teach young girls something besides content, it is critical to disentangle the other strands of this social intervention in order to understand its impact on health status. One of these strands might be the ancillary benefits that accrue from the very "experience" of going to school. Another is the fact that education may make a woman more desirable as a spouse, thereby leading to marriage to a wealthier man, greater economic resources, and, as a result, improved health status for her children. Attending school may keep a young girl out of a dangerous work environment, thereby preserving her health for future pregnancies and increasing the birth weight (and consequent health) of her children.[7] Data from Malaysia suggest that education for women may result in postponed marriage, meaning that a mother will be older when her children are delivered. This also promotes child survival (DeVanzo 1984).

In their review of maternal education and child survival in developing countries, Cleland and van Ginneken conclude that "health beliefs and domestic practices" are essential to an explanation of the relationship between maternal education and child mortality (1988). Citing data from the United Nations and the World Bank, they show that, on average, each one-year increment in women's education corresponds to a 7 to 9 percent decline in deaths of children under five years of age. The effect is more pronounced in childhood than in infancy. After considering a number of mediating factors that might account for this effect, the authors conclude that increased education has little impact on such changes in reproductive behavior as birth spacing or nutritional practices during pregnancy. Rather, they argue that about half of the gross effect of maternal education actually reflects the economic advantages associated with education, such as clothing, housing quality, and other ancillary benefits.

Overall, however, Cleland and van Ginneken seem to agree with other authors that exposure to Western medicine necessarily results in improved health, the implication being that maternal education enhances health by increasing the use of biomedical health services. For example, the authors assume that substitution of modern drugs sold in pharmacies for traditional herbal remedies results in improved self-care.

At the same time, Cleland and van Ginneken conclude that the effect of maternal education "transcends access to modern health services" and that "it appears probable that domestic behavior is the key to the enhanced survivorship of children born to educated mothers" (1988:1365). They postulate a number of effects of maternal education upon attitudes, including two that are not supported by the anthropological literature. These are, first, that compared to the uneducated, educated mothers "attach a higher value to the welfare and health of children," and second, that they are "less fatalistic about disease and death."

In fact, considerable empirical evidence supports the contention that maternal education has a broad range of effects upon illness behavior aside from fostering the use of biomedical services. Moreover, these effects may themselves work to improve health status.

Maternal education influences each of the following aspects of the help-seeking process: symptom definition, treatment action, adherence to treatment, evaluation of outcome, and social networks and lay consultation.[8] Maternal education influences symptom definition in a number of ways, some of which have been documented in developing world settings. Spending some time in school, even if what is taught there is not immediately relevant to health and disease, can help to develop certain cognitive abilities in ways that facilitate the identification of bodily symptoms. Learning new modes of categorization, for example, can mean that symptoms will be more readily classified as indications of illness or not, and that categories of illness will tend to be distinguished from one another (Tsui, DeClerque and Mangani 1988).

The ability to recognize the presence of illness may also be enhanced by education, as research by Das Gupta (1989) in rural Punjab, Levine et al. (1987) in urban Mexico, and McClain (1977) in Mexico suggests.

Often, the content of education is ineffective in changing beliefs about disease causation and health maintenance. In some situations, however, the content of education has been shown to have a meaningful impact in such diverse areas as nutrition, sanitation, and family planning (Das Gupta 1989).

Maternal education is also related to treatment action. Changes in this aspect of illness behavior, influenced by maternal education, have been claimed to result in the increased use of biomedical services (Caldwell 1979; Cleland and van Ginneken 1988).

Most examinations of the impact of maternal education on health practices have focused upon only a small part of treatment action. The education of mothers may contribute to a change from the more person-oriented view associated with peasant and working classes to an institution-oriented view found in professional and managerial circles. As a result, maternal education can bring about an increased ability to negotiate with medical institutions.

Schooling may increase a woman's ability to procure health care in a number of ways. For example, it may foster an appreciation of institutional time, which in turn may increase access to knowledge and assistance (Lindenbaum 1990). Educated women may also be more familiar with, and therefore better skilled in handling, the interrogatory style of health care providers, especially biomedical practitioners. And education may function as a form of assertiveness training, making women more likely to leave the local area in search of health care for their dependents (Caldwell 1986).

On a practical level, maternal education influences treatment action insofar as it makes educated women better financial managers. Good financial management expands options for therapy in times of sickness (Cosminsky 1987). The content of what is taught may also help mothers to choose appropriate healers and therapy (e.g., oral rehydration for diarrhea, spiritual healers for possession) and to understand disease causation (which might lead to better hygiene).

Maternal education affects adherence to treatment. Education may increase mothers' abilities to comprehend medical recommendations and to remember them or write them down accurately. With respect to cognitive development, education may modify a patient's construction of reality so that it is easier for her to assimilate and accept medical recommendations (McClain 1977). A woman's experience in school may make her more comfortable with outsiders, thereby increasing her trust

in health care workers and her willingness to follow potentially efficacious medical advice.

Evaluation of treatment outcomes may vary with mothers' educational levels. A mother with little education may mistakenly decide a child
is no longer ill, seriously ill, or in need of further therapy. Such decisions
may result in inappropriate termination of certain potentially effective
forms of care. Chronic diarrhea, for example, may be accepted as normal
and therapy may be arrested.[9]

Education also has a number of predictable and documented effects
upon a mother's social networks and practices of lay consultation. In
many developing countries, women marry and have children when they
are still very young, often by age 16. In such settings, providing even two
years of primary schooling for girls is a relatively recent innovation. For
these women, being in school may increase the size and sophistication
of the social network, giving them access to more resourceful lay
consultants.

Borrowing the terms of social network theory, school experience
may increase the range and decrease the insularity of a woman's network
by improving her marriage prospects and taking her into the outside
world (Lindenbaum 1990). Through its effect on social networks, school
experience may increase the size of the therapy management group
(Janzen 1978). A woman's rhetorical competence (based on a sense of
self-efficacy) at communicating her concerns regarding her own illness
or those of her dependents to members of her social network or family
may benefit from education. For example, in Bangladesh, educated
women have higher status within the family and are better able to
marshal resources for the care of the ill (Lindenbaum 1990).

Maternal education has a number of predictable and demonstrated
effects upon the home environment. Educated women have been shown
to maintain cleaner households (Bertrand and Walmus 1988), to be better
financial providers, and to provide better nutrition for their children, all
of which potentially decrease disease incidence. Literacy may also
facilitate the use of sanitary facilities, such as piped water, in a way that
reduces the onset of disease (Esrey and Habicht 1988). Das Gupta (1989)
found that better educated mothers provide more hygienic conditions for
their children.

Evidence that maternal education may lead to increased illness should
also be noted here. For example, educated mothers have been shown
to breastfeed less (Caldwell and MacDonald 1982; Goldberg 1984). They

are also more likely to seek employment outside the home (Farah and Preston 1982; Hobcraft, McDonald and Rutstein 1984), which might adversely affect child health if there were less direct supervision of children as a result.

Our intention here has been to lay out some of the ways in which maternal education, one of many possible examples of large-scale socioeconomic change in modernizing societies, can be expected to modify health and illness behavior. All of these behavioral changes may in turn work to improve health status. Quicker identification of symptoms and more accurate recognition of disease, recourse to more appropriate or effective healers, improved compliance with recommendations that increase efficacy and reduce iatrogenesis, more appropriate evaluation of outcome, and favorable modifications of risk factors, such as diet, hygiene, and parenting practices, may all exert a positive influence on health. We now look at ways in which Western biomedicine, as it becomes an integral part of indigenous cultures, is itself modifying illness behavior.

Changing Patterns of Illness Behavior are Part of the Health Transition

An integral part of the health transition is an ongoing evolution in illness behavior. The health transition involves not only change in the patterning of health indicators, but also a transition in the use of health services. This is often best appreciated at the local level.

The transition in illness behavior is driven by particular aspects of traditional and cosmopolitan medical practice in the modern world. These include the proliferation of Western pharmaceuticals and convergence in the content of traditional and cosmopolitan medicine in many developing societies. Stated in general terms, illness behavior is changing under the pressure of the same social changes and health inputs that have given rise to the health transition.

Pharmaceuticals

The widespread distribution of Western pharmaceuticals, the proliferation of pharmacies throughout the developing world, the growth of indigenous pharmaceutical companies, and the fact that these companies often conduct their own research have all had a dramatic impact upon illness behavior in developing societies.

For many of the rural and urban poor in the developing world, the pharmacy is the only contact with the Western health care system. In El Salvador, for example, 55 percent of poor families and 23 percent of upper-class families in one study were shown to rely on commercial pharmaceutical practitioners as their primary source of health care (Ferguson 1988). The implications of this are clear. The easy availability of "prescription" drugs in the developing world and the ordinarily poor training of pharmacists who stand to benefit financially from the sale of their wares can lead to significant iatrogenesis and inappropriate drug use. This has been documented both in the highly urban setting of Seoul, Korea (Kim 1989), and in a more rural setting in Taiwan (Kahane 1987).

Pharmacists in the developing world dispense more than drugs. They also offer medical advice and function as comprehensive health care providers. As a result, pharmacists are perceived as being very similar to doctors. For example, Logan reports that in urban Mexico, "many people routinely consulted the local pharmacist 'almost like a doctor' [*casi como doctor*]. They presented their physical complaints and described their symptoms, expecting the pharmacists to diagnose their illnesses and to prescribe treatment. The pharmacists obliged their clients by labelling their illnesses and by selling them the pharmaceutical preparations they recommended...[Moreover], many people self-diagnosed their illness and medicated themselves..."(Logan 1988).

Pharmacists are often preferred as care providers for some of the same reasons folk healers are preferred over physicians: they treat patients more politely, offer faster service, are more convenient, and have adequate supplies on hand. Both the care and the medications provided by pharmacists are often regarded as superior. Lay pharmacists in Guatemala, for example, are highly regarded as care providers; they are popular because of their easy accessibility, familiarity with the local people, and the fact that they extend credit (Cosminsky and Scrimshaw 1980). In El Salvador, Ferguson argues, village pharmacy personnel "serve as interpreters between different medical care traditions, gleaning what they can from information they receive regarding Western medi-cations and relying to a large extent on shared cultural understandings of the nature and treatment of illness" (Ferguson 1988:31). The informa-tion pharmacists rely on, in general, is provided by sales representatives of local distributors.

The rampant misuse of pharmaceuticals in the developing world takes many forms. A recent study of self-medication practices in Brazil and the Philippines reveals that in both countries, antibiotics are applied as crushed powder to wounds and skin lesions, as well as taken internally (Haak and Hardon 1988). Ferguson (1988) reports having observed mothers giving babies a teaspoon of tetracycline daily "as a preventive measure," despite the fact that the drug is contraindicated for use in small children. Pills are often packaged individually in the developing world. Patients may buy no more than four pills, regardless of their complaint or the medicine's effect. Injections tend to be highly regarded in developing societies; they are felt to be intrinsically stronger and preferable, especially for serious illness. In fact, the last few decades have seen the emergence of a wholly new type of health care provider: the itinerant injectionist. Patients demand injections (Cunningham 1970; Kleinman 1980; Good 1987).

Western medicines are available not only through biomedical practitioners and pharmacists. Traditional healers throughout the world are increasingly using Western drugs. In one study in Bangladesh, for example, 30 percent of homeopaths and 5 percent of traditional healers were found to be using allopathic drugs; 44 percent and 3 percent, respectively, were giving injections (Sarder and Chen 1981). Ninety percent of Indian traditional healers in another study made some use of Western drugs (Bhathia et al. 1975). Wolffers (1988, 1989) found that 50 percent of traditional practitioners in a rural community in Sri Lanka used Western drugs such as narcotics, antibiotics, and steroids. These practices are rationalized as being a response to the growing demand for pharmaceuticals from patients who are increasingly familiar with the procedures of biomedicine, and who expect comparable interventions from traditional healers.

Finally, we should note those instances in which the distribution of pharmaceuticals has moved beyond the domain of biomedical practitioners, pharmacists, and even traditional healers, into the hands of local entrepreneurs. For example, Whyte (1991) reports that in Uganda, hospital workers (not only doctors, but also nurses, aides, drivers, and janitorial staff) supplement their income by setting up small businesses, or "private clinics," for dispensing Western medicines that they may have appropriated from the government clinics where they work. Those who manage to procure a steady supply of drugs develop a reputation as informal medical practitioners in the community. Untrained and eager to make a profit, these practitioners tend to furnish medicines indiscriminately, invoking local cultural knowledge, if not actual misinformation, in distributing their goods.

A well-developed network for the distribution of Western drugs makes them easily and widely available for self-treatment, even in remote areas (Hardon 1987; Abosede 1984). Self-medication is the most common way of using medicines in most developing societies; this is the main impact, the most prominent inroad, that biomedicine has made in traditional communities throughout the world. For example, Whyte (1990) has also reported that in Uganda, residents prefer to purchase medicines in the marketplace rather than in a professional setting, in part because they already know what medicines they wish to use and are therefore interested neither in diagnosis nor prescription.

Studies of pharmaceutical use in Ethiopia (Kloos et al. 1988) and Mauritius (Sussman 1988) suggest that the proportion of patients who practice self-medication in a sophisticated way with Western drugs varies according to type of illness. A pharmacist in Sri Lanka described the situation thus: "The patient knows what he wants, I know what it costs, and I don't see the need for any additional information" (Wolffers 1988).

Thus, in the developing world, biomedicine is yielding control of one of its most powerful and distinctive features — its pharmacopoeia— to local pharmacists, traditional healers, and patients themselves. Owing to international and local commercial practices, the proliferation of pharmaceuticals is responsible for the commodification of stress and distress, as well as the practice of taking medicines for every problem. It is certainly responsible for a considerable amount of pharmacogenic illness in developing societies.

Convergence of Traditional and Biomedical Practice

The use of Western drugs by traditional healers is one major way in which the spread of biomedicine is changing traditional medical practice. It is just as important to realize, however, that traditional and biomedical practice are now part of a system of mutual influence in which each is being shaped by the other. Evidence suggests that in medically pluralistic settings, the differences in the therapies recommended by different types of healers are steadily decreasing. It is not unrealistic to expect, in fact, that these two systems of healing may eventually converge.

For example, in a study of Ayurvedic vaidyas and their biomedical colleagues in Sri Lanka, Waxler (1984) found that doctor-patient interaction styles, physical diagnostic techniques, and prescribing patterns were all remarkably similar. The efficacy of their work was also perceived to be comparable. Waxler argues that the persistence of distinctions between Ayurveda and biomedicine, despite this convergence of practice, is attributable to the fact that the two systems provide opportunities for social mobility to different segments of the population. Nevertheless, she considers the futures of these medical practices to be interdependent.

Similarly, Ladinsky and colleagues (1987) show that contemporary Vietnamese medicine is a "harmonious merging of Chinese, Vietnamese, and Western medical systems." For example, traditional medicines are often taken together with antibiotics to protect the patients from the possible side effects of Western medicines. A similar situation has been observed in Northern Thailand (Weisberg 1982, 1984).

The changing patterns of illness behavior documented in these examples further corroborate the argument being advanced in this chapter. Pharmacists' role as caregivers as well as drug dispensers in the developing world, the adoption of Western pharmaceuticals by traditional practitioners, the increasing reliance on Western medicines for self-treatment, and the convergence of traditional and biomedical systems of healing are all indications of the variety of ways in which Western biomedicine is being integrated into indigenous cultures. This variety is additional evidence of the complexity of the relationship between biomedical interventions and changes in health status and underscores the importance of attending to local cultural differences. In any given case, one cannot simply assume that biomedical treatment is effective, while traditional health care or self-care is ineffective.

Implications for Research and Health Policy

A number of significant gaps in our knowledge of illness behavior in the developing world remain to be filled by additional research. These may be divided into the following categories: (1) the nature and efficacy of biomedical services in developing countries, (2) the precise impact of social change, such as improved maternal education, on health and illness behavior, (3) the problem of suffering, (4) illness behavior in chronic illness in Third World settings, and (5) the ways in which particular types of illness behavior work to influence health status.

An illness behavior perspective directs our attention away from abstract, idealized representations of health and health services, toward a concern with people's actual experiences as they seek, receive, and deliver health care within the give-and-take of real-life contexts. To fully understand how biomedicine is practiced in developing societies and to ascertain how effective it is, we should adopt not only the bureaucratic gaze of the public health official, but also the ethnographic gaze of the anthropologist. The anthropologist's perspective takes us well beyond formal systems of biomedical care, to the realms of traditional healing, lay practice, and self-treatment. Because most of these have not been well studied, they should figure prominently on the agenda for future research on the health transition.

The effect of specific socioeconomic changes, such as increased education of mothers, upon illness behavior also requires further study. Needed are basic descriptive and analytic studies of the actual content of education for children. The existence of parallel systems of schooling (e.g., secular and religious schools) may help to reveal the relative contributions of content and process to the effect of education upon health. How does schooling affect the illness behavior of the students themselves? Do children with more or less education vary in the kinds of health behaviors they exhibit? Under what circumstances does education change illness beliefs?

While we tend to associate traditional healing with the developing societies of the Third World, it is important to recognize that nonbiomedical approaches to health care survive and even flourish in highly industrialized nations (McGuire 1988; Sonoda 1988). Why might this be? One reason is that unlike biomedicine, whose focus is narrowly biological, traditional healing seeks to relieve not only bodily distress, but also suffering, the psychic pain that ensues from an assault on the social, psychological, and moral worlds of the self. In ascribing meaning to the seeming pointlessness of illness, or symbolically reconnecting a sick person to his or her social world, or simply witnessing, and therefore validating, the existence of pain, the traditional healer confronts illness as human experience, not just as organic pathology. The survival of traditional healing in "developed" countries, and of "traditional" functions of the healer within biomedicine itself, testifies to the value and importance of this orientation toward the provision of care.

Like illness and death, suffering is universal to the human condition. Yet research on the health transition in developing countries has focused almost exclusively on morbidity and mortality. A responsible and humane approach to the study of health problems in the Third World requires that suffering be included as an object of analysis. An illness behavior perspective allows us to incorporate this other fundamental aspect of human experience into our evolving program of research.

As we have seen, the changing composition of morbidity in the direction of increased chronic illness is one of the defining characteristics of the health transition. Yet very little is known of the nature of illness behavior in chronic disease in the Third World or of the social factors that affect it. The wide variety of choices and practices we have described suggests that the outcome of chronic illness reflects a "social" course more than a "natural" one.

Additional research should illuminate the burden of disability in developing societies. The role of traditional healers in attending to the suffering of chronically ill individuals is of particular significance here, but so is the way in which social supports at the family and community levels amplify or dampen disablement.

Finally, we need to know more about the mechanisms and processes through which illness behavior influences health status. What are the implications for the health transition of the widespread misuse of oral antibiotics and parenteral drugs? Evidence has accumulated that in optimal circumstances, preventive services, such as vaccination and water purification, can improve the health of people in the developing world. But do curative biomedical services also make a difference in mortality at the local level? In settings of medical pluralism, do families that choose different healers for a given disease differ on objective measures of health status? Does adherence to recommended biomedical treatment affect the ultimate outcome?

The major implications of illness behavior for health policy can be indicated in a series of questions: How can health programs promote lay recognition of disease states so that appropriate action is taken quickly? How can they foster social networks instrumental in supporting and referring patients to appropriate health care providers? How can they eliminate obstacles to help seeking? How can they foster compliance with medical regimens?

Government officials, public health experts, and health care workers in international health all tend to define their policy concerns too narrowly, focusing almost exclusively on how the quality and frequency of interactions between biomedical professionals and patients might be improved. But, as we have seen, illness behavior encompasses much more than those aspects of help-seeking that result in patients' interactions with biomedical practitioners. The components of help-seeking in

Figure 11-1   Illness Behavior

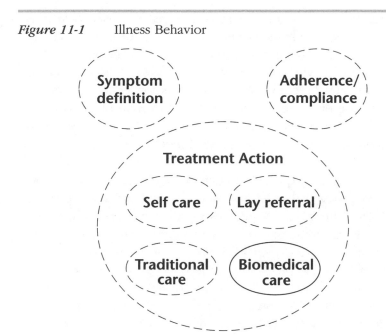

Illness behavior encompasses many purposeful actions by people confronting illness. Most attention to date has been devoted to the study of the interaction of patients with biomedical practitioners (solid line). But, as we have seen, such a focus is too narrow; many other aspects of illness behavior are relevant to the health transition, especially in the developing world (dotted lines).

relation to other aspects of illness behavior are represented diagrammatically in the illustration above.

Pharmaceutical policy is an especially important area where illness behavior has implications. More attention must be devoted to the ways in which pharmaceuticals are used (and misused) in developing societies. As we have seen, the use of Western drugs bought from local pharmacies or drug peddlers is the principal contact most people throughout the developing world have with biomedicine. Too many assumptions are made, however, about drug-use behavior. For example, it is sometimes wrongly assumed that the replacement of traditional pharmacies by their biomedical counterparts is partly responsible for the health transition. From a policy perspective, much should be done to foster more appropriate use of drugs, to educate drug users and prescribers, and, where it is shown to be dangerous, to constrain drug availability (e.g., through government sponsored essential drug lists or through more stringent regulation of international pharmaceutical firms). Attempts must also be made to tame the craving for injections and to foster more patience in those who expect an immediate response from Western drugs (and who stop taking them if they do not get one). Finally, communities must be empowered with the knowledge necessary for appropriate use of the technology that is already in place. How can families and communities, in other words, be encouraged to use pharmaceuticals in ways that constitute a more effective mode of self-care?

The near-veterinary quality of much biomedical care in developing societies, coupled with the pharmaceutical abuses that place populations at high risk for iatrogenesis, require responses at different levels. Control of the commercial abuse of caregiving in clinics, pharmacies, and mass media advertisements is essential. But also essential are efforts to increase lay and professional appreciation of the value of core cognitive tasks, such as careful elicitation of a history (responsible in and of itself for 80 percent of accurate diagnoses in primary care), explanation of the reasons for treatment (a cost-effective way to increase compliance and participation in preventive programs), and communication aimed at improving health education for health maintenance.

Conclusion

The basic point we have established is that any attempt to explain the social and behavioral roots of the health transition is incomplete unless it takes local cultural variation into account. To advance this argument, we have isolated a particular theoretical formulation — the notion that the health transition is the product of the combined forces of biomedical intervention and modernizing social change — and illustrated some of the different meanings and impacts these forces have when they are introduced into indigenous cultural settings around the world. The conceptual medium for carrying out this exercise has been illness behavior.

The decision to adopt an illness behavior perspective brings with it a number of advantages, such as the reorientation of attention away from mortality, toward the less-studied problem of morbidity. A focus on illness behavior can also be misleading for our purposes, however, unless the scope of the concept is made clear.

Because it highlights processes such as symptom identification and help-seeking, illness behavior may be mistakenly interpreted as a purely individual-level phenomenon. In fact, illness behavior is social as well as individual, because economic and political forces, socially-defined relationships, and cultural meanings are all reflected in the ways individuals respond to the perception and experience of illness.

It is this capacity to span macro- and micro-levels of analysis that makes illness behavior particularly useful as an organizing framework for social science research on the health transition. Because it illuminates the social nature of the individual, an illness behavior perspective offers a valuable alternative to large-scale epidemiological studies in tracing the social origins of changes in health status. Research that approaches the social through the individual — that defines as the object of analysis particular people within a particular cultural setting — offers a valid, empirically grounded, and comparatively inexpensive approach to understanding the social and behavioral determinants of health change.

Notes

1   The first two of these three aspects will be taken up in this chapter. For a discussion of behavioral pathologies in relation to the health transition, see Sugar, Kleinman and Heggenhougen, in this volume.

2   In fact, the classification of conditions as more appropriate for treatment by indigenous healers or biomedical practitioners varies considerably across cultures. In the case from Singapore cited above, for example, traditional Chinese medicine was strongly preferred for rheumatism, fractures, menstrual irregularities, and anemia, and significantly preferred for diarrhea, measles, worm infestations, influenza, and constipation. In Nigeria, traditional healers have been found to be strongly preferred for psychiatric disease, fractures, snake bites, and convulsions. Nnadi and Kabat, 1984.

3   See also Sokoloff, "The Proud Midwives of Huchitan," Honors Thesis, Harvard Medical School, 1986.

4   There is further the troubling problem of the meaning of "efficacy." Is this phenomenon to be understood in terms of subjective or objective improvements — or both?

5   We recognize that important distinctions among the many different types of traditional healers found around the world are glossed over in this report. These distinctions have been subsumed under the larger category of "traditional" healer in the interest of focusing attention on the issues of primary interest for this discussion.

6   McCormack (1988)has argued, however, that maternal education in the absence of other favorable societal features, such as female autonomy and control of wealth, may not have the desired effect upon health.

7 For a more extensive discussion of the mechanisms which may link women's education to child health, see LeVine et al., in this volume.

8 Virtually all of the following discussion could apply equally well to fathers. However, mother's education has repeatedly outweighed father's education as a predictor of child health status, presumably because of mothers' greater role in health care and child-rearing.

9 It is worth noting that termination of treatment may paradoxically result in better health care. For example, mothers might accept the persistence of low-grade symptoms after a course of otherwise effective therapy, thereby avoiding exposure to a new and potentially dangerous drug. Nations and Rebhun, 1988.

References

Abosede, O.A. 1984. "Self medication: An important aspect of primary health care." *Social Science and Medicine*, 19(7): 699–703.

Ahern, E. 1978. "Sacred and secular medicine in a Taiwan village: A study of cosmological disorders." In A. Kleinman, P. Kunstader, E.R. Alexander, and J.L. Gale, eds. *Culture and Healing in Asian Societies: Anthropological, Psychiatric, and Public Health Studies*. Cambridge, MA: Schenkman Publishing Company.

Annis, S. 1981. "Physical access and utilization of health services in rural Guatemala." *Social Science and Medicine*, 15D: 515–523.

Ayeni, B., G. Rushton, and M.L. McNulty. 1987. "Improving the geographical accessibility of health care in rural areas: A Nigerian case study." *Social Science and Medicine*, 25(10): 1083–1094.

Bertrand, W.E., and B.F. Walmus. 1988. "Maternal knowledge, attitudes and practice as predictors of diarrheal disease in young children." *International Journal of Epidemiology*, 127: 1079–1087.

Bhatia, J.C., et al. 1975. "Traditional healers and modern medicine." *Social Science and Medicine*, 9: 15–21.

Caldwell, J.C. 1979. "Education as a factor in mortality decline: An examination of Nigerian data." *Population Studies*, 33: 395–413.

Caldwell, J.C. 1986. "Routes to low mortality in poor countries." *Population and Development Review*, 12(2): 171–220.

Caldwell, J.C., and P. McDonald. 1982. "Influence of maternal education on infant and child mortality: Levels and causes." *Health Policy and Education*, 2: 251–267.

Chrisman, N. 1977. "The health seeking process." *Culture, Medicine and Psychiatry*, 1(4): 351–372.

Cleland, J.G., and J.K. van Ginneken. 1988. "Maternal education and child survival in developing countries: The search for pathways of influence." *Social Science and Medicine*, 27(12): 1357–1368.

Cominsky, S. 1987. "Women and health care on a Guatemalan plantation." *Social Science and Medicine*, 25(10): 1163–1173.

Cominsky, S., and M. Scrimshaw. 1980. "Medical pluralism on a Guatemalan plantation." *Social Science and Medicine*, 14B: 267–278.

Cunningham, C.E. 1970. "Thai injection doctors: Antibiotic mediators." *Social Science and Medicine*, 4: 1–24.

Das Gupta, M. 1989. "Death clustering, maternal education and the determinants of child mortality in rural Punjab, India." Discussion Paper Series, Center for Population Studies. Harvard University, Cambridge, MA.

DeVanzo, J. 1984. "A household survey of child mortality determinants in Malaysia." In W.H. Mosley and L.C. Chen, eds. *Child Survival*. New York: Cambridge University Press.

Esrey, S.A., and J. Habicht. 1988. "Maternal literacy modifies the effect of toilets and piped water in infant survival in Malaysia." *American Journal of Epidemiology*, 127: 1079–1087.

Farah, A.A., and S. Preston. 1982. "Child mortality differentials in Sudan." *Population and Development Review*, 8: 365.

Ferguson, A. 1988. "Commercial pharmaceutical medicine and medicalization: A case study from El Salvador." In S. van der Geest and S.R. Whyte, eds. *The Context of Medicines in Developing Countries, Studies in Pharmaceutical Anthropology*. Boston: Kluwer.

Finerman, R. 1987. "Inside out: Women's world view and family health in an Ecuadorian Indian community." *Social Science and Medicine,* 25(10): 1157–1162.

Fosu, G.B. 1981. "Disease classification in rural Ghana: Framework and implications for health behavior." *Social Science and Medicine*, 15B: 471–482.

Goldberg, H.I., et al. 1984. "Infant mortality and breastfeeding in north-eastern Brazil." *Population Studies*, 38: 105.

Good, C. 1987. *Ethnomedical Systems in Africa*. New York: Guilford Press.

Haak, H. and A.P. Hardon. 1988. "Indigenised pharmaceuticals in developing countries: Widely used, widely neglected." *The Lancet*, 8611: 620–21.

Hardon, A. 1987. "The use of modern pharmaceuticals in a Filipino village: Doctor's prescription and self medication." *Social Science and Medicine*, 25: 277–292.

Ho, S.C., K.C. Lun, and W.K. Ng. 1984. "The role of Chinese traditional medical practice as a form of health care in Singapore—III. Conditions, illness behavior, and medical preferences of patients of institutional clinics." *Social Science and Medicine*, 18(9): 745–752.

Hobcraft, J.N., J.W. McDonald, and S.O. Rutstein. 1984. "Socio-economic factors in infant and child mortality, A cross-national comparison." *Population Studies*, 38: 193.

Janzen, J. 1978. *The Quest for Therapy in Lower Zaire*. Berkeley: University of California Press.

Justice, J. 1986. *Policies, Plans and People—Culture and Health Development in Nepal*. Berkeley: University of California Press.

Kahane, J.D. 1987. "The Role of the Western Pharmacist in Rural Taiwanese Medical Culture." Ph.D. Dissertation. Department of Anthropology, University of Hawaii.

Kim, J. 1989. "Pharmaceutical industry in Korea." Presentation delivered to the Harvard Seminar on Medical Anthropology. Harvard University, Cambridge, MA.

Kim-Farley, R.J., et al. 1984. "Outbreak of paralytic poliomyelitis, Taiwan." *Lancet*, (2): 1322–1324.

Kleinman, A. 1980. *Patients and Healers in the Context of Culture*. Berkeley: University of California Press.

Kleinman, A., and J.L. Gale. 1982. "Patients treated by physicians and folk healers: A comparative outcome study in Taiwan." *Culture, Medicine and Psychiatry*, 6: 405–423.

Kloos, H., et al. 1986. "Utilization of pharmacies and pharmaceutical drugs in Addis Ababa, Ethiopia." *Social Science and Medicine*, 22(6): 653–672.

Kloos, H., et al. 1987. "Illness and health behaviour in Addis Ababa and rural Central Ethiopia." *Social Science and Medicine*, 25(9): 1003–1019.

Kloos, H., et al. 1988. "Buying drugs in Addis Ababa: A quantitative analysis." In S. van der Geest and S.R. Whyte, eds. *The Context of Medicines in Developing Countries, Studies in Pharmaceutical Anthropology*. Boston: Kluwer.

Ladinsky, J.L., N.D. Volk, and M. Robinson. 1987. "The influence of traditional medicine in shaping medical care practices in Vietnam today." *Social Science and Medicine*, 25(10): 1105–1110.

Leslie, C. 1978. "Pluralism and integration in the Chinese medical systems." In A. Kleinman, P. Kunstadter, E.R. Alexander, and J.L. Gale, eds. *Culture and Healing in Asian Societies*. Cambridge, MA: Schenkman Publishing Company.

LeVine, R., et al. 1987. "Schooling and maternal behavior in a Mexican city." The Population Council Fertility Determinants Research Notes, No. 16.

Lindenbaum, S. 1990. "The education of women and the mortality of children in Bangladesh." In A. Swedlund and G. Armelagos, eds. *The Health and Disease of Populations in Transition*. South Hadley, MA: Bergin and Garvey.

Locke, M. 1980. *East Asian Medicine in Urban Japan.* Berkeley: University of California Press.

Logan, K. 1988. "*Casi Como Doctor:* Pharmacists and their clients in a Mexican urban context." In S. van der Geest and S.R. Whyte, eds. *The Context of Medicines in Developing Countries, Studies in Pharmaceutical Anthropology.* Boston: Kluwer.

McClain, C. 1977. "Adaption in health behavior: Modern and traditional medicine in a west Mexican community." *Social Science and Medicine,* 11: 341–347.

McCormack, C.P. 1988. "Health and social power of women." *Social Science and Medicine,* 26(7): 677–683.

McGuire, M. 1988. *Ritual Healing in Suburban America.* New Brunswick, NJ: Rutgers University Press.

Mechanic, D. 1978. "Illness." In D. Mechanic, ed. *Medical Sociology.* New York: Free Press.

Nations, M.K., and L.A Rebhun. 1988. "Angels with wet wings won't fly: Maternal sentiment in Brazil and the image of neglect." *Culture, Medicine and Psychiatry,* 12(2): 141–200.

Nnadi, E.E., and H.F. Kabat. 1984. "Choosing health care services in Nigeria: A developing nation." *Journal of Tropical Medicine and Hygiene,* 87: 47–51.

Rahaman, M.M., et al. 1982. "A diarrhea clinic in rural Bangladesh: Influence of distance, age, and sex on attendance and diarrheal mortality." *American Journal of Public Health,* 72: 1124–1128.

Reid, J. 1984. "The role of maternal and child health clinics in education and prevention: A case study from Papua New Guinea." *Social Science and Medicine,* 19(3): 291–303.

Sarder, A.M., and L.C. Chen. 1981. "Distribution and characteristics of non-government health practitioners in a rural area of Bangladesh." *Social Science and Medicine,* 15A: 543–550.

Sargent, C. 1982. *The Cultural Context of Therapeutic Choice: Obstetrical Case Decisions among the Bariba of Benin.* Hingham, MA: Kluwer.

Sonoda, K. 1988. *Health and Illness in Changing Japanese Society.* Tokyo: University of Tokyo Press.

Stock, R. 1983. "Distance and the utilization of health facilities in rural Nigeria." *Social Science and Medicine,* 17: 563–570.

Sussman, L.K. 1988. "The use of herbal and biomedical pharmaceuticals on Mauritius." In S. van der Geest and S.R. Whyte, eds. *The Context of Medicines in Developing Countries, Studies in Pharmaceutical Anthropology.* Boston: Kluwer.

Tsui, A.O., J. DeClerque, and N. Mangani. 1988. "Maternal and sociodemographic correlates of child morbidity in Bas Zaire: The effects of maternal reporting." *Social Science and Medicine*, 26(7): 701–713.

United Nations. 1985. *World Population Prospects: Estimates and Projections as Assessed in 1982*, Populations Studies. No. 86. Department of International Economic and Social Affairs, ST/ESA/SER.A/86. New York.

Waxler, N.E. 1984. "Behavioral convergence and institutional separation: An analysis of plural medicine in Sri Lanka." *Culture, Medicine and Psychiatry*, 8(2): 187–205.

Weisberg, D.H. 1984. "Physicians' private clinics in a northern town—patient-healer collaboration and the shape of biomedical practice." *Culture, Medicine and Psychiatry*, 8(2): 165–186.

Weisberg, D.H. 1982. "Northern Thai health care alternatives: Patient control and the structure of medical pluralism." *Social Science and Medicine*, 16: 1507–1517.

Weisberg D., and S.L. Long. 1984. "Biomedicine in Asia." *Culture, Medicine and Psychiatry*, 8(2): 117–205.

Welch, R. 1980. "Illness and Sorcery among the Ningerum of Papua New Guinea." Unpublished Ph.D. Dissertation, Department of Anthropology, University of Washington.

Whyte, S. 1990. Presentation to the Department of Anthropology, Harvard University, Cambridge, MA, October 30.

Whyte, S. 1991. "Medicines and self-help: The privatization of health care in eastern Uganda." In H.B. Hansen and M. Twaddle, eds. *Structural Adjustment and the State of Uganda*. London: James Curry.

Wolffers, I. 1988. "Traditional practitioners and western pharmaceuticals in Sri Lanka." In S. van der Geest and S.R. Whyte, eds. *The Context of Medicines in Developing Countries, Studies in Pharmaceutical Anthropology*. Boston: Kluwer.

Wolffers, I. 1989. "Traditional practitioners' behavioural adaptations to changing patients' demands in Sri Lanka." *Social Science and Medicine*, 29(9): 1111–1119.

Young, J.C. 1981a. *Medical Choice in a Mexican Village*. New Brunswick, NJ: Rutgers University Press.

Young, J.C. 1981b. "Non-use of physicians: Methodological approaches, policy implications, and the utility of decision models." *Social Science and Medicine*, 15B: 499–506.

———. 1983. *Morbidity and Mortality Weekly Report*, 32(29): 385.

12

Schooling and Survival: The Impact of Maternal Education on Health and Reproduction in the Third World

Robert A. LeVine
Sarah E. LeVine
Amy Richman
F. Medardo Tapia Uribe
Clara Sunderland Correa

A growing body of evidence suggests that maternal education has played, and continues to play, a uniquely important role in the reduction of child mortality and fertility throughout the world. Continued improvement in survival chances for children as well as the long-term survival of the human species through population control may well depend on expanding female school enrollments in those Third World countries where they remain low. In this chapter, we attempt to deepen our understanding of the maternal schooling phenomenon and its policy implications through a consideration of the processes intervening between school attendance and reproductive change. An overview of the demographic and epidemiological evidence is followed by discussion of the social processes that might account for it; in the final section, pathways from schooling to diminished mortality and fertility are illustrated with data from our Mexican research, and some general conclusions are formulated.

The school attendance of women is consistently associated with reduced child mortality and fertility, as well as other changes in health and child care, across a wide range of populations past and present — including those of the United States and many contemporary Third World countries. As it becomes clearer through multivariate analyses of cross-sectional and time-series data that women's schooling is often a better predictor of health and reproductive outcomes than other household-level variables such as family income and husband's occupation, the expansion of female school enrollment seems to offer an attractive policy solution to the reduced pace of improvement in life expectancy, child health and fertility control in the Third World.

Caldwell (1986) has introduced a note of caution into consideration of this policy option. His historical analysis of child mortality reduction in the low-income populations of Sri Lanka, Kerala, Cuba and Costa Rica suggests that the most dramatic benefits of maternal schooling may be reaped only under certain cultural and political conditions that are less controllable than school expansion, viz an indigenous tradition of female autonomy and a politically organized local demand for health services. Furthermore, his case studies demonstrate that maternal schooling should be treated not as a form of medical technology with a known influence on health but as an aspect of locally variable social processes that are far from completely understood. Among the least understood processes are those that mediate the effects of school experience during childhood on the behavior of adult women as mothers and reproductive decision makers in Third World countries. This is the "black box" in survey data linking years spent in school with demographic and health outcomes; it is often covered by speculative assumptions and interpretations, but rarely investigated. Our purpose in this chapter is to shed some light from empirical research into this dark area, on the assumption that knowledge of the processes involved is essential to policy analysis.

An Overview of the Evidence

Analyses of national censuses and large-scale sample surveys in developing countries since 1960, including the World Fertility Survey (WFS) of 41 developing countries, show the school attendance of women to be negatively related to their fertility and the mortality of their offspring, even when other socioeconomic factors are controlled (Caldwell 1979. 1982, 1986; Cleland and Hobcraft 1985; Cleland and van Ginneken 1988; Cochrane 1979 1983; Cochrane, O'Hara and Leslie 1980; Kasarda, Billy and West 1986; United Nations 1986). This is one of the most widely and consistently replicated findings from quantitative research into the relationships between socioeconomic and demographic variables in the populations of Asia, Africa, Latin America and the United States. Recent reviews of the evidence support the following generalizations:

1. The assumption that maternal schooling affects birth and death rates *merely* through economic and geographical access to health care and other resources has been laid to rest, suggesting (largely by default) that schooling exerts an *educational* influence on maternal behavior.

2. Mortality between 1 and 5 years of age rather than in the first year of life is robustly related to maternal schooling when other socioeconomic factors are controlled, suggesting that child care in the *post-infancy* period is most influenced by the mother's education (Cleland and van Ginneken 1988).

3. Similarities in the links of maternal schooling to reduced child mortality, reduced breastfeeding and increased contraceptive use in many populations suggest that the mother's use of health services is involved.

Thus a good deal has been learned from large-scale studies, but much of the evidence is too indirect to resolve fundamental questions about the significance of this highly predictable and widespread statistical association. The major unanswered questions concern the determinants of differential schooling, the pathways through which the schooling of women is translated into changing patterns of reproduction and health, and the nature of the person-institution interactions involved. Differentials in school attendance among women in a population do not represent random assignment and therefore raise questions about why some left school earlier than others (or did not attend at all) and whether the determinants of school-leaving had independent effects on reproduction and health. The pathways through which school effects operate within the lifespan of the individual woman have been subject to a considerable amount of speculation and a modest amount of research, including our own. Figure 12-1 shows our working model (based on Mosley and Chen 1984) of the pathways mediating the influence of maternal school attendance on risks to child survival and health. In the present context, it is most important to bear in mind that the variables in boxes 3 through 9 have hardly ever been assessed and that the assumption that girls acquire skills, attitudes and knowledge in school that remain with them as mothers has not been directly tested. Finally, the ways in which institutional factors such as health services and family relationships operate with or against the school effect on individual women remain unclear.

These problems are considered in each section of the chapter. In this overview of the existing evidence, we provide some examples of its

Figure 12-1 A Model of Hypothetical Relationships between Maternal Schooling and Child Health

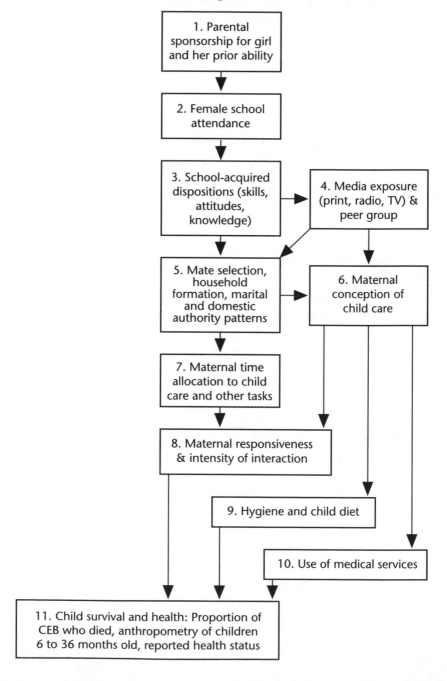

strengths and limitations, as a basis for theory and research on the processes that connect schooling to reproductive rates.

One strength of this evidence is that most of it was not produced by investigators seeking to demonstrate the value of female schooling. For example, Merrick (1985) set out to study the effect of access to piped water on child mortality in Brazilian cities during the early 1970s, when a concerted effort was made to provide all parts of the urban population with safe water. Regression and path analyses of the survival rates to age three of children born to 10,000 urban mothers aged 20-29 in the national census of 1970 and a survey of 1976 revealed the importance of parental education as well as access to piped water, with household income controlled. Merrick concludes:

> 1. That exogenous household variables (education of mothers and husbands) had the greatest total effect on differences in child mortality and that most of this effect was direct.
> 2. That access to piped water had a significant but secondary impact on differences in child mortality, accounting for about one-fifth of such differences...
>
> Examination of changes from 1970 to 1976 indicated that most of the decline in child mortality could be accounted for in terms of changes in the composition of the study population rather than changes in the parameters of the causal model, with increased education of both mothers and husbands playing a prime role, and increased access to piped water a secondary role (Merrick 1985:19).

This finding is especially striking in light of the fact that the replacement of contaminated water by safe, piped water acts directly and automatically to protect children from lethal infections, whereas the effects of parental education — though termed "direct" in this analysis — are mediated through (unspecified) behavioral pathways that would seem to be a great deal less reliable. As Merrick points out, the difference in the relative impact of parental education and access to piped water may have been exaggerated by historical timing, viz. that schooling was expanded earlier than the water supply, though even this argument suggests an increasing cumulative impact of parental education on child mortality.

Another strength of this body of evidence is that its central findings have been replicated by investigators of diverse backgrounds, working in diverse regions with diverse sources of data. Child mortality again provides a telling example. One of the most intensive studies is in the Matlab village area of Bangladesh, where demographic-epidemiological surveillance covering many household variables has been conducted for over twenty years in a population that has not known the school expansion of urban Brazil. D'Souza and Bhuiya (1982) report that for a sample of 1,522 rural mothers in Matlab during 1975-77, the mortality of children aged 1 to 4 years was more than five times greater among mothers who had never gone to school than among those who had attended for seven or more years. A similar finding emerged independently from analysis of the WFS of 28 developing countries in Asia, Africa and Latin America, viz. that the mortality of children aged 1 to 4 is strongly related to maternal schooling. After adjustment for rural-urban residence and household socioeconomic factors, the rate for children of mothers with no schooling was about twice that of mothers with seven or more years of school (Cleland and van Ginneken 1988:1360; Hobcraft, McDonald and Rutstein 1984). Diverse analysts also agree that the relationship of women's schooling to reduced fertility in the WFS and other data sets that have been subjected to multivariate analysis does not simply reflect socioeconomic access variables, but points to an educational or psychosocial impact of schooling (Cleland and Hobcraft 1985; Kasarda, Billy and West 1986; Jain and Nag 1986; United Nations 1986). This generally confirms the earlier analyses and theoretical formulations of Caldwell (1979; 1982). Thus the evidence linking maternal schooling to reproductive outcomes has achieved a level of robustness and generality that is rare in the social sciences.

Finally, a growing strength of the evidence is that the links intervening between female school attendance and fertility/mortality are being empirically identified. Three of these links are apparent in the self-report data from large-scale surveys: husband's school attainment, contraceptive use and breastfeeding. It is virtually universal that mothers with more schooling are more likely to be married to more educated men, to use contraceptives and to breastfeed their babies a shorter period of time (if at all). Marriage to a man with more schooling may not only give the woman better access to health care and other resources but provide her with interpersonal support for translating her school-acquired skills and attitudes into actions that decrease child mortality and fertility. The ubiquitous association between women's schooling and reported contraceptive use, and its statistical independence of other socioeconomic factors (United Nations 1986), indicates that the fertility-reducing effect of female education among *married* women operates through contact with health services (hospital, dispensary, pharmacy) rather than through abstinence or withdrawal. And the equally ubiquitous association with diminished breastfeeding, which increases risks to child survival, suggests that mothers with more schooling are more "medicalized" in their approach to infant care, relinquishing or reducing a highly beneficial folk practice in favor of bottle-feeding and/or infant formula, which carry the prestige and authority of modern medicine. These trends in the data point to marital choice and the influence of Western-style health services and medical technology as key factors in the processes intervening between school and reduced child mortality and fertility.

There is also more direct evidence on differentials by maternal school attainment in health-related child care practices. Cleland and van Ginneken (1988: 1361-63) have reviewed studies from a wide variety of countries demonstrating maternal schooling to be related to preventive practices such as prenatal care, medically attended delivery, infant health care and immunization, even with socioeconomic factors controlled. The burden of evidence shows that in most places, mothers with more schooling use available health services more frequently or more effectively for child health than those with less education. In a rare observational study of domestic health-related care by 185 mothers of children aged 4 to 27 months in rural Bangladesh, Guldan (1988) found a wide variety of feeding and hygiene practices predictive of better health to be associated with the mother's having attended school, controlling for family wealth; for many practices, school attainment of the husband and other members of the family was also associated with these outcomes, although not as strongly. Thus the maternal practices accounting for reduced child mortality and fertility among more educated women are becoming known.

In evaluating this evidence, we view it as part of a larger body of findings from social and developmental research demonstrating differentials by parental schooling in the care and characteristics of offspring, e.g., maternal attitudes, patterns of mother-child interaction, cognitive skills during the preschool years and achievement in primary school (e.g. Crockenberg 1983; Laosa 1982). The child development studies, conducted largely in English-speaking and Latin American countries, tend to show that the schooling of mothers affects their responsiveness to their preschool children, with a greater emphasis on verbal responsiveness among the more educated mothers and better performance on cognitive tests by their children. While this literature needs further analysis, it seems generally consistent with the findings from cross-national demographic and health research and calls for a unified explanatory model.

Despite the overall consistency of the evidence, its strengths are counter-balanced by significant limitations: (a) There are exceptions to the overall pattern, "deviant cases" that need to be examined. (b) It is not clear how much of the apparent effect of maternal schooling on child mortality and fertility is due to (usually unmeasured) background factors that might account for both a mother's level of school attainment and her reproductive and child care activity, without a causal link between the school experience and maternal behavior. (c) Most of the evidence was collected between 1950 and 1980, and its patterns might reflect conditions specific to that historical period rather than constituting a universal impact of schooling on health, reproduction and child care. We now turn to an examination of these limitations.

Exceptions. The school-mortality relationship is virtually universal across developing societies, including India and China (Cleland and van Ginneken 1988), but school-fertility patterns exhibit significant regional and country-specific divergence. In sub-Saharan Africa, women's schooling tends to show a curvilinear relationship with childbearing, i.e., women who have attended primary school bear *more* children than those with no schooling, and fertility is lower only among those with postprimary school attainment. Given the infrequency of contraceptive use in these populations, the explanation seems to be that the primary school leavers have shorter birth intervals than the unschooled — due to abbreviated breastfeeding and the quicker resumption of menses — while it is only among those with the most schooling that contraception has made inroads on fertility. The cultural attitudes that keep high fertility in place among the majority are much slower to change than health practices improving child survival, which require no deviation from traditional reproductive goals. This regional pattern has been described and analyzed by Caldwell and Caldwell (1987), Cleland (1985), Bongaarts, Frank and Lesthaeghe (1984) and Lesthaeghe (1989); accounting for it remains a problem for anthropological research (LeVine et al. in press). For the moment, the African fertility situation remains a qualified exception to the generalization that maternal schooling reduces fertility, and it remains to be seen whether this reflects an early, temporary stage of demographic transition or a longer-term historical reality.

Thailand represents a different kind of exception, in which fertility has fallen drastically to levels that are uniform across most segments of the population, eliminating educational differentials in cross-sectional surveys (Knodel et al. 1987). This does not mean that women's schooling played no part in the spread of contraceptive use and consequent reduction of fertility. Indeed, Thailand's early investment in four-year rural schools, attended by girls as well as boys, seems to have been involved both in creating the widespread conditions for reproductive change and in preventing the development of the large inequalities in schooling that cross-sectional demographic surveys usually tap.

The dominant Theravada Buddhist culture of Thailand, and its domestic organization — in which women are relatively autonomous from their husbands and older kin in matters of reproduction — are also reported to have facilitated fertility decline (Knodel et al. 1987), and they probably facilitated as well the enrollment of girls in primary schools when they were first built. Like the exceptional case of the sub-Saharan populations, Thailand implies that the school effect on fertility decline can be impeded or accelerated by cultural conditions and domestic relationships affecting the ability of women to translate attitudinal change into reproductive performance.

Selectivity. The possibility that a woman's level of school attainment reflects background factors that could affect her fertility and offspring mortality *directly*, rather than through educational influence, has rarely been taken into account in the research on which most of our evidence is based. There are two specific possibilities: (1) The sponsorship factor, i.e., that women who go further in school have parental families who are more (economically) able or (attitudinally) willing to provide them both more formal education in childhood and more support for their health-seeking behavior (including access to maternal and child health services) in adulthood. (2) The selection factor, i.e., that girls who are more manifestly intelligent during their preschool years are selected by their parents for more schooling (or select themselves by doing better in school), and that their superior cognitive skill manifests itself also in more effective adaptation to health and family planning services during their reproductive years. In the first case, more schooling and its reproductive correlates are successive outcomes of advantages in the parental generation, rather than being linked as cause and effect; in the second case, they are both outcomes of the women's prior cognitive skill.

There is little information from the WFS and other demographic surveys bearing on these hypotheses, as Cleland and van Ginneken (1988) point out. One exception concerning the sponsorship hypothesis is the Nigerian study of Caldwell (1979), in which the occupational status of the woman respondent's father was entered into the regression equation for child mortality; with father's occupation controlled, the respondent's level of schooling was still significantly related to the mortality of her children. Among the Yoruba population of Ibadan, Nigeria, then, the association of women's schooling with reduced infant and child mortality cannot be attributed simply to the prior socioeconomic advantage of the woman as measured by her father's occupational status. But this hypothesis remains an important candidate for future research elsewhere.

The selection and sponsorship hypotheses were examined by Irwin et al. (1978), who administered the INCAP Preschool Battery of 22 cognitive tests to 387 children at age 7, prior to school entry, in three of the villages involved in the longitudinal INCAP nutrition study in highland Guatemala. Subsequently, 92 of the children did not enroll in school and another 45 dropped out during the first year, while the rest completed between one and six years. The schooled children, i.e., those who completed at least one year, had scored significantly higher on the Preschool Battery than the unschooled, suggesting that prior ability played a part in their being sent to, or being kept in, school. The differences between schooled and unschooled were greater for girls than boys. A variety of family variables, indicating economic status, parental schooling, maternal modernity, and maternal stimulation/teaching, were significantly higher for the schooled than the unschooled, indicating that sponsorship was also involved in differential school attendance. Indeed, family economic status and maternal stimulation were also significantly correlated with years of school attendance for both sexes — more strongly than preschool test scores for boys, though not for girls, for whom multiple regression analysis showed the test score to be an independent predictor of length of schooling. Thus both sponsorship and selection on the basis of prior ability emerged from this study as probable determinants of schoolgoing.

These results support the position that differential school attendance in a sample of mothers reflects background factors and cannot be treated as if they had been randomly assigned to schoolgoing and non-schoolgoing groups or to groups attending school for varying lengths of time. And if their levels of schooling are due to prior advantages of personal skill or family resources, could not these same advantages continue to influence their behavior as mothers without being mediated through formal education? There is little doubt that they could and that this at the very least raises questions about how to interpret evidence linking women's schooling with reproductive rates when it does not include data on the distribution of prior advantages. In the Guatemalan study, however, two qualifying factors must be considered. First, the amount of variance explained:

> Multiple r^2 values for the composite [preschool test] score plus all family SES and values variables with length of attendance are relatively modest for both boys (r^2 = .16) and girls (r^2 = .08), indicating that most of the variance in length of attendance is not explained by variables employed in our regression analysis (Irwin et al. 1978, p. 421).

In other words, most of the variance in length of school attendance might be explainable by factors unrelated to prior advantage. Second, the mean levels of schooling for parents in this sample were two years or less, and their children had no more than 6 years of school, indicating that the population was at an early stage of educational development. If expansion in enrollment continued across succeeding cohorts, then the rising average level of schooling across cohorts might become a larger source of variation than intra-cohort variation in schoolgoing and would outweigh effects due to prior advantage. This brings us to the problem of historical change.

Historical specificity. The thirty years (1950-1980) from which most of the survey evidence linking women's schooling with reproductive rates is derived, was an exceptional period of socioeconomic and demographic change in virtually all the developing as well as developed countries. One question this raises is whether the associations found then are temporary characteristics, reflecting a pattern of change specific to that period, or to a particular phase of socioeconomic development and demographic transition through which many countries were going at that time, rather than being indicative of a more general impact of schooling on mortality and fertility. Answering this question requires a conception of how the macrosocial changes of the post-World War II decades affected the individuals interviewed in demographic and health surveys.

Between 1950 and 1980, the populations of many countries in Asia, Africa, Latin America and the Pacific changed dramatically in their aggregate indicators of health, education and material welfare. Incomes and school enrollments rose, and death rates and (after 1965) birth rates fell, as access to transportation, communication and medical facilities also expanded. These aggregate trends reflected structural change and growth of the economy, which drew many more men and women into formal employment and often into urban centers, and the expansion of public institutions and economic infrastructure in both rural and urban areas, creating new conditions for family life and individual development. But the changes were unevenly distributed within and across countries, so that even as average national levels (e.g., income, literacy, life expectancy) improved, disparities at the subnational and international levels became greater. Thus estimated adult female literacy in the developing world rose from 28 percent in 1960 to 50 percent in 1985, but at the latter date the school enrollments of females aged 5 to 19 years ranged from 65 percent in Latin America to 42 percent in sub-Saharan Africa and 30 percent in South Asia (Sivard 1985). Infant mortality and fertility showed similar patterns, with cross-national and rural-urban gaps increasing in many cases even as overall levels declined.

The rapidity of change means that samples of women aged 15 to 49 in cross-sectional surveys conducted in recent decades have usually included wide variations across age cohorts: The women over 35 or 40 came to maturity when fertility was high, chances of child survival low, and schooling (especially for women) rare. The younger cohorts in the same population were more likely to have attended school, to have borne children who survived, and (in many parts of the world) to have curtailed their fertility. In other words, age is often confounded with schooling and reproductive rates in such samples, and it is necessary to control for age (or an age-linked variable such as duration of marriage) to disentangle the influence of membership in a birth cohort from that of schooling in the analysis of reproductive change. Most analyses have used such controls and have still found a strong effect of schooling, but it remains possible that the pathways through which schooling influences reproduction and child care vary by cohort within a population, requiring investigation at the level of the particular cohort.

Under transitional conditions, each cohort is virtually a distinct culture in terms of the meanings that schoolgoing, childbearing and child survival have for its members. The expectations and normative standards governing a woman's personal reproductive and educational experience are so conditioned by the levels of mortality, fertility and school attendance prevailing in her own cohort that one cannot assume her experience or behavior to be replicating that of her mother, or even her older sisters. Thus the ways in which schooling alters her behavior as a mother may be correspondingly different but remain hidden in the available survey evidence.

A given population can be seen as located in a space defined by the intersection of a local cultural tradition (regulating nuptiality, marital sexuality, lactation, birth interval, standards of child care) with a set of transition parameters (fertility and child survival rates and school enrollment ratios) that vary across local birth cohorts and create the distinctive conditions under which each cohort responds to traditional norms of reproduction and child care. By describing a sample already investigated in Mexico with one to be studied in Bangladesh in terms not only of its traditions but also its location on the transition variables, it may be possible to assess the relevance of one study to another.

This model permits conceptualization of the historical context in which correlations between school attendance and reproductive rates are expectable. In the earliest cohorts, women's schooling is too rare to be correlated with fertility and mortality; it is only when female school enrollment has become sufficiently widespread, and child mortality and fertility have begun to drop, that they can be correlated. This is evident in Jejeebhoy's (1985) analysis of demographic change during the decade 1970 to 1980 in the state of Tamil Nadu in south India. From 1971 to 1981, the female literacy rate rose from 26.9 percent to 35.0 percent, contraceptive prevalence increased from 15.76 percent to 28.3 percent, and the crude birth rate dropped from 31.3 percent to 28.1 percent. Examining change among married women aged 35 to 44 in the 1970 and 1980 family planning surveys, Jejeebhoy shows that the mean years of schooling in this age group was 2.50 (S.D. = 3.30) in 1970 and 2.91 (S.D. = 3.73) in 1980. The relationships between schooling and socioeconomic factors such as employment and ownership of modern goods increased between the two surveys, as did the correlations of schooling with desired family size (from -.04 to -.20, p<.05), children ever born (from -.02 to -.11, n.s.) and proportion of child mortality (from -.12 to -.17, both p<.05). As female school enrollment grew and birth and death rates fell in Tamil Nadu, then, the correlations of women's schooling with socioeconomic, attitudinal and reproductive outcomes increased in magnitude, from near zero to significant levels in one decade. Given the early stage of this population in its educational transition for women, it seems likely that the correlations will increase in succeeding cohorts as female schooling becomes more widespread.

The eventual trajectory of this trend may depend on the distribution of resources, including access to health care and schooling, within the population. According to one line of thinking, if a high level of equality of access is achieved, then the correlations will reach an asymptote and then decrease with each succeeding cohort until they return to zero; if distributions remain unequal, then strong correlations between maternal schooling and reproductive rates will become a stable feature of the population. The first case can be illustrated by Thailand, where educational differentials in fertility characterized the transitional period of fertility decline but were wiped out later, when access to contraception (and primary schooling) had been provided to most women (Knodel et al. 1987). The second case could be exemplified by Brazil, Colombia and other Latin American countries in which inequalities in the distribution of resources, including education and health care, within and between rural and urban communities and socioeconomic strata, have persisted to a point that could be called permanent. (A similar contrast is possible between some of the northern European countries with small, homogeneous populations and strong welfare states, and the United States, with its large, heterogeneous population and unequal distribution of resources.) Thus the temporary or permanent character of the correlations between schooling and reproductive rates in a particular country may depend on its distributional policies and the size and composition of its population.

However, the question of whether it is the expanding availability of services (primary health care, family planning) or the improved ability of mothers (through more income and schooling) that drives reproductive change remains an unsettled and controversial issue in international health policy research (Mosley 1989), and the lack of a definitive answer from the existing evidence represents a limitation that needs attention in future research. Thus the problem of whether the correlations between maternal schooling and reproductive rates are temporary or permanent cannot yet be resolved.

The overview in this section has shown that the evidence relating female school attendance to reproductive rates in developing countries, though one of the most robust and consistent bodies of findings in comparative social science, is not without a number of significant limitations that render its theoretical meaning and policy implications unclear. In the following section we consider the meaning of these findings, with particular attention to the processes by which schooling could lead to reproductive change.

Processes of Social Change

In order to interpret the evidence and generate new research that will resolve remaining obscurities, it is useful to develop theoretical accounts consistent with the extant findings, focusing on macrosocial processes that link schooling with reproductive change in historical time, as well as on microsocial processes that mediate the impact of school attendance on maternal behavior in the context of a particular cohort's lifespan. Our formulation of three viewpoints that provide differing (though not necessarily contradictory) perspectives on the problem is predicated on the assumptions that there is a global trend toward lower birth and death rates, as specified in demographic transition theory (Caldwell 1982), and that this trend is a function of changing social and economic conditions. Each view provides an account of the process by which women's schooling facilitates or accelerates demographic transition in the context of changing socioeconomic conditions.

Bureaucratization of the life course. From this perspective, a pervasive tendency of social change is toward spending more of the average lifespan in bureaucratically organized settings: schools, clinics, corporate workplaces, commercialized markets — all part of a public social world explicitly detached from kinship and other prior ties and designed to serve specialized functions according to standardized and impersonal models of action, role relationship and personal career. The individual begins in school, progresses to a bureaucratic workplace, seeks health in bureaucratically organized hospitals and clinics. Schools acquaint children with patterns of speech, work and interaction useful for participating in other bureaucracies: the use of decontextualized language, in which mutual familiarity with the subject of conversation is not taken for granted; work routines involving attention to the procedural details of formally defined tasks; norms for interaction with an unfamiliar superior, e.g., the asking of questions to clarify assigned tasks. The longer one attends school, the more one acquires these skills as habitualized or automatized patterns of behavior and the better one is prepared to participate in other bureaucratic settings as an adult.

When girls from agrarian families attend school, their acquisition of these skills influences their later interactions with the health bureaucracy, particularly in understanding and following instructions, learning novel procedures, getting the attention of medical personnel, asking appropriate questions and generally being able to function strategically in an institution that often ignores or neglects its clients. Women who have not attended school are correspondingly disadvantaged. This affects birth and death rates because one aspect of the bureaucratization of the life course is the medicalization of reproduction, i.e., the replacement of indigenous customs of birth spacing, midwifery, home delivery, lactation and traditional healing for mother and infant by a network of bureaucratic and/or commercial health services providing curative and preventive medicine, contraception and hospital delivery based on Western biotechnology. As this process is extended within a population, it is the women with more years of schooling who use these services more frequently and effectively, other things being equal, and they are consequently more likely to survive childbearing, to bear fewer children who have better survival chances, and to follow perceived medical advice even when (as in Caesarian delivery and reduced breastfeeding) it may be of dubious value for health. Thus schooling confers behavioral skills critical to participation in a bureaucratized health care system, and educational differentials in births, deaths and the use of medical services are a ubiquitous consequence of mass schooling.

Socioeconomic transformation. From this perspective, the most fundamental change in developing countries since World War II has been the penetration of economic markets and pecuniary values into sectors of social organization and culture that were formerly insulated from commercial transaction, including the family and education, as a consequence of the transformation of economic production, exchange and distribution. Economic production changed from subsistence agriculture to industry or commercial agriculture, involving formal employment and oriented to world as well as local markets. Economic exchange became increasingly monetized and extended to goods and services that never before had monetary value, including the domestic labor of women and children, making cash the universal standard of value. Income and wealth distributions became increasingly differentiated, as unprecedented economic growth provided more monetary benefits to some than others.

Schooling played a critical role in this process. In the agrarian community, the life course and adult social identity of each person was organized by a local, gender-specific age hierarchy, and he or she looked forward to a predictable enhancement of status and other benefits with advancing age and reproductive accomplishment, in the context of a local reference group. A cultural model of the life course provided symbolically elaborated conceptions of these adult social identities that each child acquired through participation in family and community. As the market economy expanded, however, with formal employment as one of its components, a new conception of the life course and adult social identity arose; it was based on the academic occupational hierarchy, in which level of school attainment determined one's place in the occupational prestige hierarchy and thus in the social strata emerging from economic development (LeVine and White 1986).

In the new social order dominated culturally by the academic occupational hierarchy, schooling was the primary vehicle of hope for enhanced status and wealth, particularly for those who had little, and parents concerned themselves as never before with their children's careers — the occupational careers of the boys in a competitive labor market, the marital chances of the girls in what might be a competitive market for men of higher status. There were wide cultural variations in the extent to which girls had access to schooling and occupations of their own, but their schooling, no less than boys', represented the aspirations of parents legitimized by the state.

Thus the school attainment levels of women in a cohort are symptomatic of parental aspirations for a daughter they might help in many other ways as well, even during her adult years. Furthermore, the girl's own aspirations and sense of control over her life might reflect the amount of parental support she has received as a child for her career (broadly conceived), and higher aspirations and a greater sense of control would lead her to be more active in taking advantages of health services and health information for herself and her offspring. Thus this view tends to support the idea that a woman's school attainment and her reproductive and health behavior are outcomes of preschool advantages conferred by her parents.

At a more general level, the widespread association of reproductive change with women's schooling in developing societies is an inevitable product of advantage-seeking among people for whom access to resources is not equally distributed through central control. If it is inevitable that income, health care and schooling are differentially distributed in a population, it is equally certain that they will be clustered, as those who gain access to one will already have better access to the other or have the resources to improve their children's access.

This view accounts not only for the differential distribution of socioeconomic advantages and reproductive rates in a population, but also for improvements in average levels over time as the aggregate outcome of individual and family advantage-seeking behavior in a context of economic growth. What counts most is the universal pecuniary calculus of personal advantage introduced by a monetized market economy and an academic-occupational hierarchy, e.g., increasing parental awareness of their economic costs and benefits in raising a child and of what would most benefit their children in economic terms.

Changing parental strategies. This perspective, while not entirely independent of the other two, is distinctively focused on the microsocial processes by which the school experience of a woman alters her behavior as a mother and her concept of the parent-child relationship. Schools implicitly teach that children are publicly valued as citizens (Benavot 1989; Meyer 1977) and as resources worth developing; thus school attendance *per se* introduces the girl in an agrarian community to the idea that each child, even if female, is a full person rather than an adjunct to another person and represents a potential worthy of long-term development through education. This favors a shift from *quantity* to *quality* in the goals of childbearing and child care. In the agrarian setting, the primary goal for parents is to maximize the number of surviving children, so as to gain as much child labor in the short term and risk insurance in the long run as is possible when child mortality is high; in urban-industrial societies, the primary goal is to optimize the development and life chances of a small number of children, each of whom is virtually guaranteed to survive but costs much and contributes little to the parents in economic terms and faces a competitive labor market in adulthood.

These goals dictate divergent strategies for investing parental resources, including time, energy, and attention. For agrarian parents, resources are invested in repeated childbearing and a protective (or "pediatric") pattern of care, with attention being concentrated on the child during infancy, when survival risks are greatest. For urban-industrial parents, resources are invested in a more "pedagogical" pattern of care extending maternal attention throughout childhood as preparation for and accompaniment to schooling; health care is delegated to medical specialists. In agrarian societies undergoing socioeconomic transformation and bureaucratization, the expansion of female schooling facilitates the transition from quantity to quality in child care by providing models of teaching and learning through verbal interaction that influence a mother's earliest behavior toward the child and foster a greater intensity of mutual interaction. The more active child produced by such intense interaction demands a continuing commitment of maternal attention that ensures child survival after infancy and raises the energy costs of high fertility to a level that motivates contraception. This theoretical perspective is derived from cross-cultural research on child care and development and has guided our research on the impact of maternal schooling on reproductive change.

Research Design

An ideal research design for investigating the processes by which maternal schooling affects child mortality and fertility would include a number of successive cohorts in a local population, obtaining background data on each girl and her family and assessing prospectively for each cohort the levels at which they left school, subsequent experiences that might change their knowledge and attitudes toward reproduction and child care, and their situations, behavior and attitudes as mothers. To achieve generality, such a long-term study would have to be replicated in a number of diverse local settings.

The implementation of such a research design would be a major undertaking, requiring resources on a large scale and over a longer period than the working lives of some of the investigators. It seems unlikely that such a study will be mounted, except as part of national surveys or epidemiological surveillance systems designed primarily to monitor mortality, morbidity and fertility over time, nor is it certain that research on this scale will be necessary (to resolve questions raised by the existing evidence and models) or useful (given the time needed for its completion). It is nonetheless important to bear in mind that deviations from this ideal, in the interests of obtaining a manageable amount of data in a relatively short period of time, mean the substitution of indirect for direct measurement of the variables and processes involved, and reduce the certainty and clarity of the findings.

Without a prospective study conducted over a long period of time, it is impossible to know if the prior ability of the girls in a cohort is correlated with their subsequent levels of school attainment and reproductive activity. Furthermore, without longitudinal assessment it is necessary to rely upon respondents' *post hoc* reconstruction of their experiences intervening between school and childbearing as well as of the reproductive events themselves, thus diminishing the validity of the data. It is nonetheless possible, if one is aware of the biases, ambiguities and other defects in designs that are less than optimal, to compensate for some of them and estimate the effects of others, thus salvaging valid findings from research conducted within a few years rather than a few decades.

One way of investigating the impact of female schooling on demographic change in general and the risks to child survival in particular is to examine a population in which change has already occurred and the impact has been experienced by living cohorts of women. Differences by cohort, and individual variations within a cohort due to the uneven spread of schooling, provide the possibility of detecting what difference schooling has made in aspects of reproductive behavior and maternal care that affect the lives of children. This was the strategy we pursued in selecting for our first field study a country — Mexico — in which the expansion of female school enrollments and demographic change were advanced. Initial exploration suggested that the study should be carried out in an urban area in order to find enough mothers who had completed primary school, and we decided to select a city — Cuernavaca — small enough to be approached by anthropological methods, which had grown through industrial and commercial development to about 230,000 by 1980. We subsequently discovered that there were substantial populations of women with primary and higher schooling in certain rural communities of southern Morelos where *secundarias* (junior high schools) had been established many years ago, and we initiated a second study there in 1987. Results from these Mexican studies will illustrate our discussion of pathways of influence in the next section.

Pathways of Influence: Models and Evidence

In this section we examine in more detail the links between schooling and reproductive change within the life history of the individual woman. Figure 12-2 presents three simple models of the ontogenetic processes involved, i.e., the woman's acquisition during childhood and adolescence of skills, motives and cultural (normative) models that can influence, through direct and indirect paths, her maternal behavior in ways that affect child survival and fertility. Each pathway is supported by

Figure 12-2   Pathways from Schooling to Reduced
Mortality/Fertility

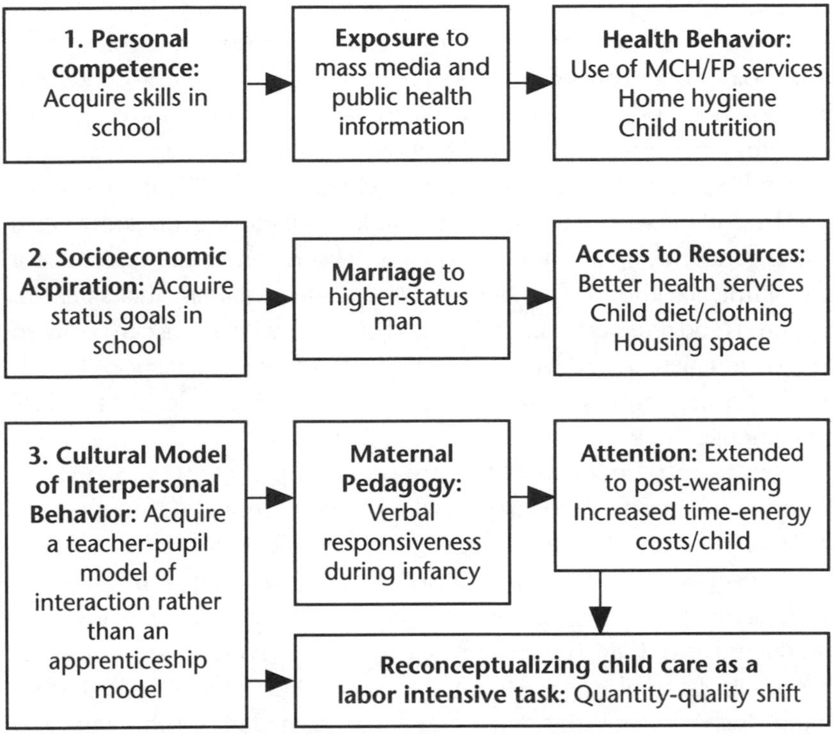

| 1. Personal competence: Acquire skills in school | Exposure to mass media and public health information | Health Behavior: Use of MCH/FP services Home hygiene Child nutrition |

| 2. Socioeconomic Aspiration: Acquire status goals in school | Marriage to higher-status man | Access to Resources: Better health services Child diet/clothing Housing space |

| 3. Cultural Model of Interpersonal Behavior: Acquire a teacher-pupil model of interaction rather than an apprenticeship model | Maternal Pedagogy: Verbal responsiveness during infancy | Attention: Extended to post-weaning Increased time-energy costs/child |

Reconceptualizing child care as a labor intensive task: Quantity-quality shift

Additional Complexities

1. Synergy: Pathways interact and jointly amplify school effects
2. Accumulation: Intergenerational magnification of school effects
3. Institutional facilitators and inhibitors of school effects

some empirical evidence from our Mexican research and other sources, as indicated in the following discussion. Noted at the bottom of the chart are additional complexities that bear on the policy implications of these pathways, particularly as they operate over time.

The first model, "Personal Competence," represents the common-sense assumption that girls acquire cognitive skills, including literacy, in school, permitting their greater exposure to media messages that favor more adaptive health behavior. Thus the more years they attend school, the more likely they are to use maternal and child health (MCH) and family planning (FP) services frequently and effectively and to improve the child's home environment according to officially recommended public health standards of hygiene and nutrition. While this pathway is plausible if one assumes that schools transmit the skills for which they are designed, there are grounds for skepticism. In many Third World communities, schools lack basic instructional equipment (books, seats, blackboards), teachers are inadequately trained and the absenteeism rates of both pupils and teachers are high, resulting in very poor academic performance by international standards (Heyneman and Loxley 1983). Yet the effect of women's schooling on child mortality does not depend on school quality and is quite evident for even a few years of attendance at apparently low quality schools. Since the effect is not due simply to other socioeconomic factors, the possibility that skills are acquired (and retained) cannot be ruled out any more than it can be taken for granted, without direct measurement of differentials in specific skills and exposure to the media among mothers varying in level of school attainment.

Our Mexican findings (1991) support some parts of this first model. Research was conducted (from 1983 to 1985) among 300 mothers of young children, with one to nine years of schooling, in two low-income neighborhoods of Cuernavaca, Morelos, a city of about 250,000 at the time, located 50 miles south of Mexico City; a second study was conducted from 1986 to 1987 among 177 mothers, with zero to nine years of school, of a rural Morelos town of about 8,000 located 30 miles farther south. In both the urban and rural samples, maternal schooling was strongly associated with the use of maternal and child health services (e.g., prenatal care, use of clinic for child illness) and with fertility adjusted for age or duration of marriage, indicating the use of family planning services. In the urban setting, women with post-primary schooling responded more rapidly to signs of serious illness in their children and reported less frequent episodes of diarrhea. In the rural community, mothers with more schooling more frequently reported washing hands after toileting and before food preparation or handling the infant. The involvement of exposure to the mass media is suggested by the facts that the more schooled urban mothers knew more about current events and more frequently reported having seen a child development program on television, and those with more schooling in the rural sample reported reading and watching television more frequently. As for skills acquired in school, a test of decontextualized language (the language of classroom instruction), applied only to the rural sample, correlates strongly with maternal school attainment ($r = .48$, $p<.001$). This pattern of findings is generally supportive of the personal competence model, but it is fragmentary; much more research is needed on the academic skills retained by mothers and their exposure to media messages regarding health behavior.

The second model shown on Figure 12-2, "Socioeconomic Aspiration," represents the conception (presented above) that the school introduces a girl from an agrarian background to the academic-occupational hierarchy that is becoming dominant in her society. She learns that a higher level of school attainment leads to a higher, more desirable status in the social order, and she acquires the motive to seek a higher status. In most Third World contexts, she has less opportunity for status enhancement through entry into a higher occupational role herself than through marriage to a man with more schooling, occupational status and wealth, which gives her and her children more access to resources: better quality health services, more food and clothing, and less crowded housing — all of which improve their survival chances. Analysts like Caldwell and Cleland have emphasized that the impact of a woman's schooling on her children's mortality is not *merely* due to a better economic situation, but it is partly so, and not only because her parents have married her off to a higher-status man; the woman's own aspirations have been elevated by schooling toward improving her status and that of her children.

In the Cuernavaca study, the strongest attitudinal correlate of a mother's schooling is the level of schooling she would like to have attained; this correlates .44 ($p<.01$) with actual school attainment among the women 25 years old or younger and .50 ($p<.01$) among the mothers over 25. The more schooling these women had had, the more they wanted. Those with more schooling also had significantly higher educational-occupational aspirations for their children, particularly sons, suggesting that their blocked desires for themselves had been diverted into hopes for their offspring. Furthermore, they had married better-educated men ($r = .41$, $p<.001$), whose formal employment permitted family membership in a social security health system (IMSS or ISSSTE) with greater access to effective maternal and child health services. Thus the second model receives some support from the Mexican urban study.

The third model of Figure 12-2, "Cultural Model of Interpersonal Behavior," represents our current way of formulating the impact of classroom interaction on mother-infant interaction and its sequelae. The school classroom as a learning environment offers the prototype of an adult expert verbally instructing child novices in a setting dedicated to instruction. This contrasts with the traditional learning environment of agrarian societies in which young apprentices learn through graded participation and observation of adult masters in a setting dedicated to production. The norms of interpersonal behavior differ between these two learning environments, particularly in the importance of teacher-pupil attention and verbal communication: The primary task of the schoolteacher is to talk to young children, while the primary task of the master craftsman, cultivator or herdsman is craft or food production, which may require little attention and even less verbal communication directed to the novice. The girls in an agrarian community who go to school thus acquire a model of interpersonal behavior in which adults talk to children with a pedagogical intent, a model unavailable elsewhere in the community.

Insofar as the girls identify with the role of teacher as they have experienced it in the classroom, they become "teachers" to their children, beginning in infancy, when they respond verbally to infant babbles and other initiatives. This creates a verbally interactive mother-child relationship unlikely to diminish in the second and third year of life when the child becomes fully capable of speech. In the context of such a relationship, the child will be more demanding, eliciting more maternal attention to its needs after infancy and thus improving its survival chances during the period (1 to 5 years of age). Cleland and van Ginneken (1988) have shown maternal education to make the biggest difference in mortality. Such a child also increases the mother's time and energy expenditure and convinces her (or reinforces the conviction she may already have had) that pedagogically-oriented child care is too labor-intensive to be consistent with the high fertility of her mother's generation, thus providing a motive for limiting the number of her children.

Home observation was carried out in Cuernavaca in a subsample of 72 mother-infant pairs who were observed when the babies were 5 and 10, or 10 and 15, months of age, on two occasions at each age point (see LeVine et al. 1991). (Comparable observations are currently being made in the rural Morelos town.) Figure 12-3 shows findings from the observations at five months (n = 29). The three lines represent variables of contingent responsiveness associated with levels of maternal school attainment. The top line shows that responsiveness to the infant's

Figure 12-3   Patterns of Maternal Responsiveness to 5-Month-Old
Infants by Schooling of Mother, Cuernavaca
Urban Sample

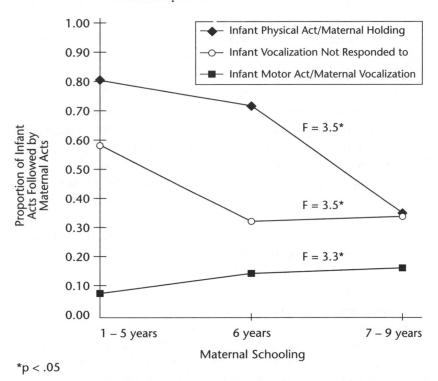

*p < .05

physical act by holding is inversely associated with maternal schooling, i.e., the less educated mothers respond to a significantly greater proportion of infant motions by holding. The middle line shows that the less educated mothers are also more likely *not* to respond at all to a (nondistress) vocalization by their 5-month-old infants. The bottom line shows that vocalizing in response to an infant's motor act is associated with a higher level of maternal schooling. Thus the mothers with more schooling are less likely to respond to infant motions with holding, more likely to respond with speech, and more likely to respond at all to babbling. (Schooling is correlated .37, p<.05, with proportion of infant babbles responded to by maternal speech). In other words, the trend is for the women with more education to treat their five-month-olds as if they were capable of carrying on a conversation, i.e., as if their babbles called for a response and as if the infant could understand maternal speech.

This is particularly interesting because this observed responsiveness to infant vocalizations at five months (the middle line on Figure 12-3) is positively correlated ($r = .41$, $p<.05$) with the mother's estimating (in the interview) a younger age at which an infant can recognize the mother's voice. And the belief that young infants are capable of recognizing their mothers' voices is strongly associated with maternal schooling ($F=12.8$, $p<.001$; for women with seven or more years of school, the mean estimated age is 3.1 months). Thus schooling is related to believing that very young infants are capable of recognizing their mothers' voices, which is in turn correlated with responsiveness to babbling at 5 months in naturalistic observations. Mothers who have gone further in school believe young infants to be more capable of knowing the mother's voice, and they act on the assumption that infants at 5 months are able to communicate.

This outcome of schooling is not limited to early infancy but increases with age. More educated mothers spoke more frequently to their infants at every age: five months, $r = .31$, n.s.; 10 months, $r = .33$, $p<.05$; 15 months, $r = .38$, $p<.05$. Table 12-1 shows that the tendency of the more educated mothers to respond more communicatively — with speech or looking — to infant acts is at least as strong at 10 and 15 months as at the earlier age. At 15 months, all the categories of verbal and visual responsiveness are positively correlated with maternal schooling, and frequency of holding is negatively correlated. None is correlated with the father's schooling. As the baby moved into the second year of life, with increasing competence to participate in conversational routines, the mother with more schooling was increasingly attentive to signs — visual, verbal or motoric — that the toddler was initiating a conversation. This is what we interpret as a pedagogical style based on experience in the classroom. She granted the child a claim on her visual and verbal attention that was measurably greater than that of the mother with fewer years of school and had less physical contact with the child. Thus maternal schooling is associated with a style of mother-infant interaction that increases the time-energy cost of raising a child by making it more difficult for the mother to attend to other tasks at the same time. This evidence supports the idea that women who attend school longer acquire a conception of child care as a labor-intensive task requiring

Table 12-1 Correlations Between Responsiveness and Schooling

| | Correlations with maternal schooling Mean=6.4 years, SD = 2.4 | | | Correlations with paternal schooling Mean =7.9 years, SD = 3.7 |
	5 months (n = 29)	10 months (n = 71)	15 months (n = 47)	15 months
1. Proportion of infant vocalizations followed by maternal speech				
	.37*	.30*	.31*	.04
2. Proportion of infant looks followed by maternal speech				
	.11	.29*	.41*	.18
3. Proportion of infant looks followed by maternal looks				
	.04	.22	.37**	.10
4. Proportion of infant motor acts followed by maternal speech				
	.40*	.25*	.42**	.01
5. Frequency of mother holding infant				
	-.01	-.16	-.33*	-.22

*p<.05   **p<.01

more attention for a longer period of time, thus increasing postinfancy survival chances and reducing fertility.

However valid these three models may turn out to be as partial representations of pathways through which schooling influences child survival and fertility, they are clearly oversimplifications, in at least the three following ways:

1. Synergy. Instead of acting independently, the three pathways shown on Figure 12-2 may actually operate in concert, flowing into one another diagonally and creating a joint effect exceeding the sum of their separate ones. For example, the motivational impact of the second model may propel the woman to seek health information and expose herself to media messages that might improve the life chances of her children through adaptive health behavior (first model). The impact of the teacher-pupil model of the third model may be for the girl to identify with the pupil role as well as that of the teacher, thus adopting in adulthood the stance of a learner in relation to the mass media and health professionals, with a resultant effect on her health behavior. Furthermore, if she re-conceptualizes child care as a labor-intensive task that demands fewer children, this might permit a greater allocation of resources, including diet and clothing as well as hygienic attention, to each child. Other plausible interactions can easily be imagined, and it remains an empirical question whether the impact of maternal education is reducible to specific behavioral pathways. Perhaps, as Mosley (1983) contended, the potency of the maternal schooling effect on survival and health comes from its being diffuse and operating through multiple pathways.

2. Accumulation. Even if the net impact of these pathways on the reproductive rates of a particular cohort should be slight, it is possible that the effects not only accumulate over a decade or two (as Jejeebhoy 1985 and Caldwell 1986 have demonstrated) but accelerate in later cohorts with more schooling, resulting in both a substantial decline in overall birth and death rates and a concomitant build up in attitudes and practices that prevent a subsequent reversal of the secular trend (Murray and Chen, this volume). In the Cuernavaca study, there is evidence that the children of mothers who have gone farther in school perform better academically, thereby indicating a cumulative impact of maternal schooling on educational advancement. Thus the educational development of a population through the spread of schooling may result in effects that are not only dramatic but irreversible.

3. Institutional facilitators and inhibitors. Even if women acquire the skills, aspirations and normative models indicated on Figure 12-2, they may be inhibited by their post-school institutional environment from translating their own behavioral tendencies into action reducing mortality and fertility. On the one hand, a mother may be prevented by the cultural norms of family life from gaining enough control over reproductive decision making or health care to express her preferences in behavior. The Cuernavaca evidence suggests that Mexican husbands are in control of fertility goals for the family, and women cannot express their preferences in actual fertility unless they marry men with more schooling whose preferences match their own. When it comes to child health care, however, the high degree of control assigned the mother facilitates the impact of maternal education on survival and health. In parts of Hindu South Asia, by contrast, the joint family organization puts childbearing women under the dominance of their mothers-in-law and other elders, curtailing their control over health practices and perhaps minimizing the impact of maternal education, at least in the early stages of female school expansion (Caldwell et al. 1985).

In addition to institutional factors affecting domestic control, there is the operation of the health care system, which affects a woman's access to maternal and child health care and family planning services regardless of her school-derived preferences and behavior patterns. In rural areas lacking health services and public health information, schooling may make only a small difference to birth and death rates, whereas the accessibility of such services in the city may increase educational differentials. In other words, there may be a lower threshold of accessibility below which maternal schooling is not so important because even the most educated cannot overcome the geographical and social barriers to health care. There may also be an upper threshold beyond which school effects, though detectable, are much less consequential because even the least educated have good access. Thus the evaluation of the impact of maternal education for policy intervention must include an analysis of the local constraints under which women function as mothers. Whatever universal effects of maternal schooling may be discovered in future research, the variable social and cultural conditions of reproduction and health care cannot be ignored.

Implications for Health Policy

This chapter has focused on the processes through which maternal schooling contributes to decline in birth and death rates, i.e., to the demographic transition, a well-defined historical phenomenon clearly associated with the schooling of women. The demographic transition is also a child health transition, since it is only through the control of infectious diseases that child mortality rates are reduced, and if each woman bears fewer children, their chances of good health as well as survival are likely to be enhanced. Furthermore, as we have seen, the differential use of maternal and child health services and linked family planning services by women of varying levels of education is one path through which maternal schooling affects reproductive rates in contemporary Third World societies. Yet when we contemplate the implications of the maternal schooling phenomenon for health policy in those societies, several warnings are necessary:

1. Maternal schooling can have negative as well as positive health consequences, primarily due to the reliance on bureaucratized medical services among women who have spent more time in school. Schooling

encourages women to follow the lead of professional experts (or those they believe to be experts), and they can be misled in matters of health care. Thus women who have been to school are less likely to breastfeed their infants, a practice they may associate more with their illiterate grandmothers rather than with the modern medical experts in whom they believe. The compliance of educated women with authoritative advice may, under certain circumstances, lead them to undergo un-needed Caesarian deliveries or to seek treatment from inadequately trained practitioners who assume the mantle of medical authority. In other words, schooling may be a necessary but insufficient condition for a healthy population.

Furthermore, it is important to bear in mind that survival is not equivalent to health, even in young children. The improved survivorship of children in families whose economic resources do not match their fertility may increase the prevalence of malnutrition and nonlethal diseases in the growing population, even with expanding female school enrollment, particularly prior to a substantial decline in the birth rate. Thus mortality may be traded for morbidity, with survivors reaching adulthood in an unhealthy state.

2. The reductions in child mortality and fertility from widespread female schooling are reliable in the long run and may even be irreversible, but they do not represent quick solutions to any health problem. Birdsall's (1989:3) question, often heard in policy circles, of "whether there are short-term substitutes (for mother's education) more amenable to short-term program efforts (specific information programs, growth monitoring as a mechanism for informing mothers)," remains, as she suggests, a problem for future research. There are, however, grounds for skepticism about whether the effects of primary and intermediate schooling at ages 6 to 15 can be obtained through a short course for adult mothers. Even without the assumption that childhood and adolescence are privileged periods for cognitive and psychosocial development or that childhood experience necessarily affects adult behavior, it seems more plausible that schoolchildren will be shaped toward new ideas, habits and attitudes during six or nine years under the authority of a teacher, than that women, who are already busy participants in family life, will acquire new ways in a brief, part-time experience. Children are still in the process of forming social identities, and insofar as what is learned in school becomes part of an identity as a literate or educated woman, it is far more likely to inform future practice than a lesson learned

by someone whose identity has already been formed. Furthermore, women who attended school in childhood often have years between leaving school and giving birth to amplify their knowledge, e.g., through the mass media, before practicing it.

Perhaps most important in many places is the possible impact of schooling on mate selection, i.e., the girl's choice of a husband who not only has more education himself but shares her school-acquired preferences and will at least tolerate her subsequent implementation of these preferences in the reproductive and health behavior of their new family. Short courses for mothers cannot replicate these advantages of schooling; they might supplement but not substitute for the expansion of female school enrollment.

3. The impact of schooling on reproductive change does not operate through the same pathway or at the same pace in all populations. For example, some school-induced reductions in fertility are due primarily to an increased age at marriage (where women formerly married very early), others to the use of contraception by married women. Similarly, an association of reduced child mortality with maternal schooling might be due in one case to the use of medical services, in another to geographical or economic access or child care practices. Although this problem would reward further investigation (see Figure 12-1), enough is known to suggest that diversity in socioeconomic and cultural conditions generates a variety of pathways and velocities of change. Policy makers considering expansion of female schooling as an instrument for improving family health have to take these diverse local conditions into account to arrive at realistic expectations of outcomes.

This point can be illustrated by the problem of whether the school impact on reproduction and health care is mediated by a woman's enhanced sense of control or her perception of self-worth as the result of going to school. It has long seemed to many observers that this process must be involved, i.e., that women from agrarian communities gain from school an elevated sense of control, self-worth or confidence sufficient to assert themselves in situations of health, reproduction and child care where women have been conventionally expected to be passive, and that such assertion on behalf of themselves and their children results in lower fertility and child mortality. Demonstrating this, however, is inherently difficult because the methods available to assess such psychological variables depend on verbal elicitation techniques effective with secondary school and university students but not with rural women of lower school attainment in many parts of the world. This problem will eventually be solved through the construction of locally valid procedures. In the meantime, a comparative perspective on the social roles of women (Oppong and Church 1981) can help clarify the processes that might be operating.

Let us compare two hypothetical rural communities in Asia. In one, a South Asian village, women are married young (10–13 years old) and absorbed into their husbands' extended families in distant villages, where their roles as wives and mothers involve strict subordination to elders, particularly mothers-in-law, in matters of health care and reproductive decision making. The school attendance of girls is seen by parents and potential parents-in-law as freedom from domestic work during childhood that might make them less compliant wives and mothers later on. Nonetheless, some girls are permitted to attend school. In this context of female deference and servitude, girls are likely to experience schooling as partial liberation from the constraints of role obligations, affording a sense of control not otherwise possible for a young woman, and might indeed renegotiate their roles as wives and mothers so as to perpetuate the greater autonomy experienced in school.

In the second hypothetical community, located in Southeast Asia, the traditional roles of wives and mothers are less restrictive and permit married women control over matters of their own (and their children's) health and reproduction; parents have no qualms about sending girls to school. In this context of greater female autonomy, girls do not experience schooling as liberation from the constraints of conventional roles and are unlikely to gain a greater sense of control or self-worth from (primary) schooling than they would if they did not attend. On the other hand, however, they may acquire skills, information and sophistication in school that they are free to use in the relatively unconstrained domestic roles of their adult lives. The school effect on their reproductive and health behavior may be conveyed through such skills and information rather than through the enhanced sense of control that is more important in the hypothetical South Asian community, and the outcomes in birth and death rates may occur more rapidly. Thus the impact of schooling on a woman's sense of control derives in part from its contrast with traditional female roles in a particular setting, and it cannot be assumed to represent a universal pathway mediating the effect of school on reproduction. The meanings of schooling to women, and the ways in which it affects their lives, vary with the social and cultural conditions in which those lives are led.

The subjective meaning of the female school experience and its impact on a woman's sense of control is, then, culturally mediated and variable across the diverse social situations of women's roles in developing countries. The same is true of the other pathways through which the school-reproduction relationship operates, the speed at which change occurs, and the range of consequences — negative as well as positive — that accompany declining birth and death rates. In other words, the robustness of the statistical associations between years in school and reproductive outcomes in the developing world is not matched by a uniformity of the situations in which health policy is to be carried out. Policymakers cannot afford to ignore these local complexities in the design and implementation of health programs.

There are nonetheless several reasons why the expansion of female school enrollment can be recommended as a health policy option in many Third World countries. Although schooling is only an indirect determinant of reproductive change and not inexorably connected with birth or death, the mass schooling of women has been and continues to be a precondition of decline in national fertility and child mortality rates in most settings and is also associated with practices that improve the health of mothers and children. It appears to be a necessary though not sufficient condition for large-scale health improvement. Any policy designed to achieve further improvements *without* mass schooling would have to include a strategy for replacing the impact of maternal education. In some countries, like India, programs to reduce the fertility and child mortality of the rural population without widespread maternal education have had disappointing results, suggesting that a strategy of expanded female schooling (effective in some states of India) would be advisable. Finally, the expansion of female school enrollment is a step toward improving the lives of poor women in rapidly changing Third World communities, in addition to its impact on child health and family planning, and can form part of a more comprehensive policy to strengthen the adaptive capacities of a population. There remain questions for future research about how schooling affects health and population change, but the expansion of educational opportunities for women need not await the answers.

Acknowledgments

The preparation of this paper was supported by the Spencer Foundation. The field research reported in it was funded by the Population Council (Fertility Determinants Awards Program, Subordinate Agreement No. CP 82. 47A), the Rockefeller Foundation (Population Sciences Division), the Ford Foundation and the MacArthur Foundation. Analyses of data were funded by the Population Council and the Spencer Foundation.

References

Benavot, A. 1989. "Education, gender and economic development: A cross-national study." *Sociology of Education*, 62: 14–32.

Birdsall, N. 1989. "Understanding health and development: Does research matter?" Paper presented at workshop on the health transition, Harvard University Center for Population Studies, June 27–30.

Bongaarts, J., O. Frank, and R. Lesthaeghe. 1984. "The proximate determinants of fertility in sub-Saharan Africa." *Population and Development Review*, 10:511–537.

Caldwell, J.C. 1979. "Education as a factor in mortality decline: An examination of Nigerian data." *Population Studies*, 33: 395–413.

Caldwell, J.C. 1982. *Theory of Fertility Decline*. New York: Academic Press.

Caldwell, J.C. 1986. "Routes to low mortality in poor countries." *Population and Development Review*, 12: 171–214.

Caldwell, J.C., and P. Caldwell. 1987. "The cultural context of high fertility in sub-Saharan Africa." *Population and Development Review*, 13: 409–437.

Caldwell, J.C., P.H. Reddy, and P. Caldwell. 1985. "Educational transition in rural South India." *Population and Development Review*, 11: 29–51.

Cleland, J., and G. Hobcraft. 1985. *Reproductive Change in Developing Countries: Insights from the World Fertility Survey*. New York: Oxford University Press.

Cleland, J., and J.K. van Ginneken. 1988. "Maternal education and child survival in developing countries: The search for pathways of influence." *Social Science and Medicine*, 27: 1357–1368.

Cochrane, S.H. 1979. *Education and Fertility: What Do We Really Know?* Baltimore, MD: Johns Hopkins University Press.

Cochrane, S.H. 1983. "Effects of education and urbanization on fertility." In R. Bulatao and R.D. Lee, eds. *Determinants of Fertility in Developing Countries*, Vol. 2. New York: Academic Press.

Cochrane, S.H., D.J. O'Hara, and J. Leslie. 1980. "The effects of education on health." World Bank Staff Working Paper, No. 556. Washington, DC: World Bank.

Crockenberg, S. 1983. "Early mother and infant antecedents of Bayley Scale performance at 21 months." *Developmental Psychology*, 19: 727–730.

D'Souza, S., and A. Bhuiya. 1982. "Socioeconomic mortality differentials in a rural area of Bangladesh." *Population and Development Review*, 8: 753–759.

Guldan, G. 1988. "Maternal Education and Child Caretaking Practices in Rural Bangladesh." Unpublished Ph.D. thesis. Tufts University School of Nutrition.

Heyneman, S., and W.H. Loxley. 1983. "The effect of primary school quality and academic achievement across 29 high and low income countries." *American Journal of Sociology*, 88(6): 1162–1194.

Hobcraft, J.N., J.W. McDonald, and S.O. Rutstein. 1984. "Socio-economic factors in infant and child mortality: A cross-national comparison." *Population Studies*, 38: 193–227.

Irwin, M., P. Engle, C. Yarbrough, R. Klein, and J. Townsend. 1978. "The relationship of prior ability and family characteristics to school attendance and school achievement in rural Guatemala." *Child Development*, 49: 415–427.

Jain, A., and M. Nag. 1986. "Importance of female primary education for fertility reduction in India." *Economic and Political Weekly*, 23: 1602–1608.

Jejeebhoy, S. 1985. "Women's status and fertility: A time-series analysis of Tamil Nadu, India, 1970–1980." Paper presented at Rockefeller Foundation Workshop on Women's Status and Fertility, Mount Kisco, NY.

Kasarda, J.D., J. Billy, and K. West. 1986. *Status Enhancement and Fertility.* Orlando, Florida: Academic Press.

Knodel, J., A. Chamratrithirong, and N. Debavalya. 1987. *Thailand's Reproductive Revolution: Rapid Fertility Decline in a Third World Setting.* Madison, WI: University of Wisconsin Press.

Laosa, L. 1982. "School, occupation, culture and the family: The impact of parental schooling on the parent-child relationship." *Journal of Educational Psychology*, 74: 791–827.

Lesthaeghe, R., ed. 1989. *Reproduction and Social Organization in Sub-Saharan Africa.* Berkeley: University of California Press.

LeVine, R., S. Dixon, S. LeVine, A. Richman, P.H. Leiderman, and T.B. Brazelton. 1994. *Child Care and Culture: Lessons from Africa.* Cambridge, U.K.: Cambridge University Press.

LeVine, R., S. LeVine, A. Richman, F.M. Tapia Uribe, C. Sunderland Correa, and P.M. Miller. 1991. "Women's schooling and child care in the demographic transition: A Mexican case study." *Population and Development Review*, 17: 459–496.

LeVine, R., and M. White. 1986. *Human Conditions: The Cultural Basis of Educational Development.* London: Routledge and Kegan Paul.

Meyer, J., F. Ramirez, R. Rubinson, and J. Boli-Bennett. 1977. "The world education revolution." *Sociology of Education,* 50: 242–258.

Merrick, T.W. 1985. "The effect of piped water on childhood mortality in urban Brazil 1970 to 1976." *Demography,* 22: 1–22.

Mosley, W.H. 1989. "Will primary health care reduce infant and child mortality?" In J.C. Caldwell and G. Santow, eds. *Selected Readings in the Cultural, Social and Behavioural Determinants of Health. Health Transition Series No. 1.* Canberra: Australian National University.

Mosley, W.H., and L.C. Chen. 1984. "An analytical framework for the study of child survival in developing countries." In W.H. Mosley and L.C. Chen, eds. *Child Survival: Strategies for Research.* A supplement to Volume 10 of *Population and Development Review.* Population Council.

Oppong, C., and K. Church. 1981. "A field guide to research on seven roles of women: Focussed interviews. Population and Labour Policies Programme Working Paper, No. 106. Geneva: International Labour Organization

Sivard, R. 1985. *Women: A World Survey.* Washington, DC: World Priorities.

United Nations. 1986. "Education and fertility: Selected findings from the World Fertility Survey data." United Nations Population Division Working Paper.

13

Patriarchy, Gender, and Family Discrimination, and the Role of Women

John Caldwell
Pat Caldwell

Much of this chapter will aim at showing how and why differential care and utilization of health resources can occur within families (major sources are Caldwell 1982, 1986b, 1988; Caldwell and Caldwell 1987, 1988). Subsequently, we will examine the relatively small amount of quantitative data now available to measure these impacts. The initial focus will be on the traditional family, although, later, an examination of social change will be made. This approach is based on two assumptions.

The first is that families are not indivisible emotional and economic units (cf. Caldwell 1982). Although there are good reasons for societies to claim that families act so as to maximize the good of all members and to share labor and consumption equally according to need, this is not what actually occurs. In fact, some members are relatively privileged and others correspondingly exploited. The study of such differential treatment is difficult precisely because of strong social convictions that justify the existing patterns and attempt to make the family a viable unit by convincing all members of the fairness of their lot. This means that the only objective measures must be quantitative ones of outcome such as hours of work, condition of clothing, food consumed, height and weight, morbidity and mortality. Even here there is a problem in agreeing on standards for comparison.

The second assumption is that differentials in treatment, such as allocation of food, care or health resources, result in health differentials such as morbidity and mortality levels. This second assumption is not a difficult one to accept, for, although there are few satisfactory community data on morbidity, there is accumulating evidence of differentials in mortality that cannot be explained solely by economic levels and the extent of medical intervention but that must have social origins. The ranking of Third World countries by mortality level results in a vastly different order than that predicted by their per capita incomes and levels of medical intervention (Caldwell 1986a).

It is of interest that those countries that do relatively badly are concentrated along an east-west axis from the Mediterranean to the Arabian Sea, precisely the origin of the most rigid patrilineal and patriarchal society. It might be argued that the explanation is Islam, but the truth is undoubtedly more complex than this as is shown by greater mortality in North than South India, in keeping with greater patriarchal rigidity in the former (Dyson and Moore 1983). Excess female mortality is clearly a response to family and social structures. Visaria (1967) showed that the Indian pattern of relatively high female mortality persisted even in economically well-off overseas Indian populations. Langford (1987) demonstrated in Sri Lanka that female mortality fell below that of males not during periods when economic or health advance was most rapid but between 1953 and 1963 during the Bandaranaike Government-led social revolution from 1956. The work of Hill (1985) and colleagues in rural Mali and that of DaVanzo et al. (1983) in Malaysia show that different ethnic groups, presumably characterized by different theories of child care, exhibit very different levels of child mortality in similar conditions.

Family Systems

The dawn of European sociology in the nineteenth century was occasioned by the interest in comparing the traditional European family with the one that was emerging in the new industrial society. There is still a tendency to dichotomize societies and their families into the traditional and the modern. This division is too simple for our purposes and we will further subdivide these divisions.

First, we will examine all premodern families that are essentially systems of familial production, and we will examine their structure and its implication for the distribution of resources and the maintenance of health. Then we will contrast the very distinctive family system that emerged in the heartland of the Old World with systems found in Africa and elsewhere.

The Family of Familial Production

Most premodern production takes place in the family and most of the social relations within the family are fashioned so as to enhance that production. This is true also of hunters and gatherers, but we will concentrate on agriculturalists who have long made up the great majority of the world's population.

In our research on the traditional agricultural family and its demo-graphic implications, especially in Bangladesh and South India, the most striking finding was not how it contrasted with the modern firm but how similar it was. The real contrast is between the modern firm and the modern family. There appears to be a certain internal logic about the organization of productive units. Both the traditional family and modern firm are characterized by an emphasis on the need for their members' loyalty, by social segregation that forbids too much familiarity between those who give and those who receive orders, and by an associated hierarchical chain of command. Respect is accorded by the height achieved in the hierarchy and this largely determines the distribution of resources. The chief aim is the survival of the organization itself.

The major reason for the rigidity of the family system is a belief that any relaxation and any move toward more egalitarian family relations would endanger the level of production and the survival of the family. Peasant production usually does not yield large surpluses, and the production that is attained is achieved by endless work or by what Chayanov (1966:6) in Russia called drudgery. We found that farmers in Nigeria had similar attitudes and only 17 percent wished a similar job upon their children (Caldwell 1982:30).

We summarized the situation in Bangladesh and South India (cf. Caldwell, Reddy and Caldwell 1982) in the following way (Caldwell 1986b:7):

> the family is a work unit where the direction of work and subsequent obedience are of prime importance and where too close emotional relationships may both endanger efficiency and prove exhausting when directing work or imposing discipline.

Most directions are given by older to younger persons, usually of the same sex and usually relatives. In Bangladesh we found that 80 percent of waking hours were spent working in such relationships (Caldwell, Jalaluddin, Caldwell and Cosford 1980 1984). In a study in South India of conversation during work we found that 90 percent of conversation took the form of directions or was in some way related to family controls and the morality that encapsulated them (Caldwell, Reddy and Caldwell, n.d.).

The family hierarchy is stabilized by a veneration for the old, especially the patriarch. It is this that drives the wealth flows upward (cf. Caldwell 1982) and gives the patriarch a large share of resources, including care. In Brazil, Rosen (1982:21) noted a parallel between extrafamilial relations of the patron-client type and intrafamilial relations between the patriarch and his dependants. In neither case was the relationship characterized mainly by force and resentment, for the weaker "legitimate their claims by being respectful, submissive, obedient and, above all, loyal." Once there is such veneration, the patriarch usually has abundant additional sources of control such as land, housing, inheritance, and the power to arrange marriages. Even where there is no land, artisan fathers control the tools and often the right to work in the occupation, while landless laborers may control their children's right to work with the patron.

The patriarch is often credited with superior knowledge, sometimes of secret lore, and of religious powers in this world or in the afterlife, as well as receiving credit for having granted the gift of life itself. Sons rarely unite against their fathers, but are typically rivals for his affection and benevolence. The allocation of the greatest care and health resources to the patriarch is not mere blind devotion but is also based on the realities of an agrarian society with this type of organization. The death of the patriarch can convert his powerful wife into a weak and pathetic widow. Cain (1978) has shown how defenseless a whole family can be in the transition period after the patriarch's death and how likely it is that some of their land will be stolen.

There is a degree of pretense about the actual work that old patriarchs do and the value of their knowledge and management skills. The latter often amount to no more than repetitive nagging about things that have been done a thousand times and where the routine is known to all. The reason that the old are not overthrown, except possibly in some hunting or nomadic societies where a premium is placed on strength, is the need to retain stability by a simple system where at every age the younger defer to the older. The exploited in the family are not a proletariat tempted to revolution, because they know that the investment they have already made in subservience will pay off as they age and the younger will have in their turn to be subservient to them.

The central loyalty is to the family, which provides an all-inclusive protection in return for an acceptance of one's place and one's share of resources. So inclusive is the family that in rural areas there is no one else to whom the weakest, the women and children, can turn. When dealing with other families, it is the patriarch who represents the family in negotiations. This tends to weaken the self-confidence of others when dealing with extrafamilial bodies, be they other families or health services.

The structure of the larger family depends on first loyalties being to the family hierarchy. Typically the marriage of a young couple is arranged and, in keeping with the tenets of a patrilineal and virilocal society, they then take up residence with the groom's parents. This keeps the young wife in a subdued position, which is further accentuated in North India by the practice of village exogamy whereby she loses nearly all contact with her own relatives. Her husband is usually substantially older than her, which allows him to treat her somewhat paternally and to give his greatest loyalties to his parents. The traditional family is well aware that its greatest point of potential weakness is the priority that the young mother gives to her own children and her attempt to convince her husband that he should do likewise. Her strongest weapon is her sexual relation with her husband, and consequently the family attempts to downplay the importance of this relationship and to make it difficult to express conjugal affection. In doing this, they have to counter the young woman's belief that her children come first and that her husband should see things this way. This has implications for the use of health resources, except where there are family priorities at stake, such as the survival of the only grandson. It also has implications for how much attention she can devote, in what might be regarded as a selfish and self-centered way, to her own children rather than to the general labor of the household and farm.

To a substantial degree, family stability is achieved by an extraordinary degree of segregation by age and sex. The chief instrument of control in the large family is, as is the case in many firms, a high degree of segregation of tasks. This is not always clear when broad precoded categories are used in surveys to describe labor. However, when we employed the families' own terms to describe work inputs in Bangladesh, we found that every job was regarded as being most suited only to a specific sex and age group (Caldwell, Jalaluddin, Caldwell and Cosford 1980 1984). Daughters-in-law also undertook different work, and more onerous work, than unmarried daughters of the same age, and were in a worse position to communicate their views to the older generation. However, although females worked somewhat longer hours than males, those who had more powerful positions by virtue of being men or by being middle-aged did not receive advantages from their position in terms of marked remissions from work. There was, indeed, pride in being able to perform tasks that they felt only they could do. The advantages they did receive were greater control over their own lives and those of others, more conscientious care, a greater freedom to rest from work when sick, and more material benefits. D'Souza and Chen (1980) also found in rural Bangladesh that males received more food, clothing and conscientious care. These extra advantages are apportioned by convention and manners rather than by a continued series of decisions.

In most traditional agrarian societies, there is no simple division by generation and no symmetry by age and power between the sexes. A single-sex apex, in the form of the patriarchy, is achieved in the family by having the husband much older than the wife. Thus, the latter is, with regard to age and rights, intermediate between the husband and the children. This prevents a close conjugal relationship from developing and restricts the communication between wife and husband. It also means that, when change does occur in the traditional family, it is not merely along generational lines. When improvement occurs in the situation of either wife or children, the condition of the other is also likely to change.

The weak point in the traditional agrarian family, at least when change occurs, is the position of the daughter-in-law. Within the society, a strong belief in blood relationships, the institution of exogamy, the age gap between spouses, and the husband's first duty toward his parents, the young woman feels for years extremely isolated. The only relationship where this is not the case is that with her children. In one sense she is dependent upon them because their existence is her ticket to respectability in the family and it is they who will give her deference and greater power as they grow up. The family tries to counter this by insisting that she give greater attention to family work, and they attempt to make a direct claim upon the children by, for instance, making their own health treatment decisions in regard to the children without delegating the major responsibility to the younger woman. The daughter-in-law counters, especially as society changes, by attempting to see that her husband regards the children as not only hers but also his, and that he gives them greater attention relative to his parents and siblings.

The major implications of the agrarian, patriarchal family for health are that resources, including health care, go to the old rather than the young, and that daughters-in-law are prevented from giving too much care to their children, or diverting family resources to them through their husbands, in order to maintain family stability and priorities.

The Eurasian and Non-Eurasian Families

The traditional family, or that of familial production, is not the same everywhere. It has long been known that the family that developed in the old farming areas from the Mediterranean to South Asia is distinctly different from that, for instance, of sub-Saharan Africa. The former, compared with the latter, is characterized by a greater emphasis on marriage, on female sexuality being confined within marriage, and on monogamy. In Africa there is more emphasis on reproduction than on female chastity outside marriage. The important social institution is the descent lineage. Polygyny and child fostering are common. The African situation is found, at least in part, in Melanesia, in some of its aspects in parts of Southeast Asia, and among some indigenous populations of the Americas and Australia.

Goody (1976) has identified the Mediterranean-South Asian family, which he terms Eurasian, as an innovational and rather peculiar development. He regards it as being essentially an attempt by societies that could produce agricultural surpluses once the plow had been invented to retain the all-important land holdings by controlling marriage, achieving it monogamously within a social class where others were equally well-off, and by devolving property upon the next generation through dowry and inheritance. In contrast, African bridewealth did not go to establish the younger generation but instead was passed, as a kind of revolving fund, to the parental generation to allow more marriages to take place.

Africa was insulated from the Eurasian system by its poor, upland, lateritic soils, which were unsuited to the plow, and which were largely cultivated by women with digging sticks or hoes. As a result, it was protected from the development of real class or caste systems.

From the health stance, the important point was that the Eurasian system placed enormous emphasis on the right kind of marriage and on marriage arrangements not being imperiled by pregnancies to unchosen males or by any males claiming rights to women through the fact of sexual relations. This produced an emphasis on premarital and extramarital female chastity that became so strong that it was often identified as the core of both individual and family morality. In order to preserve it, women were made dependent on men and confined so that their behavioral and decision making options were limited. This morality was codified in religion, which both intensified the situation and allowed it to be exported by diffusion to marginal parts of Europe and East Asia and by settlement to the Americas and Australasia. These aspects of the Eurasian family are widely regarded as being traditional in the sense that they follow logically from the family structure dictated by the needs of familial production, but this, as sub-Saharan Africa clearly demonstrates, is not the case.

The Eurasian family system has two additional implications for health. The first follows from the restriction of women's movements and decision making. This restriction means that women often can neither make quick, self-confident decisions about their own health or that of their children, nor easily act upon decisions once made. The second implication is that such seclusion restricts the value of women's work outside the home, especially for employment in the cash economy, and it constrains the roles that they can play in protecting families and negotiating with other families and the broader society. Thus in areas like South Asia, daughters may be of less value than sons, and, if numerous, a direct threat to the family's economy and survival. This is reinforced where it is customary to pay very high dowries and to celebrate marriage lavishly. The result may be a greater allocation of resources to ensure the survival of sons, or even the deliberate neglect of daughters.

The African system, especially the West African one, does not discriminate so strongly against females. Nevertheless, the relative unimportance of marriage compared with the lineage means that there is not a strong conjugal family to pool resources for the protection of children's health (cf. Abu 1983; Vercruijsse 1983). Often, children are dependent, especially in the towns, almost solely on their mother's earnings, and this can mean skimping health treatment because of the cost.

The African system has another implication for health. The lineage places tremendous emphasis on generational succession. Its religious counterpart is the cult of the ancestors, and the old are given great deference and superior treatment not only for social reasons but also for theological ones. Thus, health and other resources are directed toward the old in sub-Saharan Africa to a greater extent than is probably true even in South Asia despite the fact that the death of a patriarch does not endanger the lineage to the same extent that it may endanger the joint or extended family of Eurasia.

The Eurasian and sub-Saharan African systems can in many ways be contrasted. Beyond them lie intermediate cultures. Northern Europe and its settlement areas in North America and Australia were frontier lands with a shorter tradition of preserving land and a less clear-cut division between valuable high-quality and often irrigable land and the rest. They imported Eurasian religions but often modified them. Women were never so secluded as in the heartland of Eurasia, nor were the old given such deference as in sub-Saharan Africa. The picture is not dissimilar in most of Southeast Asia. The Chinese situation is yet another modification of the Eurasian system. The Chinese religious systems were only partly imported, and deference for the aged was essentially the product of the secular Confucian creed, which was taught at least as much to ensure the stability of the state as that of the family. However, great emphasis was placed on female premarital and extramarital chastity without the Eurasian stress on seclusion. Nevertheless, postmarital residence was strongly virilocal, and aging parents depended on sons for support. In these conditions, and in one where there tended to be surplus labor for agriculture, daughters were not highly valued, and female infanticide has been noted in China over the ages.

The Demographic Impact of Family Structure

Much of the discussion so far has implied that the multigenerational, hierarchical family of familial production, and its Eurasian and African subtypes, are normally coresidential. Now that we are about to examine real data, it should be noted that more often than not, this is not the case. Nevertheless, when examining agrarian populations in their locality of origin, the multigenerational model is not far from the truth. In our research area in rural South India, the usual residential system, except among the Brahmins, is on one hand the stem family consisting of the old parents, their unmarried children, plus one married son together with his wife and children, and on the other hand those additional nuclear families formed by the marriage of the other sons (Caldwell, Reddy and Caldwell 1984). Indeed the latter formed 59 percent of all families. Nevertheless, three points should be noted that tend to mitigate the extent to which this residential separation leads to sufficient emotional nucleation to modify substantially the description given above. Firstly, much of the movement is only to adjacent housing so that the family continues to work in many ways as a continuing unit. In rural India that is likely to be, at the furthest, still within the caste subsection of the village (cf. on Andhra Pradesh, Raju 1988). Secondly, when the children are young and subject to the highest mortality risk, they and their parents are still likely to be living with the grandparents. In the South India study, 88 percent of couples were still with the husbands' parents five years after marriage, and on average they spent the first 16 years of marriage there. Even in Kerala (Sushama 1989b) and Sri Lanka (R. Freedman, personal communication 1989) around one-third of young couples were still with their parents five years after marriage. Thirdly, in South India, and doubtless elsewhere, the situation is changing toward more coresidence as a result of the decline in the birth rate. In Karnataka the birth rate fell from 40 to 28 per thousand between the late 1960s and the late 1970s, with the likely average number of sons surviving to marriageable age per household falling from around 2.1 to 1.6. This trend will almost certainly continue without any relaxation of the insistence that the old parents must live with a married son, and with greater survival levels among those parents.

Health Decision Making

Much of our health work in rural South India centered on the nature of health decisions (Caldwell, Reddy and Caldwell 1983 1988). The social context was that of the Eurasian family, but in a less stark form than in Northern India. There was no demand for village exogamy, although the difficulties faced by smaller castes in finding suitable caste partners meant that many wives were obtained from other villages. Half of all marriages were to relatives, so that wives often had their own blood relatives in the same household, in a neighboring house, or at least in the village. Wives were not secluded, but forward caste wives did not work in the fields, and only the lower caste women worked for wages as agricultural laborers. Nevertheless, even in these circumstances, there remained a strong feeling about the place of the young wife and the impropriety of her being too strident in her spoken thoughts and decisions.

This had important implications for health decision making. Because of the existence of a larger family, whether coresidential or not, and because of an age gap between spouses that averaged almost ten years, the father was not nearly as close to his young children as was the mother.

The result was that sickness in children was detected first by mothers in 80 percent of all cases. Yet the majority did not even draw attention to the fact until others, particularly their mothers-in-law and husbands, had done so. Only one-seventh of mothers sought treatment of their own volition as soon as they noticed the illness.

In health terms, this deference and the lag times it involves have serious implications. A study (Khan et al. 1987) in North India found that wives without schooling or outside employment lacked so much autonomy that they had no confidence in their own ability to detect sickness or to make treatment decisions. This was not so extreme in South India, but the less educated wives were less certain of going to the health center, were less likely to describe fully the case once they were there, and were less likely to carry out the full treatment course (Caldwell, Reddy and Caldwell 1983). The latter was also affected by their financial situation. However, their lack of autonomy and self-confidence did emerge most strongly in their reluctance to report back to the health center and the doctor if the treatment did not seem to be improving the condition of the children or of themselves. This problem appeared to be a significant explanation for continued high mortality.

We carried out similar work in Sri Lanka (Caldwell, Gajanayake, Caldwell and Peiris 1989) where there has never been the same degree of pyramidal, patriarchal family organization and where women have greater autonomy than in any part of India except Kerala. In these circumstances, mothers made health decisions on their own in half of all cases compared with fathers doing so on their own in one-tenth of cases. This was an important factor in the unusually rapid rate of sickness detection and of treatment action in Sri Lanka, a process which helped to achieve a life expectancy of around 70 years despite a per capita income only one-thirtieth of that of industrialized countries or one-fortieth of the United States. In Kerala, female autonomy had been nurtured in conditions where half the population had traditionally lived in a matrilineal system, and mothers took a great deal of responsibility over their children's health (Sushama 1989a).

In the African lineage system, especially in its attenuated form in urban areas where the family system tends toward matrifocality (P. Caldwell and J. Caldwell 1987b), frequently gives mothers almost a monopoly of health decision making power. Their problems are resources and time, and it is this which frequently forces them to seek cheaper indigenous treatments or to place their hopes in faith-healing religion (Orubuloye, Caldwell, Caldwell and Bledsoe 1991).

Evidence from Mortality Differentials

There are no published studies of the impact of kinship, family type, relationships within the family, or marriage type on mortality. As yet, we are forced to search for rather tangential evidence and to seek its implications. We are in an even worse situation with regard to morbidity, and hence differential illness will not be discussed here.

Age. The Princeton Model Life Tables (Coale and Demeny 1966) are based on real experience, and those with a life expectancy of 40 years refer to traditional agrarian families, while those of 75 years refer to urbanized industrial society. In the former case, one-third of all deaths in a life table population occur before 15 years of age (and two-thirds each year in a society growing at three percent per annum) compared with one-fiftieth in the latter. This may merely show that the only way to low mortality is to eradicate childhood diseases. However, it may also incorporate evidence that the only path to really low mortality lies through a change in family priorities toward children that allows a successful attack on childhood sickness and death. There is some evidence of this. In a single society with a fixed level of access to health facilities, such switches of emotional and wealth flows in families tend both to precede the decision to restrict family size and to follow its accomplishment. In 1973 we examined the consequence of limiting family size in Ibadan, Nigeria, and found that those who had done so experienced only half the proportional child loss of those who had not taken this step (Caldwell and Caldwell 1978). In China, the death rate in one-child families appears to be abnormally low even by current Chinese standards (Caldwell and Srinivasan 1984).

In the work undertaken by Hill and colleagues (Hill 1985) in the West African savanna, two adjacent ethnic groups, the Tamasheq (or Tuareg) and the Delta Fulani, experienced similar adult mortality, although the former lost only 30 percent of their children by five years of age compared with 50 percent for the latter. The researchers regarded this as evidence of the importance of cultural factors for care (Hilderbrand, Hill, Randall and van der Eerenbeemt 1985), and, if this is the case, it is also worth noting that the Tamasheq are matrilineal while the Fulani are patrilineal. A nagging doubt must remain that part of the explanation lay in a higher incidence of malaria and water-borne diseases among the riverine Delta Fulani.

DaVanzo et al. (1983) reported marked differences between the three ethnic groups in Malaysia with regard to child mortality even when income and other socioeconomic indices were controlled. It was unclear whether this arose from differences in the roles of women or children or both, or from more or less pressure on women to devote themselves to child care or to take the blame for child deaths. Wherever the explanation lay, it clearly had its impact through different cultural interpretations of family priorities, which themselves reflected different family structures.

One can obtain even more indirect evidence of the likely impact of relatively low levels of care for children of certain age groups by examining the differential impact of less care for female children. This differential between female and male mortality must arise from different levels of care and is accordingly evidence of what could happen to either sex with less care.

Much of the Third World evidence on gender differentials in mortality is derived indirectly using such techniques as the proportion of children of each sex surviving to mothers in each age group, followed by the use of formulae for allocating the deaths to specific ages of the children. However, the World Fertility Survey recorded detailed life histories that appear to provide adequate, direct data by single years of age of the children at death (Rutstein 1984). These data demonstrate that where there is excess female child mortality, it is most likely to occur after infancy but in the first years of life. Other evidence from North India and Bangladesh (D'Souza and Chen 1980) shows that the protection in infancy may last only for the first months and that, by six months of age, female mortality is rising above that of males. This is evidence of a peculiarly vulnerable period of life when quite modest differences in priorities given to the young relative to the old can make important differences in survival chances. It is likely that the relatively high female child mortality is an index of all child mortality. A comparison of child mortality between Indian states employing Sample Registration Survey data shows that the states with the highest ratio of female to male child mortality are also those where male child mortality is unusually high (P. Caldwell and J. Caldwell 1987a).

Further evidence for the vulnerability of the age group 1 to 4 years comes from the studies of India's National Institute for Nutrition (1987), which demonstrated that parents with no or little education experienced much higher mortality among their children in this age range than did more educated parents. They concluded that the explanation was not deliberate lack of care but insufficient feeding based on a misunderstanding of nutritional needs of very young children.

In the Princeton (West) model life tables the majority of all deaths in populations growing at 3 percent per annum occur under five years of age for all populations with life expectancies below 50 years. Accordingly, the overall mortality rate is very sensitive to the exact survival level at these young ages. If this survival level is determined by quite subtle differences in levels of care, and these emerge from family priorities, then clearly different family structures are likely to have substantial impacts not only on child mortality but also on total mortality.

One way of examining the relationship between adult and child mortality is to group states or countries with similar life expectancies at 15 years and to compare mortality below that age. This is attempted in Table 1 for the relatively few Third World countries for which measures of age-specific mortality rates are available for adult ages. Even so, not all of even these data are trustworthy. The table is dominated by Indian states because of the existence of the Sample Registration System. Most estimates are for 1985, but the exact date is not of particular significance because of the grouping by level of adult mortality.

Table 13-1 demonstrates how stable adult mortality levels are compared with child mortality. Among the Indian states, the lowest life expectancy at 15 years is only 15 percent below the highest, but the highest child death rate is 468 percent above the lowest. If we exclude the listed country with the highest mortality and that with the lowest, the range in life expectancy at 15 years is 9 percent compared with 1,336 percent for the child death rate. Indeed, achieving high life expectancies at birth is clearly a case of controlling child mortality.

If, in India, we exclude Punjab and Haryana from the Hindu heartland, and retain Uttar Pradesh, Rasjasthan, Bihar and Madhya Pradesh, we find life expectancies at 15 years ranging from 49.8 to 52.7 years and child death rates from 17.8 to 21.0; while in the four southern states, Kerala, Tamil Nadu, Karnataka and Andhra Pradesh, life expectancies at 15 years range from 52.9 years to 57.7 years and child death rates from 3.7 to 10.4. Prosperous Punjab and Haryana are at the top end of the latter range. Examining the age bands separately, there is moderately strong evidence that the northern austerely patriarchal and village exogamous states do relatively badly in terms of child mortality compared with adult mortality. But it might be fairer to conclude that they do worst in terms of all mortality, but that rising incomes can reduce both adult and child mortality.

If we examine the whole world, but at first exclude sub-Saharan Africa, it is clear that children do relatively badly in the Eurasian heartland: Egypt, Bangladesh, Pakistan and Algeria (but Tunisia is a partial exception, probably because of relatively low mortality among girls). Eurasian settlement areas in Latin America fall in an intermediate position. The countries that do well are the fringe Asian areas with a less depressed female situation — Thailand, Peninsular Malaysia and Sri Lanka — plus the two prosperous East Asian societies: South Korea and Hong Kong.

There is limited evidence, supplied admittedly only by Malawi and Mali, that sub-Saharan Africa does spectacularly badly. The loose lineage system, with its great responsibilities thrown on mothers, does not appear to provide children with as much protection as the Eurasian patriarchal family, let alone more egalitarian conjugal families. Nevertheless, Malawi and Mali are high mortality African countries (and may also be affected by the data being from an earlier year) and it would be unwise to conclude that the children's case against the lineage has yet been fully made.

Gender. The occurrence of excess female mortality is of importance both in itself and because it is likely to raise overall child mortality because of the probability that the surplus of female child mortality will be greater than the resultant reduction in male child mortality. Excess female mortality is also an indicator of relative adult female disadvantage, which will almost inevitably result in higher child mortality in the case of both sexes because of limitations on mothers' ability to provide maximum care.

The World Fertility Survey (WFS) showed excess female child mortality throughout the Middle East and North Africa with the exception of Tunisia and mainland South Asia (P. Caldwell and J. Caldwell 1987a). This pattern is found in some Latin American countries such as Colombia, Mexico and Panama. However, distinctly higher female toddler and child mortality is found in Southeast Asia only in the Philippines. In sub-Saharan Africa, female child mortality is substantially below that of males, except in Senegal and Nigeria, where it is around parity.

These patterns clearly reflect the underlying nature of the society and its family structure. The Eurasian family system, with its focus on female

Table 13-1 The Relationship between Adult and Child Mortality in the Third World (within each group in order of increasing child death rate)

Adult mortality grouping (range of life expectancy at 15 years)	Countries (various dates)						Indian States (1985)				
	Country	Year	Life expectancy at birth	Life expectancy at 15 years	Death rate 0–14 years (per 1000)	No. of births resulting in deaths by age 5 years (per 1000)	State	Life expectancy at birth	Life expectancy at 15 years	Death Rate 0–14 years (per 1000)	No. of Births resulting in deaths by age 5 years (per 1000)
(a) High adult mortality (less than 52 years)	Malawi	1977	39.6	45.0	51.5	412	Orissa	50.4	49.6	16.5	208
							Assam	50.0	48.8	17.8	195
							Bihar	49.4	49.8	18.7	217
							Uttar Pradesh	48.5	50.1	21.0	239
(b) Medium adult mortality (52–55 years)	S. Korea	1983	65.8	54.7	1.4	12	Maharashtra	61.6	54.9	8.9	110
	Thailand	1984	60.5	53.9	1.6	16	Tamil Nadu	59.1	52.9	9.6	121
	Ecuador	1981	60.6	53.8	6.2	67	Andra Pradesh	58.2	53.0	10.4	136
	Bolivia	1977	50.8	a	8.7	98	Himachal Pradesh	59.3	53.8	10.5	125
	Egypt	1981	58.1	a	10.4	130	West Bengal	57.7	52.3	10.6	128
	Bangladesh	1982	54.8	53.9	14.2	163	Jammu and Kashmir	57.8	52.9	10.7	142
	Mali	1976	48.3	53.2	29.4	272	Gujarat	55.9	53.4	14.1	171
	India	1985	54.6	52.4	14.6	176	Rajasthan	53.0	52.7	17.8	205
							Madhya Pradesh	50.9	52.6	19.8	236

Table 13-1 (continued) The Relationship between Adult and Child Mortality in the Third World (within each group in order of increasing child death rate)

Adult mortality grouping (range of life expectancy at 15 years)	Countries (various dates)						Indian States (1985)				
	Country	Year	Life expectancy at birth	Life expectancy at 15 years	Death rate 0-14 years (per 1000)	No. of births resulting in deaths by age 5 years (per 1000)	State	Life expectancy at birth	Life expectancy at 15 years	Death Rate 0-14 years (per 1000)	No. of Births resulting in deaths by age 5 years (per 1000)
(c) Low adult mortality (over 55 years)	Hong Kong	1985	76.4	62.3	0.7	8	Kerala	68.7	57.7	3.7	50
	Peninsular Malaysia	1984	70.1	57.2	2.2	25	Karnataka	61.3	55.1	9.0	117
	Mexico	1982	64.0	55.9	3.7	47	Punjab	62.6	57.2	9.8	124
	Sri Lanka	1982	69.7	58.1	3.9	45	Haryana	61.0	56.4	11.4	139
	Brazil	1984	63.4	a	4.3	52					
	Tunisia	1980	60.6	a	4.8	58					
	Pakistan	1979	59.1	56.5	9.1	111					
	Algeria	1982	62.4	56.4	13.4	150					

a No exact estimate, but estimate within this mortality band.

purity and the resultant lesser female economic value, is abundantly clear in the pattern of excess female mortality stretching from Morocco to Bangladesh. It is noteworthy that a WFS survey was also done in Portugal, which revealed substantially higher female mortality between two and five years of age. The Latin American pattern largely reflects the export of Mediterranean family patterns. It is noteworthy that, where Mediterranean influences were least, namely in Jamaica, female mortality was relatively the lowest.

In sub-Saharan Africa, the lineage structure of society places responsibilities rather than protection and seclusion on women. In these circumstances, female child mortality is substantially below that of males except in Senegal and Nigeria. The explanation is the Islamization of Senegal and Northern Nigeria with the importation of Eurasian family priorities and even structures. Southeast Asia was also not part of the original Eurasian system, as is demonstrated by a continuing tradition of uxorilocality after marriage. The result is female mortality levels between one and five years of age in Indonesia and Malaysia 20 percent or more below that of males.

Higher female than male mortality has been studied more intensively for the northern region of the Indian subcontinent than anywhere else in the world, beginning with the census takers of British India a century ago and reinforced by a great deal of attention in the last 30 years (Visaria 1961 1967; Mitra 1978 1979; D'Souza and Chen 1980; Miller 1981; Dyson and Moore 1983; Social Science Research Council 1987).

The age structure of excess female mortality is available from the Indian Sample Registration System (P. Caldwell and J. Caldwell 1987a) and from the International Diarrhoeal Diseases Research Centre for the Matlab Surveillance Area in Bangladesh. The patterns for India as a whole and Matlab are very similar and show excess female mortality from after the first months of infancy until almost ten years of age. Then female mortality is at parity with that of males for at least the next five years, probably demonstrating that by this age the child is capable of largely caring for itself rather than being almost wholly dependent on the family.

Female mortality is relatively higher even than in childhood during the subsequent reproductive span, although the actual number of deaths is fewer. Between 15 and 35 years of age, female mortality in India is 60 percent above that of males, and 150 percent higher on most of the Gangetic Plain. This pattern does not appear to be as extreme in any other major region of the world. It may owe much to the poor physical condition of the women, and possibly, in largely vegetarian conditions, to low levels of animal protein. The latter possibility is supported by evidence of very high levels of anemia.

How firm is the evidence that family structures and family priorities play a significant role in these patterns? With regard to North India the colonial census-takers, all believed that the relatively low value of females in highly patriarchal families, feeling the need for at least a partial seclusion of females, provided the explanation(Visaria 1967, Mitra 1978, Miller 1981, and Das Gupta 1987). Chen, Huq and D'Souza (1981) found in the Matlab surveillance area in Bangladesh that girls suffered more from malnutrition, had lower levels of intake of both calories and proteins, and were much less likely to be taken for treatment when experiencing diarrhea. Dyson and Moore (1983) argued that the extreme patriarchal nature of the family and the tendency toward female seclusion were less pronounced in South India, and that this was reflected in lower levels of excess female mortality. They drew on the work of Sopher (1980) for contrasting social and behavioral indices between North and South India and concluded that South India was a different, softer and less patriarchal society. They believed that key elements were the South Indian lack of insistence on village exogamy and the related factor of high incidence of marriage between close relatives.

The publication by the Sample Registration System of age-specific death rates by five-year age groups allows the testing both of this hypothesis and of how closely related the peaks of female mortality in early childhood and during the reproductive span are. The following conclusions are drawn from an analysis (Caldwell and Caldwell 1987a) for aggregated data spanning three years 1976 to 1978. The comparisons are made for the age groups showing the greatest excess female mortality, 5 to 9 years, for which the all-Indian excess was 26 percent, and 25 to 29 years, when it was 53 percent.

With regard to childhood mortality, the North-South contrast holds up well. If we confine ourselves to the major states, where the sample size was sufficient not to produce improbable fluctuations, female excess mortality was less than 25 percent above that of males in the four Dravidian states (Tamil Nadu, Kerala, Karnataka and Andhra Pradesh), plus the two neighboring states of Gujarat and Madhya Pradesh. Indeed, in Tamil Nadu, female child mortality is never above that of males, in contrast to Kerala, where, from 5 to 14 years of age, it is about 20 percent higher. Further north, female child mortality is everywhere much higher, being 59 percent above that of boys in Haryana, 77 percent in Punjab and 81 percent in Orissa. These are cultural and not economic differences, as is clearly brought out by the figures for the prosperous states of Haryana and Punjab.

In the age range 25 to 29 years, the all-Indian figure for excess female mortality is 53 percent. Lower figures are recorded for three of the four Dravidian states, Karnataka being the exception, and for Gujarat and Punjab. Elsewhere the excess is above the Indian average, being highest in all mountain areas where presumably there are difficulties in getting obstetric assistance. Elsewhere, the excess reaches 147 percent in Orissa and 97 percent in Haryana. Even in the reproductive span, female mortality in Kerala is consistently below that of males, while in Tamil Nadu it is around parity. The southern states and Punjab are substantially assisted by lower fertility, but this does not explain the whole difference. The most interesting case is that of Punjab, where prosperity appears to have improved the situation of women once married, but where it does not avail girls who are yet to face expensive marriages and high dowries. Das Gupta (1987) differentiated between relatively low mortality for the first daughter in Punjab and much higher mortality for successive daughters.

A more complex issue arises when we consider mortality at older ages. In India, the patriarchy does not seem to protect older males. Indeed, Indian mortality at older ages is surprisingly high when comparisons are made around the world with countries with similar mortality up to early middle age. Even between 40 and 60 years of age, female mortality is about 30 percent lower than male mortality. In general, the north-south patterns that we have observed still hold good with females doing less well than the Indian average in Haryana, Punjab and Uttar Pradesh. However, there are some interesting exceptions. Older Tamil Nadu women do not follow the pattern of their younger sisters, and exhibit mortality levels not much below those of males, although the Tamil Nadu pattern could be interpreted as showing near-equality between the sexes at all ages. In contrast, Rajasthan women at older ages unexpectedly perform as well as the Indian average.

Langford (1987) provides, as outlined at the beginning of the chapter, valuable information about gender differences in Sri Lanka and the conditions of change. Up to 1953 there was excess female mortality across the whole age range of 1 to 44 years. Indeed, relative female mortality had been worsening since at least 1921. Between 1953 and 1963 the situation suddenly changed, with a dramatic trend toward relatively better female mortality, so that by 1981, females exhibited lower mortality at every age except between 1 and 4 years. The timing is important. The change did not take place during the steep mortality decline in the half-dozen years following World War II; indeed, in several age groups the worsening of the relative female situation accelerated during that time. Nor did it stem from declining fertility, which largely occurred after 1963. Indeed, the improvement was relatively greater, or at least as great, in those age groups where few Sri Lankans bore children, 15 to 19 and 35 to 54 years compared with the 25 to 34 year span. It is difficult to avoid the conclusion that major social change occurred during this period. It was, in fact, a period of immense social upheaval, as the Solomon Bandaranaike government sponsored the Sinhalese language and the Buddhist religion. Among the Sinhalese, at least, this inevitably produced a political and social appeal to the individual as distinct from the family and, together with rising educational levels, changed family relationships and hence female mortality.

One mechanism whereby the patriarchy is translated into higher mortality has been so intensively studied that the evidence cannot be repeated here. In patriarchal societies there tends to be a substantial gap between levels of male and female education. For instance, in mainland South Asia the surplus of boys over girls in primary school rises from 40 percent in India and Bangladesh to 90 percent in Pakistan, while in secondary school there are twice as many boys in India and closer to three times as many in Bangladesh and Pakistan (World Bank 1988). The Middle East has been changing rapidly with oil money, but the Yemen Arab Republic still records five times as many boys as girls in both primary and secondary schools. In contrast, the very different social and family system of Southeast Asia has resulted in near-parity in the sex ratio of students in Malaysia's primary and secondary schools and in Indonesia's primary schools, although Indonesia still has one-third more boys than girls in secondary schools. As the now considerable literature (cf. the summary in Caldwell and Caldwell 1988) on the relation between maternal education and child survival shows, such disparities invariably lead to overall higher child mortality.

The question arises as to why patriarchal societies jeopardize the health of their children, even their sons, in this way. In the more extremely gender differentiated societies the answer is partly that the investment in girls yields a lesser return. One reason is that the need to preserve their purity means that they are less likely to secure employment subsequently. Schultz (1982) found lower excess female mortality in those Indian states where females were more likely to work during adulthood (although it is likely that he identified only a single element of a larger and more complex whole). Another reason is that, in strongly patrilineal and virilocal societies, girls' subsequent earning power will be of little value to their own parents in old age. In rural South India (Caldwell, Reddy and Caldwell 1988, 177), parents were worried about keeping older girls at school, particularly after the onset of puberty, because it would imply only casual concern about their sexual purity with consequent adverse effects on their chances of a good marriage.

The patriarchy probably works both directly and indirectly to sustain high mortality levels among its children. The indirect route is through the education of mothers. The direct path is by restricting the movement and decision making of women so that they are inefficient providers of care. They cannot easily go alone with their children to seek medical help, nor can they be the primary decision makers about whether such care is needed. They tend to lack confidence with regard to their own ability to make the right decision (Khan et al. 1987). At least in rural areas, where doctors are almost always male, the reluctance of the family to allow women to have children in a nontraditional setting is influenced by the fear that a man will be involved in the delivery.

In the Old World patriarchal societies, women's roles have been largely restricted to the home and to childbearing. This means that family planning has hardly been necessary and further that the use of contraception by women is often regarded as impure. There is a strong association between the use of family planning and low child mortality (Caldwell 1986a). This is stronger than can be explained merely by increasing child mortality with higher parity and appears to be a result of the fact that a decision to plan the numbers of one's children is associated with planning their future and the family's future, and leads to greater concern about the children's health.

Education almost certainly provides a girl (as it does a boy) with a greater chance of survival during both childhood and adulthood through enhancing her ability to look after herself. However, the analysis of the direct impact of education, and more broadly of autonomy, on individuals has hardly begun, as those who die are no longer available to testify in surveys. Such information could be obtained by death registration systems that recorded education separately from occupation and urban-rural residence but, outside the comprehensive registration systems of Scandinavia, such opportunities are rare.

The five-year age-specific mortality rates by sex can also be employed to examine excess female mortality, as in Table 13-2.

Female mortality in the 20 to 29 age group is certainly influenced by the fertility level. Nevertheless, this is not the major explanation for high young adult female mortality in mainland South Asia, India, Pakistan, Bangladesh and Afghanistan. There is a clear regional influence adverse to females operating, which must be related to family systems and female preference. This influence appears to affect females during their reproductive span more than in childhood. Within India, not only are the young adult female ratios much higher in the Hindu heartland, ranging from 1.44 to 2.10 in Rajasthan, Uttar Pradesh, Bihar and Haryana, compared with a range from 0.57 to 1.28 in the few Southern states, but they are much higher relative to child mortality. For child ratios, the maximum range is from Kerala to Rajasthan, where the latter is 57 percent above the former (and in the 5-9 age group it is only 117 percent); for young adults the range among major states is from Kerala to Haryana with the latter being 268 percent above the former.

In the rest of the world the child ratio is below the young adult ratio only in Zimbabwe, Costa Rica, Mexico, Brazil, Malawi, and Mali. The sub-Saharan African lineage system does not discriminate against females, and, on the whole, little girls do better than their mothers.

Global patterns. In trying to obtain an overall picture of the impact of patriarchal structure on mortality, one could attempt to map the situation. In one sense this was done when Caldwell (1986a) compared the mortality level of each Third World country with its per capita income and hence with its ability to buy health services. Those eleven countries which, by this measure, performed worst were Oman, Saudi Arabia, Iran, Libya, Algeria, Iraq, Yemen Arab Republic, Morocco, Ivory Coast, Senegal and Sierra Leone. In contrast, the eleven best were, in order, Sri Lanka, China, Burma, Jamaica, India, Zaire, Tanzania, Kenya, Costa Rica, Ghana and Thailand (the Indian state of Kerala does better than any of them). The worst eleven had an average per capita income of almost $4,500 but nevertheless a life expectancy of only 51 years and an infant mortality of 124 per thousand. Only 7 percent of their married women of childbearing age practiced family planning. In contrast, the best

Table 13-2   The Ratio of Female to Male Mortality by Age (Same dates as Table 13-1; dates for new countries in parentheses)

Ratio of female to male mortality		Countries				Indian States			
Adult ratio (20-29)	Child Ratio (0-14)	Country	0-14 ratio	20-29 ratio[a]	Total fertility rate	State	0-14 ratio	20-29 ratio[a]	Total fertility rate
(a) Low (below 0.8)	(i) Low (below 0.8)	Costa Rica (1984)	0.79	0.39	3.5				
		Brazil	0.77	0.38	2.3				
	(ii) Medium (0.8-1.3)	Egypt	1.04	0.61	4.8	Kerala	0.84	0.57	2.4
		Tunisia	0.90	0.61	4.8	Punjab	1.22	0.72	3.5
		Zimbabwe (1982)	0.92	0.41	6.6				
		Ecuador	0.92	0.64	5.0				
		Mexico	0.82	0.39	4.6				
		Jordan (1979)	0.92	0.57	7.4				
		Peninsular Malaysia	0.80	0.48	3.8				
		Hong Kong	0.85	0.59	1.5				
		South Korea	0.95	0.60	2.0				
		Sri Lanka	0.84	0.59	3.4				
		Thailand	0.82	0.44	2.2				

Table 13-2 (continued) The Ratio of Female to Male Mortality by Age

Ratio of female to male mortality Adult ratio (20-29)	Child Ratio (0-14)	Countries				Indian States			
		Country	0-14 ratio	20-29 ratio[a]	Total fertility rate	State	0-14 ratio	20-29 ratio[a]	Total fertility rate
(b) Medium (0.8-1.3)	(ii) Medium (0.8-1.3)	Algeria	0.96	0.91	6.7	Andhra Pradesh	0.98	1.28	3.7
		Malawi	0.91	0.95	7.0	Gujarat	1.04	1.14	3.9
		Mali	0.89	1.14	6.7	Himachal Pradesh	1.11	1.30	3.6
		Bolivia	0.96	0.91	6.3	Karnataka	1.02	1.23	3.6
						Madhya Pradesh	1.11	1.21	4.6
						Maharashtra	1.17	0.91	3.5
						Tamil Nadu	1.12	1.12	2.8
(c) High (over 1.3)	(ii) Medium (0.8-1.3)	Afghanistan	0.95	1.31	6.9	Assam	0.91	1.66	4.1
		Bangladesh	1.04	1.77	6.2	Bihar	1.22	1.79	5.4
		Pakistan	0.95	2.13	5.8	Rajasthan	1.17	1.44	5.5
		India	1.14	1.34	4.3	Jammu and Kashmir	0.90	2.50	4.5
						Orissa	0.94	1.58	3.8
						Uttar Pradesh	1.30	1.57	5.6
						West Bengal	0.99	1.48	3.7
	(iii) High (over 1.3)					Haryana	1.37	2.10	4.6

a Ratios are averages of 5-year age groups.

eleven, although averaging a per capita income of only $500, enjoyed a life expectancy of 61 years and an infant mortality rate of 64. Of their married women of childbearing age, 44 percent practiced family planning.

Clearly the poor health achievers are dominated by the Eurasian patriarchy stretching from Morocco to Oman. However, these really poor health achievers were an example of an extreme form of that patriarchy, namely that which had been sanctified and protected from change by Islam accepting the Eurasian family system as being divinely favored. Thus, in India, where the Eurasian patriarchy existed, but where Moslems form only a minority, the health achievement has been good relative to the very poor incomes. Conversely, in Indonesia and Malaysia, the fact that the majority of the population is Moslem has had no critical impact on uxorilocal societies where women have traditionally enjoyed a great deal of freedom.

What is even clearer is that the eleven superior achievers in health are, with three exceptions, from the fringe lands that did not participate in the development and intensification of the Eurasian patriarchy. In Asia, Kerala, Sri Lanka, Burma and Thailand all belong to the forested periphery and none had women in a subordinate position. Similarly, Zaire, Tanzania, Kenya and Ghana lay well to the south in sub-Saharan Africa where the lineage predominated over the family formed by marriage and where women had a great deal of independence as well as economic responsibility.

There are apparent exceptions. Among the poor achievers, the inclusion of three African countries can probably be explained by strong Islamic elements in Senegal and Sierra Leone, while Ivory Coast is partly Moslem but also has had an economic system where the majority of the population did not fully share in its income. Among the superior health achievers, China, India and Costa Rica have adopted particularly strong health policies within a context of promoted social change. One might also note that Chinese society enforced premarital and extramarital female chastity without any type of accompanying seclusion.

Change

The patriarchy behaves like an autonomous state. It is weakened by any larger authority which appeals directly to its individual members granting them rights or giving rise to aspirations that are in any way at odds with the family system.

This has happened over the last thousand years in Europe because first the Church and then the State regarded individuals rather than families as their points of contact. Goody (1983) believes that the Christian Church acted in this way from as early as the fifth century with the aim of competing with the family for the inheritance and the donation of property. The State built on this and had its own reasons, including the recruitment of troops, for seeking relations with individuals.

In the 12th century the Church intervened in the family to the point of forbidding arranged marriages (Davis 1977). Similar changes have occurred in many Third World countries over the last few decades as governments have sought both to enforce their own powers and to guarantee individual freedoms.

However, the greatest assaults on the patriarchal family have come from within. The Eurasian patriarchy was really a product of a largely subsistence agrarian society. It was completely stable when its younger members had nowhere else to secure employment. However, the growth of commerce, the monetization of the economy and the rise of towns have all weakened it. The possibility of employment elsewhere not only tempts the son to seek such work but can lead his wife to encourage it.

Education has also threatened the system. Part of the strength of the patriarchy rests on the leadership of the old, and on the young conceding that the old have more experience and knowledge. A little schooling can easily lead the young man to feel that his father and grandfather are ignorant illiterates, misled by superstition, and incapable of dealing with the modern world. The educated daughter-in-law can successfully challenge her mother-in-law. We found in rural South India that health can be an area of challenge and one where uncertain mothers-in-law may give way because of their desire that their grandchildren should survive (Caldwell, Reddy and Caldwell 1983). This matter is very complex, for, although the South Indian rural family in many ways fears the educated daughter-in-law, they are increasingly likely to choose her expressly on the grounds that she will make a greater contribution to the grandchildren's education and health. Similarly, many peasant families fear the impact of education on their sons but are tempted to provide that education because it is the route to additional non farming incomes and upward social mobility.

Ultimately, the patriarchal family collapses when men give greater emotional and economic priority to their wives and children than to their parents and siblings. This is an eventuality that most younger wives desire. This weakness has long been known to the patriarchs and their wives, and this is why so much effort goes into keeping the conjugal bond weak and the young wife in her place. Almost instinctively, the young wife points out to her husband that her children are also his and he owes them affection and resources. The conjugal bond does tend to strengthen as wives too become educated and as the global message of the importance of sexuality begins to affect the conjugal relationship. Stone (1977) employed the term "sentiment" to describe the softer emotions that began to pervade the conjugal family in Europe. The message of the prime needs of their children has been powerfully reinforced by the increasing need of those children for schooling and the growing possibility that this will lead to nonfarming employment elsewhere.

Even demographic change has its impact. Conjugal relationships in Egypt have been slowly transformed as a result of increasing residential nuclearization, a process that has been accelerating over the last one hundred years, partly as a product of increasing land shortage and of migration for jobs (P. Caldwell 1977: 605).

This downward flow of wealth and attention now has to be seen in the context of a fertility transition that is affectihng much of the Third World. A study of all families in Ibadan City, Nigeria, in 1973 (Caldwell and Caldwell 1978) showed that families where fertility had been deliberately and successfully restricted to five or fewer children lost 50 percent fewer children through mortality than did other families (equal in model life tables to a mortality difference of 15 years in life expectancy). Those who had restricted themselves to four or fewer children lost 80 percent fewer (a difference of 23 years in life expectancy). It is doubtful whether the real patriarchy can survive the emergence of a small-family system.

This chapter has treated gender differentials, family discrimination and the specification of different female roles from male ones as aspects of family structure. It is argued that such differentiation reached its height in the Old World agrarian family, which was the product of both the creation of an efficient system for agricultural production and of a specifically Eurasian system for protecting property and inheritance.

The patriarchal family system was for eons agriculturally efficient, although this is probably no longer true. It was never efficient in health terms, largely because of the subordination of women and of the low priority given to the needs of the young.

One aspect in improving health is the decline in the patriarchy and the partly related decline in gender differentiation. There is little doubt that the egalitarian family, with little sex differentiation and considerable child orientation, is more health-efficient.

Acknowledgments

Research assistance has been received from Wendy Cosford and Yaw Ofosu. Typing has been done by Jyoti Nandan and Margaret Tunks.

References

Abu, K. 1983. "The separateness of spouses: Conjugal responses in an Ashanti town." In C. Oppong, ed. *Female and Male in West Africa*. London: Allen and Unwin.

Cain, M.T. 1978. "The household life cycle and economic mobility in rural Bangladesh." *Population and Development Review*, 4(3): 421–438.

Caldwell, J.C. 1982. *Theory of Fertility Decline*. London: Academic Press.

Caldwell, J.C. 1986a. "Routes to low mortality in poor countries." *Population and Development Review*, 12(2): 171–220.

Caldwell, J.C. 1986b. "Family change and demographic change: The reversal of the veneration flow." Distinguished Lectureship Address to the American Sociological Association Conference, New York, 1986. In K. Srinivasan and S. Mukerji, eds. 1987. *Dynamics of Population and Family Welfare*. Himalaya Publishing House, Bombay, 1988.

Caldwell, J.C. 1988. "Mass education as a determinant of mortality decline." Casid Lecture, October 25. Michigan State University, East Lansing. In J.C. Caldwell and G. Santow, eds. 1989. *Selected Readings in the Cultural, Social, and Behavioral Determination of Health*. Canberra: Australian National University.

Caldwell, J.C., and P. Caldwell. 1978. "The achieved small family: Early fertility transition in an African city." *Studies in Family Planning*, 9(1): 2–18.

Caldwell, J.C., and P. Caldwell. 1987. "Family systems, their viability and vulnerability: A study of intergenerational transactions and their demographic implications." Paper presented to International Union for the Scientific Study of Population Seminar on Changing Family Structures and Life Courses in LDCs, Honolulu, 5–7 January. In E. Bergo and P. Xenos, eds. 1992. *Changing Family Structures and Life Courses in LDCs*. Oxford: Clarendon Press.

Caldwell, J.C., and P. Caldwell. 1988. "Women's position and child morbidity and mortality in LDCs." In International Union for the Scientific Study of Population Conference on Women's Position and Demographic Change in the Course of Development, Oslo. Solicited Papers, IUSSP, Liège. Reprinted in S. Sognor, N. Federici, K. Mason and E. Grebenik, eds. 1993. *Women's Position and Demographic Change in the Course of Development.* Oxford: Clarendon Press.

Caldwell, J.C., I. Gajanayake, P. Caldwell, and I. Peiris. 1989. "Sensitization to illness and the risk of death: An explanation for Sri Lanka's approach to good health for all." *Social Science and Medicine,* 28(4): 365–379.

Caldwell, J.C., A.K.M. Jalaluddin, P. Caldwell, and W. Cosford. 1980. "The control of activity in Bangladesh." Working Papers in Demography, no. 12. Canberra: Australian National University.

Caldwell, J.C., A.K.M. Jalaluddin, P. Caldwell, and W. Cosford. 1984. "The changing nature of family labour in rural and urban Bangladesh: Implications for fertility transition." *Canadian Studies in Population,* 2(2): 165–198.

Caldwell, J.C., P.H. Reddy, and P. Caldwell. 1982. "The causes of demographic change in rural South India: A micro approach." *Population and Development Review,* 8(4): 689–727.

Caldwell, J.C., P.H. Reddy, and P. Caldwell. 1983. "The social component of mortality decline: An investigation in South India employing alternative methodologies." *Population Studies,* 37(2): 185–205.

Caldwell, J.C., P.H. Reddy, and P. Caldwell. 1984. "The determinants of family structure in rural South India." *Journal of Marriage and the Family,* 46(1): 215–229.

Caldwell, J.C., P.H. Reddy, and P. Caldwell. 1988. *The Causes of Demographic Change: Experimental Research in South India.* Madison, WI: University of Wisconsin Press.

Caldwell, J.C., P.H. Reddy, and P. Caldwell. n.d. "Measurement of rural conversation." Data file in Department of Demography. Canberra: Australian National University.

Caldwell, J.C., and K. Srinivasan. 1984. "New data on nuptiality and fertility in China." *Population and Development Review,* 10(1): 71–79.

Caldwell, P. 1977. "Egypt and the Arabic and Islamic worlds." In J.C. Caldwell, ed. *The Persistence of High Fertility: Population Prospects in the Third World,* Vol 2. Canberra: Australian National University.

Caldwell, P., and J.C. Caldwell. 1987a. "Where there is a narrower gap between female and male situations: Lessons on differential health and survival from South India and Sri Lanka." Paper presented to Social Science Research Council Workshop on Differential Female Mortality and Health Care in South Asia, Dhaka, 4–8 January. Reprinted as P. Caldwell and J.C. Caldwell. 1990. "Gender implications for survival in South Asia." Health Transition Working Paper No. 7. Canberra: Australian National University.

Caldwell, P., and J.C. Caldwell. 1987b. "Fertility control as innovation: A report on in-depth interviews in Ibadan, Nigeria." In E. van de Walle and J.A. Ebigbola, eds. *The Cultural Roots of African Fertility Regimes: Proceedings of the Ife Conference.* February 25 – March 1, 1987, Ife-Ife: Obafemi Awolowo University; Philadelphia: University of Pennsylvania.

Chayanov, A.V. 1966. *The Theory of Peasant Economy.* D. Thorner, B. Kerblay and R.E.F. Smith, eds (English version). Homewood, IL: Richard Irwin.

Chen, L.C., E. Huq, and S. D'Souza. 1981. "Sex bias in the allocation of food and health care in rural Bangladesh." *Population and Development Review,* 7(1): 55–70.

Coale, A.J., and P. Demeny. 1966. *Regional Model Life Tables and Stable Populations.* Princeton, NJ: Princeton University Press.

Das Gupta, M. 1987. "The second daughter: 'Neglect' of female children in rural Punjab, India". Paper presented at Social Science Research Council Workshop on Differential Female Mortality and Health Care in South Asia, Dhaka, January.

DaVanzo, J., W. Butz, and J.P. Habicht. 1983. "How biological and behavioral influences on mortality in Malaysia vary during the first year of life." *Population Studies,* 37(3): 381–402.

Davis, N.Z. 1977. "Ghosts, kin, and progeny: Some features of family life in early modern France." *Daedalus,* 106(2): 87–114.

D'Souza, S., and L.C. Chen. 1980. "Sex differentials in mortality in rural Bangladesh." *Population and Development Review,* 6(2): 257–270.

Dyson, T., and M. Moore. 1983. "On kinship structure, female autonomy and demographic behavior in India." *Population and Development Review,* 9(1): 35–60.

Goody, J. 1976. *Production and Reproduction: A Comparative Study of the Domestic Domain.* Cambridge: Cambridge University Press.

Goody, J. 1983. *The Development of the Family and Marriage in Europe.* Cambridge: Cambridge University Press.

Hilderbrand, K., A.G. Hill, S. Randall and M.L. van der Eerenbeemt. 1985. "Child mortality and care of children in rural Mali." In A.G. Hill, ed. *Population, Health and Nutrition in the Sahel: Issues in the Welfare of Selected West African Communities.* London: KPI.

Hill, A.G. 1985. "The recent demographic surveys in Mali and their main findings." In A. G. Hill, ed. *Population, Health and Nutrition in the Sahel: Issues in the Welfare of Selected West African Communities.* London: KPI.

Khan, M.E., R. Anker, S.K.G. Dastidar, and S. Bairathi. 1987. "Inequalities between men and women in nutrition and family welfare services: An in-depth enquiry in an Indian village." Working Paper no. 158, Population and Labour Policies Program. Geneva: International Labour Office.

Langford, C.M. 1987. "Sex differentials in Sri Lanka: Past trends and the situation recently." Paper presented at Social Science Research Council Workshop on Differential Female Mortality and Health Care in South Asia, Dhaka, January.

Miller, B. 1981. *The Endangered Sex.* Ithaca: Cornell University Press.

Mitra, A. 1978. *India's Population: Aspects of Quality and Control.* New Delhi: Abhinav.

Mitra, A. 1979. *Implications of Declining Sex Ratio in India's Population.* Bombay: Allied Publishers.

National Institute of Nutrition, Indian Council of Medical Research. 1987. Report for the Period April 1, 1986 to March 31, 1987, Hyderabad.

Orubuloye, I.D., J.C. Caldwell, P. Caldwell, and C.H. Bledsoe. 1991. "The impact of family and budget structure on health treatment in Nigeria." *Health Transition Review*, 1(2): 189–210.

Raju, K.N.M. 1988. "Trends in Household Types in a Coastal Village in Andhra Pradesh, India." Unpublished Ph.D thesis. Canberra: Australian National University.

Rosen, B.C. 1982. *The Industrial Connection: Achievement and the Family in Developing Societies.* New York: Aldine.

Rutstein, S.O. 1984. "Infant and child mortality: Levels, trends and demographic differentials." Comparative Studies: Cross–National Summaries no. 43, Revised Edition, World Fertility Survey, London.

Schultz, T.P. 1982. "Women's work and their status: Rural Indian evidence of labour market and environment effects on sex differences in child mortality." In R. Anker, M. Buvinic and N. H. Youssef, eds. *Women's Roles and Population Trends in the Third World.* London: Croom Helm.

Social Science Research Council and BAMANEH. 1987. Workshop on Differential Female Mortality and Health Care in South Asia, January 4–8, Dhaka.

Sopher, D.E., ed. 1980. *An Exploration of India: Geographical Perspectives on Society and Culture.* London: Longmans.

Stone, L. 1977. *The Family, Sex and Marriage in England 1500–1800.* New York: Harper and Row.

Sushama, P.N. 1989a. "Social context of health behaviour in Kerala." Paper presented to Health Transition Workshop on Cultural, Social and Behavioural Determinants of Health: What is the Evidence? 15–19 May 1989, Australian National University, Canberra.

Sushama, P.N. 1989b. "The Causes of Fertility Decline in Kerala." Unpublished Ph.D thesis, Australian National University, Canberra.

Vercruijsse, E. 1983. "Fishmongers, big dealers and fishermen: Cooperation between the sexes in Ghanaian canoe fishing." In C. Oppong, ed. *Female and Male in West Africa*. London: Allen and Unwin.

Visaria, P.M. 1961. "The sex ratio of the population of India, 1961 Census of India." Vol. 1, monograph 10, Office of the Registrar-General, New Delhi.

Visaria, P.M. 1967. "The sex ratio of the population of India and Pakistan and regional variations during 1901–61." In A. Bose, ed. *Patterns of Population Change in India, 1951–61*. Bombay: Allied Publishers.

World Bank. 1988. *World Development Report 1988*. New York: Oxford University Press.

Section V
Health, Policy and Promotion

14

Pragmatism, Robin Hood, and Other Themes: *Good Government and Social Well-Being in Developing Countries*

Nancy Birdsall

Introduction

The appropriate role of the state (or of the public sector, or of government) in the economy has been the subject of considerable concern in the developed and developing world in the 1980s. That concern is now beginning to affect public policies in the social sectors as well as in the directly productive sectors.

For the social sectors in developing countries, a major perceived problem of the last decade has been lack of adequate public resources to meet such goals as universal access to basic health care and universal primary education of reasonable quality.[1] Thus much of the policy debate in this period has centered on the merits and demerits of specific options — such as selective (i.e., low-cost) primary health care, reallocation of education spending to (low-cost) primary education, and introduction of user charges for some social services[2] — that might allow expansion of social programs without increasing the fiscal burden of such programs.

But the fiscal problem alone does not provide an adequate long-run basis for developing sound public policy on the role of the state in the social sectors. Indeed, it could be argued that the lack of funds has simply made more obvious other serious problems, including the inequity of much social spending by governments and the poor management of many government social programs. Given these problems, it is not obvious that more money alone for government programs will buy progress. But neither is "privatization" of social programs the answer: the private sector alone cannot be expected to provide such services, especially to the poor. Moreover, while the financial pressure of internal and external debt at the moment is reducing government spending on social programs in poor countries (as a share of all government spending), the long-run trend has been and probably will continue to be one of increasing government involvement in social programs, at least as financier; increasing involvement of government in social programs has historically been the pattern in the now-developed countries.

What should be the nature of this involvement? The purpose of this chapter is to set out issues that arise in considering the appropriate role of the state in social programs, particularly in developing countries, given not only the need to operate programs within financial limits, but other more fundamental social objectives, such as improving the quality of life and the income potential of the poor, and increasing people's own participation in the development process. Section I of the chapter provides background on changing views of the role of government, particularly in the social sectors. Recent financial pressures and what I call the "Robin Hood failure" are provoking some pragmatic rethinking of government's role in the social sectors. Section II lays out a simple framework regarding government's role, within which a variety of specific policy issues can be considered. The distinction between direct provision by government and public financing of services provided by the private sector is made; particular stress is put on the "consumer empowerment" functions of government (information, regulation and quality control), all of which are relatively neglected in most developing countries. Section III uses this framework to set out research and program needs in a number of specific areas: health and other forms of social insurance; public policy toward private sector provision of social services; public finance of basic research and capacity-building in developing countries; the targeting of social spending; decentralization of social services.

Changing Views of the Role of Government

In the industrial countries, the share of government spending in gross national product (GNP) had mounted steadily throughout this century, especially after World War II, and by the 1980s had reached an average of 47 percent.[3] By the 1980s, however, industrial countries were struggling to reverse this trend and to cut government spending, fearing the inflationary pressure of large public deficits (revenue growth began to fall behind expenditure growth in the 1970s) and in some countries fearing that public spending was displacing private initiatives. Politically successful leaders, including Mr. Reagan and Mrs. Thatcher, preached vigorously the rhetoric of less government (though in the case of the

United States, without any real success in cutting spending). Less government generally meant a reduction in the regulatory power of government, and a reduction in government spending on domestic social programs. The 1980s have also seen increasing interest in reducing the role of government in some highly planned socialist economies. Hungary, China and most recently the Soviet Union and most of the Warsaw Pact countries of Eastern Europe are seeking ways to imitate, if not duplicate, the apparent advantages of market-led economies in which the planning functions of government are limited. The emphasis in these countries has been on reducing the role of government in the directly productive sectors.

In developing countries, government spending also rose rapidly after World War II, though as a percentage of GNP to lower levels than reached in industrial countries (about 22 percent in 1985, excluding state and local government spending). As in the industrial countries, revenue growth fell behind expenditure growth; because most developing countries have much more difficulty financing their deficits domestically (through for example sale of government bonds) than developed countries, the resulting deficits were more likely to be inflationary and were more likely to lead to accumulation of external debt by the public sector.[4] By the 1980s, the external debt crisis had combined with internal fiscal deficits to expose the apparent disadvantages of a large public sector with substantial involvement, often through state-owned public enterprises, in industry, agriculture and finance. Involvement by the state in these economic sectors was increasingly viewed as a recipe for inefficiency and bloated spending, and as a long-term constraint to solving the problem of external as well as internal debt. The World Bank began supporting the divestiture and privatization of state-owned public enterprises through policy "adjustment" loans[5] in the early 1980s, and the Bank and other donors showed increasing interest in the private sector as a more efficient and less costly conduit for investment-led growth in the productive sectors.[6]

The apparent tendency of governments to accumulate external debt (without applying the borrowed funds to good investments) and fiscal deficits challenged the widely held view among development economists that government is (or at least can be made into) a positive force in the development process. From the 1950s on, development economists generally held what might be called the "public interest" view of government, which basically assumes that government acts in a benign way (though mistakes and failure are possible, they are not inevitable or irreversible). In this view, government needs to intervene directly or indirectly to foster development, because, given poor capital markets and entrenched economic and political interest groups, private agents alone are unlikely to address the huge unmet needs for physical and social investments in developing countries. The problems of the 1980s, however, gave greater credence to an alternative view, the public choice[7] or "private interest" school. In the private interest view, the interests of those who control government are confined to advancing their personal goals rather than the welfare of the commonweal. In this view, big government will simply mean a large bureaucracy and much lobbying (or rent-seeking) by special interest groups; these will soak up societal resources that would otherwise contribute, through productive contributions by individual workers and entrepreneurs, to raising individual and social welfare.[8]

Government and the Social Sectors in Developing Countries

But the issue for the social sectors is obviously more complicated, especially in the developing countries. Involvement of government in social sector programs is warranted for at least two reasons:

- **fairness:** social programs are often defined as ones to which society wishes to assure equal access, irrespective of ability to pay; and

- **market failure:** because of positive externalities of many social services, there are social benefits of social sector programs over and above their private benefits, and the private market alone may not provide enough of the program or service from society's point of view. In addition, other market failures may justify particular government interventions. The problems of adverse selection and moral hazard dictate a regulatory role for government in health and other insurance. Because capital markets will not generally accept future human capital as collateral, governments may need to finance the administrative costs of student loan programs.

For these two reasons, substantial government responsibility for the financing, organization and delivery of social programs has been taken as given, at least since the beginning of the 20th century, even in such market oriented countries as the United States. On the one hand, the arguments seem even more salient for developing compared to industrial countries, because more people are poor, the difference between private

Table 14-1   Government Spending on Social Programs,
Developed and Developing Countries, 1984

	Share of Central Government Spending in GDP, 1980	Share of Central Government Spending in Social Sectors	Central Government Spending on Social Programs as Percent of GNP	Central Government Spending on Social Programs in US$ per capita
Developed countries	47	50	17	500
Developing countries	22			
Middle income:		30	8	50
Low income:		<10	1	2

Source: World Bank, 1988c.

and social returns to investments in education, health and other social programs is likely to be greater, and because insurance and capital market failures are more pervasive.[9] On the other hand, any argument for more government activity in developing countries must be made in the face of growing evidence that administrative skills are more scarce, and that for this and other reasons, government itself as an institution is less efficient than in developed countries.

In any event, government spending on social programs is still much smaller in developing countries than in industrial countries, not only in absolute terms, but as a percent of total GNP and as a percent of total government spending (Table 14-1).[10] For example, industrial countries in 1984 allocated more than 50 percent of all government spending to social programs (including transfers under old-age and disability social insurance), compared to about 30 percent in the middle-income developing countries (mostly in East Asia and Latin America) and less than 10 percent in the poorest (low-income) developing countries, mostly in Africa and South Asia.[11]

Recall that overall government expenditures also represent a higher proportion of total national income in industrial countries, and of course national income itself is much higher in industrial countries. The result: in 1984 central government spending on social programs represented about 17 percent of GDP in the industrial countries compared to about 1 and 8 percent in the low- and middle-income developing countries respectively; and per capita central government spending on education and health combined (excluding transfers under social insurance programs) amounted to about $500 in the industrial countries, compared to about $50 in the middle-income countries, and about $2 in the low-income countries.[12]

Finally, there is substantial evidence that in the developing countries, government involvement in the social sectors, limited as it has been in terms of money, has been a marked success. Governments in developing countries have played a major role in the extraordinary decline in death rates in developing countries since World War II — most obviously through direct interventions such as immunizations and malaria control, but also through more general public investments in education and sanitation, and in the communications and transportation networks that have reduced the mortality toll once taken by recurring famine.[13] These kinds of government interventions, often exploiting newly available technologies, explain why mortality in developing countries has fallen more rapidly and at average income levels lower than those associated with mortality decline in the West. For example, life expectancy in India in 1980 exceeded life expectancy in France in 1930, despite incomes and educational levels much lower in India than in France at that time.[14] Similarly, government has been the major actor in the increases in access to education in developing countries. In Africa the gross primary school enrollment ratio has risen to 75 percent from 36 percent in 1960, and the adult literacy rate from 9 to 42 percent; between 1970 and 1980, public domestic expenditure on education almost tripled.[15] In Asia and Latin America, primary school enrollment ratios rose from perhaps 50 percent in 1950 to over 90 percent in 1980 (UNESCO data). Though private schooling has played a role, particularly in some countries of Asia and Latin America at the higher level, governments have been the major actors at the primary and secondary levels; in 1980 more than three-quarters of primary and secondary students in most developing countries were enrolled in public schools directly supported by government.[16] These increases in education are widely viewed as improving welfare directly — because education expands people's horizons — and as contributing to higher income and better health and nutrition by improving people's skills.

Under these circumstances, it is difficult to imagine that over the long run the developing countries will reduce the amount or proportion of government spending in the social sectors. On the contrary, publicly financed social programs seem to be highly income elastic[17] (something countries clearly want more of as average income grows), and assuming even limited income growth, developing countries are likely to go through the same phases of gradual expansion of social programs that the industrial countries previously underwent. This is likely to be the case in spite of the difficulties many industrial countries now face in sustaining high levels of spending on social programs. (The point is a positive, not a normative one.) A pertinent example is that of health insurance. Systems of national health insurance have existed for several decades in Latin America (generally as part of larger systems of social security), but have only recently expanded beyond coverage of households in the formal sector; such systems do not exist at all in most countries of Africa and Asia. But Korea and China, as well as a number of other countries, including in Africa, are now considering establishing some form of health insurance system.

The Robin Hood Failure

On the other hand, in the recent past the share of government spending going to the social sectors in developing countries has been declining — largely as a result of increasing spending on servicing internal and external debt. Between the early 1970s and 1985, the share of central government budgets in all developing countries going to health fell from 7 to 4 percent; the share going to education fell from 14 to 10 percent (World Bank 1988c, p. 110). (Data are not available on other social programs, such as housing and child care, which in most countries are much smaller.) In some countries, particularly in Africa, the fall in shares translated into real overall declines and even larger declines on a per capita basis.[18] Financial problems are apparently forcing governments to retreat, at least temporarily, from their historically successful involvement in social programs.

Moreover, the financial reality has combined with the influence of the "private interest" view of government to contribute to a shift in attitudes about what governments can and should do in the social sectors in developing countries. Recent World Bank studies have emphasized in particular the extent to which the pattern of government spending in health, education, housing and social security is inequitable, generally favoring the rich and the middle-class over the poor.[19] In health and education, the problem is often referred to as the "resource allocation" problem. In health, it is one of substantial spending of public resources on generally high-cost, curative hospital care that tends to benefit the rich, compared with low-cost primarily preventive services that tend to benefit the poor.[20] In education, it is one of substantial spending of public resources on high-cost university education, again benefiting primarily the rich, compared with low-cost primary and secondary education. Many governments thus fail to play Robin Hood, i.e., to assure that through social programs some national resources are transferred from the rich to the poor.[21]

This failure means much government spending is ineffective as well as inequitable. Because it is among the poor that health and education indicators are still low, spending that does not reach the poor has limited impact on average indicators for nations as a whole. The situation is particularly ironic because the unit costs of many programs that would reach the poor (primary health care, basic education) are relatively low.[22]

The merits of the argument that governments in developing countries are failing in their essential social tasks require inspection in particular countries and under particular circumstances. In countries in which social programs are financed by highly progressive tax systems (relatively few if any developing countries), the rich may not receive disproportionately higher benefits, given their greater tax contributions (though if the poor receive no benefits at all, government is still failing in its Robin Hood role). In some circumstances, it may make sense to allocate 70 percent of resources to urban-based hospital care directly serving a mere 5 percent of the population, given the high unit costs of hospital care and the need for such care at the summit of a referral system.[23] Finally, to assure that social programs are sustainable politically may require that the rich and middle class share in the benefits.

But even given these extenuating factors, few would question that in many countries, improvement in the Robin Hood function of government is possible. The issue is how. Does the apparent failure of government result from some of the same problems that have plagued government involvement in the industrial, finance and agriculture sectors — large and unresponsive (sometimes corrupt) bureaucracies, and lack of accountability to consumers in a noncompetitive market? Does the Robin Hood failure also reflect a difficulty with government-led "delivery" or "supply" of services that lacks mechanisms to involve recipients as consumers making their own "demands" on the system? Are even apparently adequate supply-side programs limited in their effects and difficult to sustain without the creative input of sovereign consumers (as in the cases of resistance to immunization programs and to sending children to school)?

Put another way, the Robin Hood failure poses a worrisome dilemma. On the one hand, a fundamental justification for government involvement in the social sectors in the first place is that the private market alone is not likely to provide basic ("merit")[24] goods to the poor at a price the poor can or will pay. On the other, if social programs end up as disguised subsidies for the nonpoor (or for government bureaucrats, unionized teachers or other interest groups), it is less easy to argue for their expansion.

An Emerging Pragmatic Approach

We may arrive in the 1990s at a fork in the road with respect to the role of government in the social sectors in developing countries. On the one hand, as governments in developing countries retreat from involvement in the directly productive sectors of the economy, government involvement in the social sectors is likely to grow.[25] On the other hand, that growing involvement can only really be justified to the extent that it reinforces rather than undermines the Robin Hood function of government, and reinforces other less tangible development objectives, for example the involvement of people in a participatory process at the local level.

There are already signs that a new, more pragmatic approach to development is emerging, based on improved understanding of the successes and failures of the state (or governments) in developing countries during the postwar development era, including in the social sectors. In effect, the first stage of the development era ended sometime in the last decade, when it became increasingly clear that governments could not do everything — even in terms of social programs — and that governments needed to take a position somewhere between the extremes of fully centralized planning and the free market. The new approach could be thought of as a pragmatic combination of the ideas of the "left", emphasizing the responsibility of government to provide for basic human needs, and the ideas of the "right", emphasizing the need to get government, with its taxing and potential monopoly powers, off the backs of the people, thus empowering people to exercise their inherent entrepreneurial and organizational skills to improve their lives. On the one hand, government activity in such sectors as health, education and various forms of social insurance can help ensure that basic human needs are met and that people have the tools for their own empowerment. On the other hand, to be effective in these sectors, governments need to avoid highly centralized planning and provision, and exploit the power of the market.

A Pragmatic Framework for Assessing Government's Role

Social Programs: Definition and Society's Objectives

What do we mean by the "social sectors" and "social programs?" These can be defined in terms of the two reasons for government involvement noted above: fairness and market failure. Social services can be defined as a particular class of quasi-public goods (where there is market failure) for which society is particularly concerned to assure some fairness in terms of access.

Most social services, along with other goods and services such as roads, sanitation systems and communications networks, are "quasi-public" goods; they are neither pure public goods (such as clean air or national defense), for which all benefits of use are captured by all members of society, nor pure private goods (such as apples or clothing), for which all benefits of use are captured by the individual who consumes the good. For pure public goods, there is no private willingness to pay because others cannot be excluded and everyone wants a free ride; societies must tax individuals and provide these goods at zero cost to beneficiaries through the mechanism of government. For pure private goods, individuals will purchase "enough" (neither too little nor too much) from society's point of view without encouragement, and there is no need for government involvement at all.

For quasi-public goods, there are private returns to investment, but there are likely to be social returns over and above those private returns (unless private returns are sufficient to induce optimal social behavior, e.g., to induce everyone to enroll in primary school). For example, individuals will not take into account nonprivate or "social" benefits of social programs (such as education's contribution to a more informed citizenry,[26] or health care's contribution to the reduced likelihood that others will be exposed to communicable disease), and will therefore not consume enough of these services unless encouraged to do so, for example by a subsidized price (which may even be zero).[27] Because there are private returns to investment in quasi-public goods, there will exist a private market;[28] but left to itself the private market and private consumers may not produce and consume as much of these quasi-public goods as society as a whole wants, and from which society as a whole can benefit (in terms, for example, of more rapid economic growth). Some government involvement may therefore be warranted.

Among quasi-public goods, social services are those for which society has, in addition, a particular concern about fairness. Fairness dictates that certain "merit goods" be available to all members of society, irrespective of ability to pay. What these goods and services are (and hence which should be the subject of public policy) will vary across societies, depending on income, stage of development, and values. Access to basic education and health care are almost universally included; some societies, particularly in the industrial countries, include unemployment, disability and old age insurance, decent housing, and child care.[29] Note that difficult issues of definition (and fairness) arise not only around what services should be included, but around how much of certain services (vocational and university education as well as primary and secondary education? coronary bypass operations as well as prenatal care?), and of what quality, should be included.

Interestingly, if equity in access to services for the poor is itself taken as a public good (because it is a societal end in itself, or because it contributes to social cohesion and stability), then it is possible to collapse "fairness" and "market failure" (the two rationales for government involvement in the social sectors) into one, with lack of fairness a subset of market failure, arising because the poor have insufficient income to purchase certain merit goods.

In summary, social programs as a group are quasi-public goods (with both private and social returns, for which there are social returns over and above private returns) that society deems for reasons of "fairness" should be available to all, i.e., should not be rationed on the basis of ability to pay.

Quasi-public "Social" Goods: Government Options

It follows that quasi-public social goods should be financed, at least in part, by the public sector. A societal standard of "fairness" may require that government finance (though not necessarily provide) delivery of social services to those unable to purchase such services on the private market. The nature of quasi-public goods may also require that government finance (partly but not necessarily fully) certain social services because even those able to pay will not purchase enough from society's point of view.

But it is also in the nature of quasi-public goods that private markets will exist; the private practice of medicine (including by traditional practitioners) and the existence of private schools in even the poorest developing countries (except where these are expressly forbidden) attest to this, as do social security at the village level and other forms of informal social insurance based on community reciprocity.

One way to think about the role of government in the social sectors is therefore to be concerned with the appropriate mix of inputs of government, given not only society's objectives and fiscal constraints, but also given initial conditions and potential opportunities regarding the private alternative (is there a private sector, and whom does it serve?). Given objectives such as improving health, raising educational levels, reaching the poor, protecting the vulnerable, what are governments' options regarding inputs? What combination of inputs will maximize a particular society's ability to achieve its social objectives?[30] Given initial conditions in a particular country, what policy changes by government, involving changes in government's own activities (more of some, less of others), would make people in that country better off?

Possible combinations of inputs by government, in descending order of government involvement, are:

1. Public provision of services, with full financing (through taxes) or partial financing (through a combination of taxes and user charges) by:

■ central or local governments, as in the case of fully funded public schools and health clinics;

■ quasi-independent public agencies (e.g., a publicly financed hospital or university with an independent board of trustees);

2. Public financing, full or partial, of the provision of such services by the private sector, through:

■ subsidies to individuals, including vouchers directly to potential consumers (allowing consumers to purchase directly from alternative public or private providers),[31] and reductions of personal income taxes associated with private spending on health, education or other social services;[32]

■ subsidies to private providers of services, including grants (e.g., to nonprofit organizations to run particular programs), reimbursement to providers of some costs by government (e.g., through public health insurance programs), and exemption from taxes;

3. Public regulation of private providers, including restriction of provision of services to nonprofit (vs. profit making) organizations; accreditation or other licensing of providers; control over inputs (licensing of teachers and doctors); price controls over outputs;

4. Public provision of information to consumers regarding particular services, products or providers (leaving decisions to consumers) in the public and private sector.

Guidelines in a Sea of Options

There is no single correct option or combination of options. Even if there were an "ideal", it would not necessarily be applicable in any single country, since the costs of moving from the current arrangements in any one country toward the "ideal" might be excessive compared with the benefits. Certain simple guidelines are useful, however, in considering changes (usually at the margin).

Guideline #1: **Remember the Robin Hood (or "fairness") rule.** It is better to take from the rich to give to the poor than to take from the poor to give to the rich.

Guideline #2: **Use public money for the most "public" of quasi-public services.** Fortunately these two guidelines almost always point in the same direction. For example, both these guidelines imply that in the health sector priority in use of public tax funds be given to such basic health care programs as immunizations and endemic disease control, which tend to benefit the poor and which are largely public goods. In education, both guidelines point to priority for primary education in those countries where primary enrollment rates are still not high, or where the quality of primary schooling is so poor that they are not producing literate and numerate citizens.[33] They also point to priority for primary education of girls, because many of the social benefits of primary education occur through improvements in children's health and welfare associated with better educated mothers and possibly through changed tastes for children (more educated women generally desire fewer children).[34]

Note that for these programs, with their substantial externalities, there is generally no reason or need to "target" public spending to the poor. The government can be justified in undertaking much of the costs of these anyway. Even the rich will not individually purchase antimalarial spraying. And though the private returns to primary schooling are high enough so that the rich and middle class will purchase such schooling on the private market, some of the social benefits of education that accrue when children of different social classes attend school together may be captured if public resources are used to finance all students.[35]

These examples illustrate a related point. Guideline #2, independent of guideline #1, underlines the legitimacy of governments undertaking a number of activities that are not directed primarily to the poor. One of these is a set of consumer empowerment functions, to which I give special emphasis below. A second is support for certain types of research, including basic research and some applied research (and in some fields associated graduate training). Research of certain types deserves particular support from governments because of its nature as a largely public good with potential high externalities.[36]

At the same time, guideline #1, independent of guideline #2, points to the legitimacy of government financing some "private" goods and services for the poor, because they are services that society does not wish to see rationed by ability to pay. Government can do this either by providing the service directly to the poor itself (option 1) or by subsidizing provision to the poor of the service by the private sector (option 2). With either option, government must find ways to target the services or the subsidies to the poor; otherwise public spending will simply replace private spending by the nonpoor, and social programs will be violating the Robin Hood rule at high public cost. Food subsidies are a good example of the high costs of poor targeting; in many developing countries, they take up a considerable portion of "social" budgets (and indeed of overall budgets), with limited benefits for the poor who need them most.[37] The same problem arises when government fully subsidizes all patients, rich or poor, in public hospitals, or subsidizes all students, rich or poor, in public universities.

Pragmatic approaches to targeting services do exist, including targeting by residence in rural areas or urban slums; by easily identified age or other population groups, such as pregnant and breastfeeding women and young children;[38] by subsidizing foods that only the poor consume; by requiring village or other certification of low income for eligibility for certain services, or for exemption from fees for certain services.

But only the last of these, use of means tests to exempt the poor from fees, is applicable for such costly "private" services as hospitals and universities, since these generally combine service to all income groups. For these services, only user charges provide a mechanism for targeting (by assuring that the poor but not the rich are subsidized), and only if means can be found to exempt the poor from charges. There is increasing evidence that means tests are possible and in fact widely used in varying forms (Griffin 1989), not only in middle income developing countries with reasonably well-developed tax systems and high levels of literacy (Jamaica, Costa Rica, Chile), but also in low income countries of Asia and Africa (Ethiopia and Senegal use village headman certification, for example). There is no single, simple approach; indeed most countries will need to constantly adjust to means testing approaches (as in Chile, where initially, virtually the entire population was judged eligible for certain programs).

Nor will any means test be perfect. Where targeting is concerned, there will always be tradeoffs. One is a technical tradeoff: The less rigorous the targeting, the more the leakage to the nonpoor and the higher the costs to the public purse; the more rigorous the targeting, the more likely it is that transactions costs will prevent or discourage people from consuming the service. A second is a political tradeoff: The more rigorous the targeting, the more difficult it is to obtain and sustain widespread support.[39] Unfortunately, little is known about the nature and magnitude of these tradeoffs.

Guideline #3: **Emphasize the consumer empowerment functions of government.** This is really a subset of guideline #2. Priorities such as primary health care and basic education are reasonably well established in recent policy work (though not always in the real world), in part because of concern with reaching the poor. However, guideline #2 points to other "public good" activities that are the special province of government and have been relatively neglected.

Within the health and education sectors, the empowerment functions of government, including the dissemination by government of information and associated education, are good examples of largely public goods. In most developing countries, private markets are not well developed for the production and dissemination of information about the relative effectiveness and appropriate use of various pharmaceuticals distributed by private providers; about the existence of and private benefits of certain family planning methods (especially withdrawal and rhythm methods) that have no marketable product; about the health benefits of breastfeeding or about the health risks of smoking, alcohol and poor diet.[40] In Brazil, for example, most women using the contraceptive pill obtain it at pharmacies virtually without attention to medical contraindications. Throughout the developing world, a tendency to multiple prescriptions and overuse of antibiotics hurts consumers' pocketbooks and probably their health as well. The private market for information about the quality and costs of various educational institutions (e.g., about proprietary institutions of vocational training) is also relatively poor in developing countries, especially where the average education of consumers is low.

Obviously, lack of a private market for information is itself a function of a poorly educated population; indeed the social benefits of education include the greater likelihood that an effective private market for consumer information will emerge as average education increases (see fn. 25). As investments in education increase, particularly at lower levels of education, a private market is likely to emerge, as it has in the U.S., Japan and the Philippines (where commercial publications provide information on tuition charges and success rates of private schools). As education increases, the costs to the public sector of providing consumer information will also decline.

Finally, note that the empowerment functions of government in these sectors can include promotion of the very *idea* of better health and education.

Guideline #4: **Apply guidelines #1 and #2 to the choice between public or private financing, not to the choice between public or private provision.** Note that guidelines #1 and #2 apply to how public funds are spent, not to the issue of private vs. public provision. The distinction between financing and provision is a useful one in thinking about the costs and benefits of "privatization" of social services (i.e., the turning over of the provision of public services to private providers, usually under contract). The public good criterion and the Robin Hood rule for determining the priorities for government involvement apply to *financing*, not to *pro. ....on* of services. That is, governments need to give priority to *financing* services for the poor, and to *financing* largely "public" services for the population as a whole. It is irrelevant (with respect to this point) whether such services are *provided* by the state or by private providers.

A corollary of guidelines #1 and #2 is that government can do harm if it finances largely "private" services for the nonpoor. The potential harm of substantial public financing of private services occurs even if the service is provided by the private sector.[41] Conversely, public provision of such services, if they are privately financed (through such mechanisms as user charges and, in the case of health, private insurance) need do no harm (unless there are inefficiencies inherent in government production, e.g., because of civil service wages above the market). "Market approaches," such as user charges, I return to below.

In fact, where *provision* of services is concerned, there is no simple "correct" division between the public and private sectors. It may, for example, be efficient for the public sector to provide a full range of services (as is the case with the National Health Service in England, or with the state of California's university system), even including provision of some purely "private" goods, to all income groups in a population.

There are at least three reasons that can justify public provision of apparently private goods, even to the nonpoor.

■ First, joint production and consumption of public goods with private goods may be the most cost-effective approach, particularly in relatively small and relatively poor countries.

The distinction between the private and public aspects of many social services is difficult to make at the point of production and delivery, making it difficult for a society to sustain public institutions providing public goods and private institutions providing private goods. For example, within health systems, rural health posts may provide mostly "public good" largely preventive services and hospitals mostly "private good" largely curative services. But even rural health posts provide simple curative care, much of it private in nature, and even hospitals provide care of patients with "public" communicable diseases, as well as often being critical centers of socially beneficial research on local clinical health issues. Furthermore, particularly in small countries with limited skilled personnel, it may be necessary that the limited number of hospitals that can be staffed and financed be an integral part of a single health system, accepting referrals from other parts of the system, and providing training and supervision in other parts of the system. The same problem may apply to educational systems in developing countries.

■ Second, quality of services is likely to suffer if the government takes responsibility only for providing services to the poor. Or it may be more costly to government to find and target the poor than to simply provide a service to everyone.

If services for the poor are provided by government, leaving to the private sector the provision of services for the nonpoor, the quality of the services for the poor is likely to be low — because the poor are less knowledgeable consumers and because they do not have the power of the purse. Society may wish to avoid any notable differences in the quality of the service provided to the poor and the nonpoor. Combined with the first problem above, and with the possible high costs of defining, finding and targeting the poor, the result can be a reasonable case for provision by the public sector of a service to everyone.

Of course, neither of these reasons prevents the public sector from contracting out the provision of all services to private providers, and subsidizing (via vouchers to individuals or direct payments to service providers) services that are of a public good nature or are provided to the poor. Where the public sector is likely to be highly inefficient (e.g., because public salaries are too high or placement of services is politically determined), then contracting private providers to deliver services would be better. However, contracting and/or subsidizing then generally requires that government monitor and regulate private sector provision, in one way or another.

Depending on circumstances, the difficulties of combining public financing with private provision can be formidable. For example, public financing of private provision of private curative health services is important in such countries as the United States and Brazil; both countries have substantial public financing of private health care via public insurance systems (in the case of the United States, Medicare and Medicaid). In both countries, there are problems of inequity (because not all members of the population are eligible for the public insurance, and many cannot purchase private insurance); cost escalation (because without adequate copayment and deductibles, there is no consumer resistance to providers' excessive supply);[42] and, if costs are closely monitored, rationed care (as private hospitals or physicians reject or limit attention to costly cases).

On the other hand, for governments to foreclose completely the option of utilizing the private sector to produce and deliver social programs has high opportunity costs, discussed below, particularly where the social costs of monitoring or regulation are not high. This brings us to the third possible reason for public provision of services.

■ Third, and more generally, various market failures mean government, if it does not provide a service directly, will need to monitor provision by the private sector. In some circumstances, the social costs of monitoring and regulation may exceed the social costs of direct provision.

For example, leaving health, unemployment and disability insurance solely to the private market without any public monitoring will not be socially optimal due to problems of moral hazard and adverse selection, and will mean some groups, including the poor and the already sick, will be uninsured.

Unfortunately, it is also true that even with public production, government will need to monitor itself, and this is not necessarily easier than monitoring private producers. The issue thus boils down to one of relative costs to government of monitoring itself vs. monitoring private providers.

Guideline #5: **If services are provided publicly, maximize use of "market" approaches, particularly for "private" services.** Governments in many developing countries are likely to continue to be involved not only in the financing but also in the direct provision of private services (for example, curative care in public hospitals and university training), if only for the joint production and other reasons outlined above. This is particularly the case for those developing countries in Africa and parts of Asia where private sector availability of such services is small. For health, the likelihood of growing involvement of government seems particularly high (despite the recent counterexample of Chile); Frenk and Donabedian (1987) attribute the recent trend toward greater involvement of government to the emergence of a high-technology "medical world economy," in which "the state has been called upon to take the lead as the only actor with enough resources to be an effective buyer, or with sufficient power to control the other powerful actors in the international private sector."

Use of market approaches means use of mechanisms that imitate the advantages of a free market. Two advantages of the market are critical for social services. One is the advantage of wider consumer choice; for a service such as education, consumers can benefit particularly from wider choice, given different regional, cultural, linguistic or religious views, even within single nations, which in varying degrees national governments may wish to allow for.[43] For education, consumers can also benefit from a range of price/quality choices. The second advantage is that of the greater efficiency generated by competition among providers,[44] even if all providers are public. Competition between public and private providers can also increase efficiency, as long as the public provider is not protected from the market (as is often the case with, for example, public airlines, television and postal systems).

Two market approaches are user charges and decentralization of the administration of government services.

User charges need to be selective, i.e., they should be applied only to the nonpoor (recall guideline #1) and only to "private" type services (recall guideline #2). Selective user charges are based on the idea that even though the state is providing a private service, individual consumers can finance those private services, as long as they are both willing and able to pay. As noted above, user charges provide a mechanism for targeting public subsidies to the poor (since the nonpoor, but not the poor, are paying). They can also improve internal efficiency of programs because they increase consumer power; if consumers can choose among alternative public providers or opt out of use of public services whose quality is not commensurate with costs compared to choices in the private sector, public services are likely to improve. They empower consumers as a group, and increase the likelihood that consumers will voice complaints about services through political or other processes. In addition, user charges can improve allocative efficiency, since they provide a mechanism for directing all consumers to "public" type goods with large social benefits; such services can be provided free to all, increasing consumers' incentive to consume them, and signalling to individuals their high social value. In this sense, a zero price on a particular service, such as immunizations, provides information to consumers about its value to the community as a whole (as well as to individuals).

User charges also allow government to calibrate its subsidies, depending on its budget, redistributional goals, and social goals. User charges need not cover full (marginal) costs; the government can choose to finance anywhere from 0 to 100 percent of costs by user charges instead of taxes, as is the case when students pay for books but not tuition, or clinic patients pay for drugs but not the other costs of a visit.

Decentralization of services is based on the idea that the publicly-provided service will be more responsive to and more accountable to local needs (i.e., clients) the closer it is geographically and bureaucratically to those needs. Decentralization also allows for greater competition (to a greater or lesser extent depending on the physical size and administrative limits of decentralized units); it also can increase consumer choice by encouraging heterogeneity in the types and nature of services.

Decentralization is an approach that with a few exceptions (India, Nigeria, Brazil) remains virtually untried in the developing world, perhaps because efforts at nation-building in the first few decades of the postwar era created centralist political tendencies. Though many central programs are regionalized for administrative purposes, the "market" benefits of decentralization probably only flow if social services are provided through local governments with real power to tax and allocate resources. Even in countries like Nigeria and Brazil with federal systems, the revenue-raising capacity of municipal level governments is relatively limited, and in the case of Brazil is actually deteriorating. (Obviously user charges can be one form of revenue raising, which if retained locally, would strengthen local control and accountability.) Though block grants from the center to local areas could in theory increase the accountability of local government to local populations for the use of funds,[45] in fact it is often difficult for central governments to resist the temptation for political favoritism built into any system of block grants. In turn, central governments may fear that funds provided to local governments without oversight will be used for local political purposes rather than for long-term social investments.

Complete reliance on local revenues, even were it possible, might not be desirable in any case since it would not assure adequate redistribution of public funds in countries with marked differences in the regional distribution of assets and income.

In short, it is difficult to separate the problem of improving the internal market for government-provided services through decentralization from larger questions about local governance and revenue-raising capacity in developing countries, as well as questions of earmarking of public tax revenues to particular sectors and regions.[46] In Africa and parts of the Indian subcontinent, the problem may be particularly intractable because of the reluctance of central or state governments to yield too much power to regional and local groups that may not fully endorse the view that the nation is the critical unit.

Guideline #6: If services are provided by the private sector, no matter how poorly, avoid public crowding out or takeover. Consider instead consumer information programs, monitoring of quality, and, where necessary, regulation. Wherever possible, rely on information to consumers over regulation and other direct forms of control. In the set of options for government outlined above, numbers 3 (regulation, including quality control) and 4 (consumer information) are relatively neglected, especially in developing countries. (A literature search on regulatory issues in health and education in developing countries turned up virtually nothing.[47]) The lack of government capacity for regulation and quality control is a particular problem in health, given rapidly changing technologies in pharmaceuticals, contraception, and waste control, new industrial technologies with Bhopal potential, and increases in people's exposure to air and water pollution.

Information and education have already been emphasized in the discussion above, in terms of their consumer empowerment aspect. Government information programs are probably relatively low in cost, compared with direct provision or subsidies for private provision, but little work has been done on the effectiveness of information programs (for example, public campaigns to reduce smoking) compared with other programs.

Regulation raises more difficult issues. It involves a large number of options in itself, as regulation (and quality control functions) can be combined in varying degrees with direct or indirect, and full or partial, public financing. Where the private sector (profit-making or nonprofit) is active in provision of social services (and in some countries for particular services the private sector is bigger than the public sector),[48] regulation and quality control may be the most effective way, at the least cost, for governments to maximize access to and quality of services. This will be the case particularly if governments choose to directly subsidize private sector institutions in order to reduce the administrative and fiscal burden associated with direct public provision.

The most straightforward forms of regulation are price regulation (as is done for electric power in the United States) and direct regulation of outputs (for example, restriction of the types of pharmaceuticals allowed on the market). Though some countries do regulate the prices private schools and physicians or hospitals are allowed to charge (or are allowed to be reimbursed for), price regulation is not really effective in protecting consumers of products whose quality is costly to monitor. Thus, for example, regulation of the prices of private schools is likely simply to drive down the quality of the schools (if they are profit-making) or to restrict the ability of schools to amass capital to finance expansion (if they are nonprofit).[49] The regulation thus defeats its own purpose.

In a few areas, including drugs and contraceptives, regulation of outputs can be effective, but in general because health, education, nutrition and child care programs are not simple homogeneous products, regulation of prices or output will either reduce access or drive down quality (as appears to be the case with nursing homes in the United States).

More effective than a single direct approach to regulation is a variety of indirect approaches, and flexibility in applying them. Many countries, for example, regulate the inputs to a service (e.g., teacher or physician qualifications, though such regulation may unduly restrict access to services where human capital is scarce). Developing countries often adopt regulatory standards regarding these inputs from the developed countries, even though they usually face a different tradeoff between the risks and benefits of varying qualifications (or safety or efficacy of a product) than do developed countries. Weisbrod points out that developing countries could thus be aided by the establishment of "objective" variable international standards for regulation of drugs, pesticides, health care and other social services.[50]

A second indirect approach is to regulate the types of institutions that can provide social services. A common form is to mandate that education and health services can only be provided by nonprofit organizations, or that only nonprofit organizations providing such services can benefit from direct government subsidies, where nonprofits are defined as organizations that do not distribute any profits (profits may be used only to expand or improve the quality of the organizations' services). If the costs of enforcing this kind of constraint are low (for example, the costs of monitoring salaries of nonprofit providers), nonprofits offer the possibility of an element of government control without the excessive bureaucratic demands of a government-run service. The issue then for developing countries is how to maximize the potential for nonprofits; on this issue, as with regulation, there is little empirical work.[51] Van der Heijden and others point out the potential advantages to government of assisting nongovernmental organizations (NGOs) in institutional developing and in creating incentives for NGOs to raise funds privately, for example, through tax policy and through direct assistance in grant intermediation. These and other program and research issues for NGOs are discussed briefly in Section III.

A Few Lessons from Developed Countries

On the one hand, there is something to be learned from the experience of developed countries in terms of government's role in the social sectors, particularly since developed countries as a group spend much more, in absolute terms and as a percent of all government expenditures, on social programs. This is particularly true in areas such as old age and disability insurance and health insurance, for which developing countries may be initiating new programs and can avoid at least some of the pitfalls. On the other hand, for a number of reasons, approaches taken in developed countries do not necessarily provide useful experience.

■ Tax exemptions, a popular and convenient form of indirect subsidy in developed countries, are not as useful in developing countries.

Developing countries generally have much less tax coverage. Subsidies that are confined to tax exemptions are likely to benefit primarily the higher-income groups that pay taxes in the first place, and thus to violate the Robin Hood rule. In Brazil, for example, tax exemptions for spending on private health care are estimated to represent more than 10 percent of all direct spending by government on health. In Zimbabwe, it is primarily those of higher income that benefit from tax breaks for private health insurance (World Bank 1992). Many developing countries give tax exemptions to nonprofit organizations that provide health and schooling services, but these exemptions are difficult to target to the nonrich. In the end, developing countries need to rely much more on subsidies, and thus more on some combination of government provision, or a combination of subsidies to individuals or nongovernment institutions accompanied by regulation.

■ The more successful social programs of governments in developed countries are in countries with smaller and relatively more homogeneous populations.

The Scandinavian countries, for example, have been relatively successful with direct provision of services by government. But this conceptually simple approach is less likely to work in those developing countries where there are greater differences among groups in income, ethnicity, religion and so forth. In countries such as the United States, social programs are more controversial politically and apparently less effective in reaching the poorest groups. The Netherlands, however, provides a useful example of a country in which ethnic differences have been accommodated through extensive reliance on nonprofit groups, which, with full subsidies from government, provide the bulk of primary and secondary education (James 1984).

■ The difficulties with means tests, great as they are in developed countries, provide few lessons for those developing countries where the formal monetized economy is much smaller and literacy is low.

In fact, developing countries probably have much more to learn from each other, given emerging evidence (Griffin 1989) that means testing, of one form or another, is more prevalent and more successful than formerly realized.

■ Regulatory and quality control functions and standards of developed countries are poorly developed, controversial, and often irrelevant given the different tradeoffs in developing countries.

■ Finally, lower levels of literacy, greater scarcity of skilled manpower and of administrative skills, and less well-developed communication systems make both the direct provision of services and the regulation of private services relatively more costly in developing than developed countries.

On the other hand, as noted at the beginning, for the same reasons, the social returns to investments in social programs are generally higher in developing countries.

Research and Program Needs: Selected Topics

The selection of topics outlined here is arbitrary and reflects the author's experience and interests. An issue in itself is that of priorities for research and program activity, given the large and diffuse subject this paper treats.

Health and Other Forms of Social Insurance

Health insurance is an example of a program area where increasing government involvement seems almost inevitable. Developing countries increasingly see creation of insurance as a mechanism to finance health care. The recent policy study of the World Bank (Akin et al. 1987) suggests that countries consider expansion of insurance markets as part of their overall approach to health financing; availability of insurance is necessary if there are fee charges in the public sector or provision of care by the private sector. The single greatest problem with health insurance is that of cost escalation in the health sector as a whole, if the insurance system does not include incentives to providers and patients to keep costs down. Insurance can also exacerbate rather than relieve inequities in access to care. Cost escalation and inequity have been the experience of the United States and several countries of Latin America.

Research and policy work on health financing issues in developing countries, especially on cost recovery, has grown rapidly in the 1980s, with much work financed by the World Bank and USAID, and some by WHO. Work on health insurance itself, however, is extremely limited. Empirical work on health insurance would concentrate on issues of equity (how to guarantee coverage for the poor and the already sick; whether developing countries should begin by providing or mandating insurance for those in the formal sector; whether insurance systems should be set up separately for the poor; whether premiums can be subsidized); and issues of efficiency (what aspects of insurance contribute to cost escalation; whether the insured seek too much care; how to regulate provision of insurance by the private sector; under what circumstances prepaid systems work, including health maintenance organizations, and whether they reduce costs at the price of lower quality; how various schedules of deductibles and copayments affect use of services and health outcomes; what the costs and benefits of preferred provider schemes are; how successful government efforts at cost control through such mechanisms as diagnostic related group pricing are).

Analysis of these issues could begin with comparative work on existing systems, but eventually new research and experiments (such as the California Rand experiment conducted in the 1970s), either in developing countries or with developing country needs and constraints in mind, will be needed in particular country settings, if there is to be real progress.

Because health insurance is often administered jointly with other forms of social insurance, work on health insurance would probably be of considerable use as input to more general work on the role of government in providing through various social insurance programs a social safety net. The specific issues as they relate to other forms of social insurance would be different, however, and are not outlined here.

Public Policy Toward Private Provision of Social Services

On the one hand, the discussion in Section II indicated that there is not any reason to support the nongovernment sector in and of itself. On the other hand, there are often good reasons to do so, whenever the private sector 1) reduces the fiscal burden by assuming costs that would otherwise fall to government, 2) is more efficient in the delivery of services, in terms of lower costs or higher quality at the same costs (even if fully subsidized by government), or 3) is more accountable to clients or consumers, providing a more appropriate service and contributing to the ability of the poor and other vulnerable groups to organize themselves.

The above criteria are useful whether the profit-making private sector or the nonprofit sector (the latter generally called "NGO" or "PVO" for nongovernment organization or private voluntary organization) is under consideration. Some governments are more "friendly" to nonprofit organizations than to the profit-making sector, in a few cases legally excluding profit-making groups from the provision of some social services (in some settings, a regulation that is difficult to enforce). Many make it difficult even for nonprofit groups to form and provide services — for example, through use of cumbersome procedures for acquiring a license.

In terms of research, three subjects have hardly been touched, despite a growing literature on the involvement of the nongovernment sector (particularly the NGO or non-profit sector) in delivery of social services in developing countries:

■ The internal efficiency of these organizations — i.e., their output given their unit costs, compared with the efficiency of government services. Some work has been recently done comparing private and public schools in developing countries (Jimenez, Lockheed and Paques 1988.)

■ The public policy framework within which these organizations operate, with special emphasis on the regulatory environment, the size and nature of public subsidies and the interaction with the regulatory environment, the nature of government quality control (e.g., of pharmaceuticals, schools, licensing of private physicians, accreditation, insurance commissions) and information programs (achievement testing, posting of generic drug prices). How effective are alternative approaches under varying conditions of income, income distribution, literacy, size of the private sector, etc.? What are effective mechanisms for government to use in subsidizing the private sector, in ways that avoid corruption, waste, and bureaucratization of the private sector?

■ The self-financing capacity of the nongovernment sector (referring only to the nonprofits), especially its capacity to raise money from fees and from local contributions (in the form of fundraising activities and voluntary labor, which presumably provide built-in responsiveness and reduce cost inefficiency) vs. from international donors and from government.

In addition to research, program support could contribute to the development of local umbrella organizations that would stimulate businesses and individuals to contribute voluntarily to nonprofit nongovernment social programs in developing countries, along the lines of the United Way. Lack of easy mechanisms for contributing and poor information about the merits of particular service organizations probably inhibit private giving in many countries. Program support could also contribute to creation of a policy and research base on the nongovernment sector in developing countries, comparable to the base in the U.S. provided, for example, by the Yale Program on Non-Profit Organizations. Creation of such a base is critical to improving openness to the potential of the private sector within government circles in many developing countries.

Public Finance of Basic ("Pre-competitive") Research and Related Training in Developing Countries

In only a few developing countries does spending, private and public, on basic research come close to 1 percent of GNP (these include India, Brazil and Korea). Government support for basic research and graduate training is tiny in most countries, despite the "public good" nature of such activities. Though much basic research, because it is an international public good (that is, nations cannot appropriate the benefits of findings), should not be financed in poor countries, it can be argued that some basic research must be done in countries themselves as part of graduate training if countries are to have the capacity to exploit new technologies.[52] (This is not to suggest there are not problems of absorptive capacity, and a prevalent tendency for basic research in developing countries to fail to address critical local needs.) The issue of basic research and its links to higher education merits more attention: (1) It may be an example of an area in which governments in developing countries are committing the combined errors of doing not enough of one thing (financing research) and too much of another (financing undergraduate training); (2) the intellectual dependency problem may be a critical constraint to what the Rockefeller Foundation calls "science-based development", i.e., to the use of science and technology to improve people's lives in developing countries; and (3) support for basic research and graduate training in university settings has been largely abandoned by the international donor community in the 1980s.

Research on this subject would focus on such questions as: What are the costs and benefits of investment in developing countries in basic and applied research, particularly in the area of science and technology? Have there been lost opportunities? Has lack of trained people restricted acceptance and adaptation of new technologies in many developing countries, or are there other more important barriers, such as lack of intellectual property rights, restrictions on foreign investment, or a discouraging regulatory environment? Are there critical supply constraints in developing countries, such as lack of critical mass and excessive dispersion of resources preventing creation of such mass at a few institutions? To what extent is basic research a public good with large unrealized economic returns? Is it largely an international public good, requiring intervention at the international level (as with the ozone problem), or largely a nation-level public good? What is the interaction between research and training of postgraduate students and undergraduate training? What is and should be the role of government in poor countries in the financing and management of basic research programs, taking into account the costs as well as possible benefits? Is there anything to be learned from the developed countries in this area?

In terms of action programs, the creation or nurturing of cross-national institutions that would encourage basic research (especially in the areas of science and technology) in developing countries, and support for efforts to reduce the costs of transferring ideas, e.g., for libraries, journal subscriptions, travel awards for developing country scientists, etc., seem warranted. If research findings could be shown to warrant it, seed money could be provided for a long-term (at least 10 year) commitment to program support for basic research on selected subjects (environment, biotechnology, health sciences) in two or three universities in the developing world, with financing from international and bilateral donors tied to some sort of financial commitment from participating nations.

User Charges and the Targeting of Public Spending on Social Programs

As noted above, there may be conditions under which it is more cost-effective and more equitable for government to provide a full range of services, including so-called "private" services such as curative hospital care, than for government to rely on private sector provision. Provision by government of a full range of services is widespread in industrial countries, and if anything, historical forces (and political forces in many countries) seem to be operating to encourage such provision.

Targeting of such services to the poor then becomes critical, if government is to avoid subsidizing the rich and, wherever resources are scarce, increasing the likelihood that the poor will lose out. For some services, targeting by residence, age, status (such as pregnancy), or product (subsidizing foods consumed primarily by the poor) is possible. But for other services, targeting requires exclusion of the poor, through some form of means testing, from user fees the nonpoor must pay.

Both user fees *per se* and means testing are topics on which limited research to date has been done in developing countries. Controversy over user fees in the 1980s has increased the interest of researchers in the topic; of particular interest is the effect of user fees on utilization of services by the poor, especially health services.[53] The topic has emerged as a popular one (in terms of frequency among research proposals submitted) in the International Health Policy Program (supported by the Pew Trust). But data problems are substantial and most research efforts are modest and are not building on each other. Real progress would clearly be enhanced by a more concentrated program, particularly one carried out in close collaboration with one or more governments.

Research on the costs and effectiveness of various approaches to means testing is rarer still.[54] Research questions are: What approaches to means testing have worked, under what circumstances; to what extent do the truly poor fail to take advantage of differential prices; what are the administrative and other costs of means testing?

Decentralization of Social Services

To what extent would decentralization of government services increase efficiency and quality, and make services more responsive to clients' needs? Is regionalization of centrally administered programs enough, or is local control of revenue required? Are block grants from the center to local governments enough or must revenue be generated locally to produce whatever efficiency or other gains are associated with decentralization?

Research on the efficiency and equity effects of more decentralized delivery of services requires before and after information on an actual change in the way governments structure themselves. There may be a preceding question: What constraints, including political and institutional constraints, have and do inhibit decentralization of services in developing countries?

Acknowledgments

At the time of preparing this paper, the author was Senior Advisor to Rockefeller Foundation. She is grateful to many colleagues for comments on an earlier draft, especially Jere Behrman, Willy de Geyndt, Michael Lipton, Jose Aristodemo Pinotti, Guy Pfefferman, George Psacharaopoulus and Richard Snape. The World Bank does not accept responsibility for the views expressed herein, which are those of the author(s) and should not be attributed to the World Bank or to its affiliated organizations.

Notes

1 U.S. goals for developing countries set out in UNESCO and WHO documents in the 1950s, 1960s and 1970s, including universal free education and health care, were dominant concerns of the 1980s. Only in the low-cost and more controversial area of family planning has the financial issue not been so prominent in the 1980s.

2 See for example the controversial paper on selective primary health care of Walsh and Warren (1979) and controversial World Bank studies on the financing of education (1979) and health services in developing countries (Psacharopoulos, Tan and Jimenez 1986; Akin, Birdsall and de Ferranti 1987).

3 See World Bank (1988c), especially Chapters 2 and 5. Much of the discussion of the size and growth of government expenditures in this section is based on the analysis and data in that document.

4 Public and publicly guaranteed foreign debt tripled as a percent of GDP between 1973 and 1986 for all developing countries. In 1986 medium and long-term public debt accounted for between 85 and 89 percent of all foreign debt in the developing countries. World Bank. (1988c) Chapter 2.

5 These policy or adjustment loans (covering trade and other policies as well as privatization) increased as a proportion of all lending (including "project" lending for investments) from virtually none in the late 1970s to about 25 percent by 1987.

6 In 1988, the Bank produced an internal report on ways to ensure adequate attention to the private sector in its operations.

7 For example, Buchanan (1986). Buchanan won the Nobel Prize in economics in 1986 for his development of the theory of public choice.

8 Krueger (1974) describes the characteristics and the social costs of a rent-seeking society.

9 For evidence that the difference between social and private returns is greater in developing countries for education, see Psacharopoulos, Tan and Jimenez (1986), p. 7.

10 This helps explain the generally higher social rates of return to social investments in developing compared to developed countries.

11 Transfers would ideally be netted out. Part of the difference (in transfers) is due to the higher proportion of elderly retired people in more developed countries; in addition, some portion of transfers is likely to be financed by earmarked taxes on beneficiaries. Both of these factors mean the difference between the two groups of countries is exaggerated. See World Bank (1988c) for a complete listing of "low-income" and "middle-income" developing countries.

12 These figures exclude state and local government spending, which is probably proportionately greater in the industrial than in the developing countries. The figures exaggerate real differences somewhat, since wage rates, and thus the cost of equivalent labor, are lower in the developing countries.

13 See Birdsall (1989) for discussion of past government successes in improving health in developing countries and citations to quantitative studies of the causes of mortality decline

14 Golladay and Liese (1980), p. 22.

15 World Bank (1988c), pp. 13-15.

16 World Bank (1988b), p. 12. It has recently been argued that the quality of public education has declined as a result of rapid expansion (World Bank 1989). Direct evidence of a decline in quality is hard to find because of lack of information on trends in, say, student achievement in developing countries. There is little doubt of the current low level of achievement of students at specific grades in most developing countries outside of Asia, compared to students from developed countries, and repetition rates and drop-out rates are very high (in Brazil, less than one in five students completes primary school in the standard eight years), all suggesting a low level of quality. Schultz (1987) notes that declining expenditures per student need not be a sign of declining quality, since the relative wages of teachers have fallen. Behrman and Birdsall (1983) provide evidence for one developing country that economic rates of return to school quality are as high as or higher than returns to years of schooling, suggesting the likelihood of relative underinvestment in quality.

17 The increasing involvement of government in the social sectors as income rises probably reflects the increasing taxing power of governments as economies become more monetized and the size of the formal sector increases, as well as the apparent income elasticity of demand for public services.

18 Though expenditures on social services fell, declines in the relative price of inputs with increasing availability of educated labor (e.g., declines in the relative wages of teachers) mean the real value of expenditures may not have fallen. This point is important, since the proportionate input of skilled labor may be greater for health and education services than for other types of government expenditure.

19 See for example Psacharopoulos, Tan and Jimenez (1986) regarding education; Akin, Birdsall and de Ferranti (1987) regarding health; World Bank (1988a — on Brazil, and 1988b) regarding these sectors as well as housing and other urban services. These documents have pointed to efficiency as well as equity problems arising from patterns of public spending in the social sectors. By one measure of "equity," if the rich pay higher taxes and receive proportionately higher benefits from social programs, public spending is not "inequitable." The actual extent to which governments transfer funds through social programs depends on the incidence of the taxes and other charges that finance the programs, as well as the distribution of the benefits. It is possible, particularly in those middle-income countries where income taxes are an important source of government funds, that certain social programs do involve at least some redistribution of income from the rich to the less rich.

20 It is obviously simplistic to fully equate "basic health" with cheap, efficient services for the poor and "hospitals" with costly, inefficient care for the nonpoor; but the relation, though not perfect, is there.

21 There is, of course, great variability across countries in the extent to which this statement holds. Governments differ across countries, and are shaped in part by past history and the resulting participation of and expectations of various constituencies and interest groups. It is notable, however, that even in countries with a political philosophy and rhetoric emphasizing equity such as China, the distribution of spending on social services favors heavily the urban areas, where average income is higher. See Prescott and Jamison (1984).

22 Brazil is an example. Though public spending on social programs is high (as much as 20 percent of all public spending), infant mortality in the poor Northeast region is higher than in India or Kenya, and fewer than one in four children completes primary school. See World Bank (1988a).

23 The option to use hospital care may have great value even to those who never use it because they never need to. See also Musgrove (1987), who explains why, once we take into account that an ounce of prevention is worth a lot of cure, high spending on hospital care for a few may make sense.

24 As discussed below, the definition of merit goods is likely to vary across societies; they can be thought of as those goods to which a particular society wishes to assure equal access, irrespective of ability to pay. Societies often define such goods in national legislation, or in the form of agreement to international declarations such as the declared objective of "Health for All by the Year 2000" enunciated at an international conference at Alma Alta in 1978. Neither is "ability to pay" easy to define; some poor households could "afford" schooling for their children if they gave up alcohol and cigarettes. In some cases, however, the lack of conditions for a private market is clear; doctors will not set up private practice in rural areas where average income is too low to assure adequate demand.

25 This is particularly true in the middle-income countries, where the period of very rapid growth of public investments in the development of basic physical infrastructure — roads, electric power, telecommunications — is ending; in low-income countries, particularly in Africa, rapid growth in the rate of these physical investments will still be essential to creation of national markets and development of industry.

26 Other social returns to education include any social gain associated with the lower fertility of better educated women and any social gain associated with better-informed consumers (e.g., if most consumers are well-informed, even the uninformed may benefit from safer or more effective products).

27 See Jimenez (1987) for a full discussion.

28 The notion that there are returns — private and social — to investments in education and health requires a special note. With the possible exception of schooling, most governments in developing countries continue to focus on physical investments in roads, irrigation, power, etc. when planning "investment" policy, and to treat education and health spending as "consumption." However, high economic returns to public investments in schooling, health and other human capital programs dictate such investments even aside from the "fairness" objective, and this is important when scarce resources force societies

to redefine the set of merit goods. Estimated social returns to investment in education tend to exceed returns to most physical investments (Psacharopoulos 1985; see also Behrman and Birdsall 1987). There are no comparable estimates of returns to investments in health. In addition, social programs probably contribute to social stability, trust, and development of shared values; all these contribute indirectly to economic development. High social returns to investments in social programs may even justify governments making some social services, such as schooling up to some level and immunizations, not only available but compulsory. Legislation mandating such behavior is probably only marginally effective, however. Where private returns are perceived to be low, consumers will not be willing to take on the private indirect costs (for time and travel), and government cannot make much if any difference through legislation alone.

29 Weisbrod (1988a) defines the social services this way. He cites Musgrave for the idea that social services are those which society does not wish to see rationed by ability to pay. (Unfortunately this definition fails to exclude sporting events, opera and other services that many societies subsidize to avoid rationing by ability to pay.)

30 This is a cost-effectiveness approach, in which society's objectives are taken as given. An alternative cost-benefit approach would allow benefits to shift as well as costs (or inputs). The simple framework laid out below can be applied in either case.

31 See Weisbrod (1988b) for a fuller description of the advantages and problems of vouchers. Vouchers have long been favored by economists because they allow considerable consumer choice and they increase the likelihood that competition among providers will increase efficiency.

32 These tend to be regressive, even if set as a reduction in taxes rather than taxable income.

33 Even given that the first two guidelines point in the same direction, some measure of benefits (a social welfare function) is still needed to allocate resources optimally.

34 Some of the benefits of the effects of education on women's capacity as mothers are largely captured by the educated women (e.g., in the form of healthier children); though they are not marketed, they are largely private benefits. But some of the benefits of healthier children and possibly of lower fertility accrue to society as a whole. Haveman and Wolfe (1984) provide a full listing of the social and private, marketed and nonmarketed returns to education.

35 Even with full government funding, the upper classes may resort to private schools to avoid the redistribution of human capital that occurs when more and less advantaged students are mixed together. See James (1989).

36 Support for research in university settings need not be inconsistent with the recommendation that the highest priority for government spending on "training" should go to primary education, since the institution of user charges in public universities can relieve the government of much of the burden of directly financing university training. See Birdsall (1988).

37 This is less of a problem when a staple consumed primarily by the poor can be subsidized.

38 Leakage of food and nutrition supplements for young children and women does occur, because of substitution within households. In these cases, the targeted benefit is simply an income transfer to a poor household.

39 Support of the nonpoor for targeting need not be assumed to be negligible. The nonpoor can benefit, economically and socially (e.g., reduced crime, a more stable labor market) when the poor have access to social programs. Moreover, the nonpoor will often support social programs if only because it is morally compelling to do so (Etzioni 1988).

40 Unfortunately government cannot always be trusted to give accurate information — for example on nuclear fallout, acid rain, toxic waste, the health effects of tobacco — underlining the advantages of a competitive private market for information.

41 Indeed public financing of privately provided services to the nonpoor can be a recipe for excessive and inefficient spending, as noted below in the case of health in Brazil and the U.S.

42 In addition, of course, consumers may be in a poor position to evaluate doctors' decisions, and full insurance is itself an inducement to development of new and more costly technologies.

43 See James (1984) for a discussion of the example of the Dutch educational system.

44 In health, it is often argued that competition leads to higher costs, as uncontrolled private providers, primarily doctors and hospitals, order more procedures and encourage excessive patient visits and hospital stays. This so-called supply-induced demand is a result of the consumer's relative disadvantage in evaluating options and difficulty of shopping around when he or she has a serious medical problem. "Healthy" competition can be induced, even in health, through use of capitation systems, and in health maintenance organizations, by compensating providers in a manner that is independent of inputs.

45 Block grants that are not earmarked will be treated by the recipient government exactly as would be locally-raised revenues (i.e., they will be allocated at the margin).

46 For useful discussion of the link between earmarking and decentralization, see McLeary (1988).

47 Memorandum of Rebecca Stone to Nancy Birdsall of August 16, 1988. Exceptions are papers by James (forthcoming; 1984) on public policies toward private education in developing countries and in the Netherlands, including discussion of regulation.

48 For example, more students are in private than in public postsecondary institutions in Brazil and the Philippines. Private expenditures for health care

exceed public expenditures in many developing countries (Akin, Birdsall, and de Ferranti 1987).

49 Weisbrod (1988a) and James and Rose-Ackerman (1986) explain the economic theory and provide examples from developed countries behind this assertion. See also van der Heijden (1988) regarding nonprofit organizations in developing countries.

50 An example of this is the Essential Drugs Program of the World Health Organization (WHO). In Africa, the program is meant to assure more efficient use of scarce foreign currency. But it also has a regulatory aspect; in some countries, government funds are used only for purchase of a restricted set of drugs deemed most cost-effective given the epidemiology of the country.

51 Memorandum of Rebecca Stone to Nancy Birdsall, dated August 19, 1988. The considerable literature on nonprofit organizations (NGOs) in developing countries concentrates on the internal structure and characteristics of the organizations. There has been little study of the (a) size of the NGO sector, and (b) nature of government/NGO interactions. Exceptions are James (1982) on Sri Lanka, Vogel (1988) for insights on four countries in Africa, Guhan (1986) on India, and van der Heijden (1988).

52 See Birdsall (1989) for the full argument and citations to other work in which the merits and demerits of government spending on basic research in poor countries are made.

53 For a recent study with references to other studies in health, see Gertler and van der Gaag (1988).

54 Though see Griffin (1988), prepared as background to this paper.

References

Akin, J.S., N. Birdsall, and D. de Ferranti. 1987. *Financing Health Services in Developing Countries.* Washington, DC: The World Bank.

Atkinson, A.B., and J. Hills. 1988. "Social security in developed countries: Are there lessons for developing countries?" Unpublished paper.

Behrman, J.R., and N. Birdsall. 1983. "Quality of schooling: Quantity alone is misleading." *American Economic Review,* 73: 5.

Behrman, J.R., and N. Birdsall. 1987. "Returns to education: A further international update and implications-comment." *Journal of Human Resources,* 22(4): 603-606.

Birdsall, N. 1988. "Public spending on higher education in developing countries: Too much or too little." Unpublished paper prepared for The Rockefeller Foundation. World Bank.

Birdsall, N. 1989. "Thoughts on good health and good government." *Daedalus,* 118(1): 89-117.

Buchanan, J.M. 1986. *Liberty, Market and the State.* Brighton, England: Wheatsheaf Books.

Caldwell, J.C. 1986. "Routes to low mortality in poor countries." *Population and Development Review,* 12(2): 171-220.

Etzioni, A. 1988. *The Moral Dimension: Toward a New Economics.* New York: Free Press.

Frenk, J., and A. Donabedian. 1987. "State intervention in medical care: Types, trends and variables." *Health Policy and Planning,* 2(1): 17-31.

Friedman, M., and R.D. Friedman. 1980. *Free to Choose: A Personal Statement.* New York: Harcourt, Brace, Jovanovich.

Gertler, P., and J. van der Gaag. 1988. *The Willingness-to-Pay for Medical Care: Evidence from Two Developing Countries.* World Bank, book manuscript.

Golladay, F., and B. Liese. 1980. "Health problems and policies in the developing countries." Washington, DC: World Bank Staff Working Paper No. 142.

Griffin, C.C. 1989. "Means testing in developing countries." Unpublished paper prepared for The Rockefeller Foundation. University of Oregon.

Guhan, S. 1986. "Grants-in-aid to PVOs in family welfare and health: India, Maharashtra and Tamil Nadu." World Bank mimeo (restricted).

James, E. 1982. "The nonprofit sector in international perspective: The case of Sri Lanka." *Journal of Comparative Economics,* June: 99-129.

James, E. 1984. "Benefits and costs of privatized public services: Lessons from the Dutch educational system." *Comparative Education Review,* 28(4): 605-24.

James, E. 1988. *Public Policy and Private Education in Japan.* Basingstoke: MacMillan.

James, E. 1989. *The Nonprofit Sector in International Perspective: Studies in Comparative Culture and Policy.* New York: Oxford University Press.

James, E. 1991. "Public policies toward private education." *International Journal of Educational Research,* 15:359-76.

James, E., and S. Rose-Ackerman. 1986. *The Nonprofit Enterprise in Market Economics.* New York: Harwood Academic Publishers.

Jimenez, E. 1987. "Pricing policy in the social sectors: Cost recovery for health and education in developing countries." Baltimore, MD: Johns Hopkins University Press. World Bank mimeo.

Jimenez, E. 1989. "Social sector pricing policy revisited: A survey of some recent controversies in developing countries." Paper prepared for the First Annual World Bank Conference on Development Economics.

Jimenez, E., M. Lockheed, and V. Paqueo. 1988. "Comparative effectiveness and efficiency of public and private schools in developing countries." World Bank mimeo.

Krueger, A.O. 1974. "The political economy of the rent-seeking society." *American Economic Review,* 64(3): 291-303.

McLeary, W.A. 1988. "Notes on the principles and practice of earmarking." World Bank mimeo.

Musgrove, P. 1987. "E Quanto Mas Vale Prevenir que Curar?" Economia Ponitfica Universidad Catolica del Peru.

Prescott, N., and D.T. Jamison. 1984. "Health sector finance in China." *World Health Statistical Quarterly*, 37: 387-402.

Psacharopoulos, G. 1985. "Returns to education: A further update and implications." *Journal of Human Resources*, 20(Fall): 583-604.

Psacharopoulos, G. 1988. "Welfare effects of government intervention in education." *Contemporary Policy Issues, Economic Analysis for the Decision Maker*, 4(3): 51-62.

Psacharopoulos, G., J.P. Tan, and E. Jimenez. 1986. *Financing Education in Developing Countries*. Washington, DC: The World Bank.

Schultz, P.T. 1987. "School expenditures and enrollments, 1960-1980." In D.G Johnson and R. Lee, eds. National Academy of Sciences background papers. *Population Growth and Economic Development*. Madison, WI: University of Wisconsin Press.

Sen, A. 1987. "Food and freedom." The Third Sir John Crawford Memorial Lecture, World Bank, Washington, DC, October 29.

van der Heijden, H. 1988. "The self-financing of NGO's in human resources development." Unpublished paper prepared for The Rockefeller Foundation. Seillans, France, as background for this chapter.

Verspoor, A. 1989. "Pathways to change: Improving the quality of education in developing countries." World Bank Discussion Paper 53. Washington, DC

Vogel, R.T. 1988. "Cost recovery in the health care sector." World Bank Technical Paper No. 82. Washington, DC

Walsh, J.A., and K.S., Warren. 1979. "Selective primary health care: An interim strategy for disease control in developing countries." *New England Journal of Medicine*, 301: 967-974.

Weisbrod, B. A. 1988a. "The role of government in the provision of social services in the developing countries." Unpublished paper prepared for The Rockefeller Foundation. University of Wisconsin.

Weisbrod, B.A. 1988b. *The Nonprofit Economy*. Cambridge, MA: Harvard University Press.

World Bank. 1988a. *Brazil: Public Spending on Social Programs: Issues and Options*. Washington, DC: World Bank.

World Bank. 1988b. *Education in Sub-Saharan Africa*. Washington, DC: World Bank.

World Bank. 1988c. *World Development Report*. New York: Oxford University Press.

World Bank. 1992. *Zimbabwe: Financing Health Services*. A World Bank Country Study. Washington, DC

15

The Political Economy of Health Transitions in the Third World

Michael R. Reich

The health transition, according to some social scientists, can best be understood as a social or behavioral phenomenon (Caldwell 1990; Findley 1990). They have argued that the key determinants of shifting patterns of mortality are found in the behaviors and values of society. It seems unlikely, however, that the transformations in mortality and morbidity now underway in poor countries can be reduced to theories that focus solely on bringing people to technology, changing individual behaviors, or altering social values. These societies are now undergoing complex social changes, including processes of commercialization, medicalization, and internationalization. These processes, all shaped by the distribution of political and economic resources, are affecting developments in health.

The resulting transitions are not necessarily in healthy directions for all social groups. New social risks — including environmental hazards, factory production processes, and traffic accidents — create new patterns of morbidity and mortality. As Julio Frenk and his colleagues have argued, the health transition (at least in some countries) is not unidirectional, does not follow clearly separated stages, and produces a maldistribution of health among population groups — resulting in what they call a "protracted and polarized" transition (Frenk et al. 1991) (See also this volume). An explanation of such health transitions in poor countries needs to consider the distribution of political and economic resources at both the national and international levels. This chapter's central point, in short, is that an analysis of political economy is essential to understanding health transitions in the Third World.

The approach of political economy covers many forms of analysis, including both Marxist and non-Marxist varieties.[1] In general, this perspective seeks to identify systematic relationships between economic and political processes and the resulting impact on the distribution of resources within a particular community (local, national, or global). The approach can be used to explain political and economic phenomena (such as powerlessness or poverty) as well as other conditions (such as poor health or illiteracy). Different forms of political economy give precedence to economic or political factors as primary determinants.[2] Some forms stress how power and political principles influence the behavior of markets: for example, how structure of the state affects national economic success or failure. Other forms emphasize how economic principles explain political actions: for example, how governmental decisions on policy result from rational economic calculations. The 1970s and 1980s witnessed a distinct analytic turn in the direction of political economy for the study of rich countries (Lange and Meadwell 1985) and poor countries (Chilcote 1985) and for the processes of development (Bates 1988b).

In the study of Third World health conditions, the approach of political economy has lagged behind the subdiscipline of health economics. The technocratic appeal of economic techniques, such as cost-benefit analysis and cost-effectiveness analysis, makes health economics appear desirable to governments, corporations, and international agencies. The practical problems of pricing health services, for both public and private institutions, are assisted by economic models that estimate the likely financial consequences of different decisions. By contrast, the analyses of political economy can raise uncomfortable questions for those who sit in the seats of public and private power. This inherent tension with established institutions may be one reason for the relative underdevelopment of health political economy in comparison with health economics. While health economics helps define what and how much should be allocated for health problems, political economy helps explain why a particular allocation occurred and why the actual distribution diverged from the predicted one.

Despite these difficulties, a growing number of studies are appearing on the political economy of health in the Third World (and a substantial literature exists on the political economy of health for the United States[3]). Critical analyses have been done of the health consequences of capitalist expansion in the Third World (Doyal and Pennell 1979; Elling 1981) and of the role of international agencies in advancing those processes (Navarro 1984). Case studies have analyzed the impact of political economy on health transitions in particular countries, such as India (Jeffrey 1988) and China (Sidel and Sidel 1973; Chen 1988). Studies of specific technologies and products have shown how political and economic forces, both domestic and international, shape the interaction of society and technology in producing good (and bad) health consequences in the Third World; these products include tobacco (Barry 1991), pharmaceuticals (Gereffi 1978; Lall and Bibile 1978; Reich 1987), and infant formula (Sethi et al. 1986). Analysts have also addressed the international transfer of specific organizational forms, such as for-profit hospitals operated by private multinational corporations, and the probable effects on health policy and access to health services in poor countries (Berliner and Regan 1987; Roemer 1987).

These studies on the political economy of health transitions in the Third World have implicitly or explicitly adopted one of two broad normative approaches. The first stresses the positive role of government intervention, and the second emphasizes the importance of market forces.[4] These two approaches reflect a broader intellectual division in political economy (Lindblom 1977), what Charles Wolf (1988) called the choice between the "imperfect alternatives" of governments or markets. Although advocates of these two approaches to good health do not always portray themselves in tension, they in fact pull in quite opposite directions. This lack of self-awareness is due in part to a deficiency in the political analysis of health systems. In this chapter, I use political analysis to critically review these two approaches and to identify problems with each perspective. I also argue that political analysis is essential to an understanding of health policy making and to efforts that seek to shape health transitions in the Third World.

The government intervention school advocates activist health policy to achieve advances in health conditions in poor countries. According to this school, government intervention is necessary to correct the market's allocation of health resources, biased toward the more powerful and wealthy groups in society, through technology selection, geographic location, and access criteria. Some members of this school propose that a government with the proper commitment, with "political will," can achieve good health for the entire population. For example, a conference sponsored by the Rockefeller Foundation in 1985 on "good health at low cost" (Halstead et al. 1985) concluded that "a sustained political commitment to universal health and well-being" was the major factor responsible for health success in countries with low per capita incomes

("Summary Statement" 1985). These findings were summarized as involving largely top-down "political will" in the case of China and primarily bottom-up "political and social will" in the cases of Kerala (India), Sri Lanka, and Costa Rica (Warren 1985). In this view, political will produces good government, which in turn produces good health.

The market forces school rejects the government intervention approach as inefficient, ineffective, and outdated. Good health in poor countries results from letting the market do its job; "good government" means minimal intervention, acting only when necessary. This view in support of privatization has been espoused by the World Bank (1988:48-52) and USAID (1989:47-59), and stated in a purist form by those opposing any regulation of industry (Starrels 1985). Elements of this approach have been advocated by economist Nancy Birdsall (1989) in her call for "good government and good health." The market forces approach sees inadequate performance as widespread and inherent in the nature of the public sector. Drawing on the broader views of public choice theory (Buchanan 1985), this school believes that public officials invariably serve their own personal interests more than the broader public interests. The solution to health problems in poor countries, therefore, must rely on private-sector initiatives, such as user fees and the private provision of services, and on turning things over to market forces.

Both schools, however, suffer from serious problems. Simply stated, the first sees the market as the problem and government as the solution, while the second sees government as the problem and the market as the solution. Both approaches oversimplify. Advocates present selective evidence to support their arguments. And proponents on both sides tend to ignore basic political realities that would undermine effective implementation of their ideas. Critical political analysis of the two approaches can illuminate these weaknesses and help us understand the imperfections of both governments and markets. And, as suggested in the conclusion, political analysis also points toward a third approach in the analysis of the political economy of health transitions, an approach that emphasizes nongovernmental and nonmarket organizations and recognizes political processes as integral to positive health transitions.

Government Intervention

The school of government intervention holds that health improvements can be achieved in poor countries most effectively through an administrative allocation of resources, with particular attention to the more vulnerable groups in society. This distribution might be carried out through the direct delivery of services, through government-owned and operated facilities or through other means (such as national health insurance) to assure adequate access to affordable health resources. The strategy is based on the assumptions that governments possess the knowledge and capability to improve health conditions in society and that market imperfections require government intervention. In many countries, the constitution specifies health as a basic right and mandates government action to provide and protect this right. The simplest version of this argument states that government intervention improves health in poor countries when there exists "political will." In short, if national leaders only exercised their political will, then health transitions would occur in a positive direction. This formulation, however, has multiple problems.

The Concept of Political Will: At a broad level of generality, the call for political will strikes a chord of common sense. What self-respecting public health professional would disagree with the need for political leaders to be committed to good health? — especially if commitment means increased budgetary allocations to the health sector. But what does political will really mean as a necessary condition to get good health at low cost? And which political conditions produce the "will" that leads to good (or at least better) health in poor countries? Is political will the same regardless of regime type? What role does ideology play in the adoption of political commitment to equity and good health? Are some forms of the state more likely to produce good health than others? The invocation of "political will" rarely provides answers to such questions.

But the conceptual ambiguity of political will has not stopped its use. The phrase appears frequently as an "op-ed" concept, often in articles opposite the editorial page in newspapers and with little systematic explanation. One example was the call for new public policies that could solve the problems of homelessness: "We know what needs to be done; what is lacking is the political will to do it" (Swanstrom 1989). The "failure of political will" has also been noted, in passing, as a reason for government's not implementing public policies on the export of hazardous substances (Jasanoff 1985:143). Others have called for making political will "more than a slogan," as did the authors of a study of antipoverty policies in the Third World (Lewis et al. 1988:25). Clear definitions of political will, however, are difficult to find. More commonly, the flag of political will is waved along with a tone of moral exhortation.

While the notion of political will may seem intuitively obvious to some observers, others have criticized it as an analytic concept. Lynn M. Morgan (1989) argued that efforts to explain Costa Rica's experience with primary health care, through the concept of political will, end up being misguided, superficial, and unhelpful. She questioned whether political will ever existed in Costa Rica and showed how use of that phrase has masked both domestic and international political processes. Along similar lines, Paul B. Vitta attacked the notion that African countries "simply" need political will in order to enact effective technology policies, "as though all it requires is the pure act of a polity changing its 'mind' from one state to another" (n.d.). More generally, Pranab Bardhan noted that chronic failures of policy implementation in the Third World are often ascribed to "a lack of 'political will' (whatever that means) or a lack of 'social discipline'" (1988:66). Other analysts have similarly criticized the pattern of blaming failure of policy implementation on a lack of political will. Merilee S. Grindle and John W. Thomas, for example, consider the term a "catch-all culprit" that has "little analytic content," adding that "its very vagueness expresses the lack of knowledge of specific detail" (1991:122-124).

Yet political will remains an attractive phrase. The conference sponsored by the Rockefeller Foundation in 1985 on "good health at low cost" successfully established the concept of "political and social will" as a necessary element in efforts by poor countries to improve their health conditions. The conference publication has become a basic reference in discussions of the health transition, and the conclusive phrase on "will" has percolated into international discourse. For instance, a report on health research strategy for the World Health Organization used the felicitous Rockefeller phrase without citing its source. While noting problems of incomplete conclusions, the WHO report stated that "in a Third World country which seeks to progress rapidly, an essential requirement, and in a sense the starting point, is the political and social will to bring about improvement" (WHO 1988:5).

Papers in the Rockefeller volume suggested two ways to operationalize the concept of political will. One operational indicator might be government legislation for social welfare. Patricia Rosenfield used "historical commitment to health as a social goal" as an indicator of political will. She assessed this factor by determining whether there existed early legislation, early government welfare policy, early medical systems, or Christian missionary influences. But it is unclear which aspect is most important: the historical length of the commitment (how long ago or how early in the development process legislation was adopted) or the intensity of the commitment (the degree of implementation or the level of resources invested in the program). Moreover, governments might exhibit an historical commitment to health, but without producing good or better health. Perhaps historical commitment represents a necessary but not sufficient condition.

Another way to operationalize the concept might be through an analysis of per capita health expenditure. Countries with comparatively high expenditure would be considered to show relatively high levels of political will. In his essay in the Rockefeller volume, Dean Jamison demonstrated that China came out with 25 percent above its expected per capita health expenditure for its GDP, in a comparison with 19 countries in 1975 with per capita GDP under $2,000 (Jamison 1985:31-32). China's higher than expected health expenditure, for its level of per capita income, could be interpreted as reflecting a greater than normal degree of political will. This finding, however, creates some problems for the Rockefeller volume's main theme of "low cost."

Indeed, "good health at low cost" may be the wrong phrase, since the three other cases in the Rockefeller volume also showed comparatively high government expenditure on health (Joseph 1985:226). The critical question may be how to maximize public and private expenditures on health despite extremely limited resources due to poverty. Perhaps the volume should have been titled "good health despite extreme poverty," or the phrase used in Costa Rica, "health without wealth" (Morgan 1989). In conditions of extreme poverty, the allocation of scarce government funds to health compared to other sectors could provide an indication of political will. This concept of a discrete government decision to do *x* rather than *y* fits well with conventional political analysis. One problem, however, is that a government decision to invest in health facilities rather than road construction, for example, could be interpreted by transportation advocates as illustrating a lack of political will.

Neither of these two approaches to political will is particularly persuasive. In the Rockefeller volume, the conceptual ambiguity of "political will," as with "low cost," may result partly from the format. Conference publications often suffer from uneven analysis. The Rockefeller volume lacked an introductory essay to pull together the individual efforts and critically reflect on the concepts and contributions. Although a central answer to the conference question (when does a society obtain good health at low cost?) focused on political commitment, the volume included little systematic analysis of political factors. Even at the end of the volume, the causal chain between political will and health outcomes remained cloudy. To be analytically useful, the concept of political will requires at least a clear definition.

Davidson R. Gwatkin (1979) used the concept of political will with more analytic care to explain India's aggressive pursuit of family planning in 1976. He employed the concept to mean that leaders, in pursuit of their goals, introduce incentives and sanctions to change the political costs and benefits associated with specific policies for lower-level political officials and civil servants. Gwatkin showed how the "application of political will" to family planning, as previously advocated by critics of the government in this area, produced coercion and chaos (1979:31). But his analysis tended to stress policy goals more than political goals; he understated the extent to which India's focus on family planning in 1976-77 belonged to Sanjay Gandhi's political strategy to extend personal and party power. Raising the political costs and benefits of implementing family planning achieved the policy objectives in some regions, but it also created a huge reservoir of opposition that contributed to Mrs. Gandhi's electoral defeat in 1977. The focus on family planning failed not only because it neglected other development measures and "the larger end of human well-being" (1979:51), but also because it miscalculated the political costs and benefits.

The lack of specificity for the concept of political will could be precisely its source of popularity. Politicians and journalists may think in terms of "political will" and find it a convenient slogan for criticism of opponents. But a phrase from public discourse does not necessarily produce a concept with analytic power. A better approach to assessing when government intervention is likely to occur and succeed would be to draw from a political economy model and apply a form of political cost/benefit analysis (Majone 1975). This approach would stress political feasibility rather than political will (May 1986). As discussed below, the value of this analysis would depend on an appropriate selection of cases, a full assessment of trade-offs, an analysis of political regime character-istics, and an understanding of the dominant political and economic interests.

Selection of Cases: Comparative analysis of public policy requires care in the selection of cases and the justification of choices (Przeworski and Teune 1970). A comparative study without an adequate explanation of how the cases were chosen should be treated with caution, as should any conclusions from the study.

The selection of the four case studies in the Rockefeller volume presumably resulted from an assessment of societies that have achieved good health at low cost. Yet nowhere does the volume provide a coherent justification for this four-some. Two sentences in the editors' preface address the process of selection: "In absolute dollar expenditures, the health gains of China, Kerala State, Sri Lanka and Costa Rica were achieved at relatively modest cost. Each of the success stories described has evolved, with one exception, in countries with unusually low gross domestic product per capita" (Halstead et al. 1985:5). This brief mention begs three questions.

First, what about other similar cases? One left-out case is Cuba, which has per capita income midway between Sri Lanka and Costa Rica, with similar life expectancy of over 70 years at birth (Jamison 1985:22). The conference apparently included Cuba in its initial program but then dropped the case before the meeting. Yet no explanation for Cuba's exclusion appears in the volume. The case of Cuba could have provided an important perspective on the political processes of allocating scarce resources to the health sector and the anticipated political benefits in the domestic and international spheres.

Cuba's concerted strategy to become a "world medical power," in the words of Fidel Castro, has generated both material and symbolic benefits (Feinsilver 1989). While not among the world's leaders in biomedical research, Cuba has achieved health indicators similar to those of rich countries and has provided substantial medical assistance and services to other nations, especially in Africa. According to one assessment, these activities have created "legitimacy, prestige, and influence" for Cuba in both domestic and international spheres (Feinsilver 1989:26). The case of Cuba demonstrates that health can be considered not only as an end in itself but also as a means to other political and economic goals.

Another unanswered question is the inclusion of Kerala State among the case studies. Kerala's fame as an overachiever in health within India deserves recognition. But are the conclusions of analysis at the subnational level of government applicable in other contexts for national governments? For example, is political commitment at a subnational level the same as that at a national level? Also, do similar overachieving regions (with distinctive political traditions as found in Kerala) exist in other large and complex poor countries, like China?

One paper in the Rockefeller volume on Kerala State did follow appropriate principles of comparison by focusing on two subnational governments. Moni Nag (1985) compared the impact of social and economic development on mortality in Kerala with that in West Bengal. These two Indian states have similar standards of living and share an emphasis on education and a leftist political orientation, but have diverged historically in their mortality rates. A subsequent study by Nag (1989) pursued these differences for the two states and concluded that Kerala had stronger sociopolitical movements in rural areas and had political parties more oriented toward rural mobilization. These factors gave rise to rural Kerala's greater political awareness, which contributed to more health facilities and their better utilization in rural Kerala than in West Bengal. In his concluding paragraph, Nag noted that his conclusions at the subnational level supported the findings of another analyst on political processes at the national level in developing countries. While not addressing the differences directly, Nag seemed to recognize that such generalization took him out on an analytical limb.

A third issue not addressed in the Rockefeller volume was the strategy of analysis implicit in the selection of cases. One might learn just as much from a comparative analysis of cases of poor health at high cost. Consideration of several countries with high per capita incomes but poor health performances (such as some oil-rich nations) might help illuminate the nature of political commitment in different national contexts. Exploring government failures could help explain the limits of government expenditure in improving health conditions, especially how the strategies and efficiencies of health expenditures relate to political benefits. This analysis could also provide a more critical view of calls for political will.

Trade-offs: Intervention by governments to improve health can also have trade-offs, with both political and economic consequences. The advocates of government intervention rarely address the potential trade-offs of specific public programs or of broader social changes toward greater equity. A reallocation of resources to improve the health conditions of one group can impose economic as well as political costs on other parts of society. That reallocation can occur across ethnic, class, or geographic lines. Deciding whether those trade-offs are justified depends on a broader vision of social justice. Knowing a society's limits in tolerating increased costs for particular groups requires a good understanding of political economy.

The economic trade-offs of government interventions to reallocate resources to improve health take many forms. Government efforts to improve equity may be accompanied by losses in efficiency. The allocation of resources to primary health care, for example, could improve the access of poor people to health facilities, but at the same time could reduce overall productivity, especially if the supply system is unable to provide rural health workers with adequate materials. The efficiency losses of government interventions in the market and the problems of implementation are well portrayed by the advocates of market forces (as discussed below). But advocates of government intervention tend to underestimate possible contributions of the market in allocating resources to improve health (Reich 1987).

Economic trade-offs also arise in the reallocation of resources from the hospital sector to primary health care and from urban to rural sectors, which are considered key elements in achieving good health in poor countries (Segall 1983). In most poor countries, the bias in development favors the urban sector, through policies on agricultural and food prices, food subsidies, and foreign exchange and trade (Lipton 1977). Reversing this urban flow of resources would impose increased costs on urban residents, for example, through higher food prices, or in the health sector, through higher costs or reduced availability of health services. W. Henry Mosley concluded, "This gets back to a political commitment to equity" (1985:244). While true, the statement does not help us understand when that political commitment can be implemented, or what kind of political regime can withstand the pressures of the economic trade-offs imposed on the urban sector.

The case of China poses the issues of political trade-offs. China's health advances have depended on a strategy of mass mobilization in national campaigns that were centrally initiated and organized. From the 1950s through the 1980s, China averaged four or five health campaigns a year (Jamison 1985:26). To an important degree, this strategy belongs to China's post-1949 authoritarian state with its emphasis on central control and mass mobilization. In short, the improvements in national health may have depended on the limitations in political liberty (and their costs for certain groups in the population). The national campaigns of mass mobilization for health improvement bear striking and troubling resemblance to the destructive campaigns of the Cultural Revolution. The effectiveness of China's health campaigns may have required the repressive national political economy. If so, could political and economic liberalization in China contribute to a slowdown in health advances? More broadly, to what extent are health improvements and democracy incompatible in China?

Political commitment to equity thus is not costless. The reallocation of social resources through revolutionary processes, in particular, can impose substantial costs in the restriction of personal freedoms and the loss of lives. Yet analyses of China's health achievements rarely consider the health costs of social revolution or else mention them only briefly in passing (Chen 1988:297). The experiences of the Soviet Union, with its history of gulags, illustrate similar problems, although the costs imposed in that country are more readily admitted and the health achievements are not held up today as an international model for replication.

Finally, an ideological commitment to equity may be a necessary component for government intervention to improve health (Caldwell 1986; Reich 1988b), but it rarely is sufficient. The Soviet Union provides a striking example of how political commitment to social equity through government intervention in health can fall short of the original ideals and hopes for socialized medicine. The mortality increases and quality problems in the Soviet health system are well recognized today (Davis and Feshbach 1980; Eberstadt 1988:11-33). As Mark G. Field (1990) observed, the Soviet health system illustrates how noble purpose combined with flawed execution to produce mixed results. Elsewhere as well, recommendations for government intervention and political commitment, which ignore the vast obstacles to implementation and the potential problems of centralized control, are unlikely to achieve the desired results.

The Nature of Political Regimes: Political scientists have compared regimes for quite some time in efforts to determine whether one type is "better" than others for social welfare. Studies in the 1960s and 1970s sought to relate regime characteristics, such as civil versus military, to differences in public policy or economic performance. The analyses generally concluded that other variables (such as socioeconomic factors) provided greater explanatory power (Bossert 1983). Since the late 1970s, however, studies have moved beyond the simple distinction between civil and military regimes to find more complex sources of variations in political regimes that affect the adoption and implementation of public policies in the Third World (Stepan 1978; Cleaves 1980).

The impact of regime type on health remains relatively unexplored. One analysis of the causes of sickness and well-being for nations ignored regime type almost completely (Sagan 1987). In the Rockefeller volume, only Patricia L. Rosenfield (1985) attempted a direct comparison of political regimes. She noted that the "political economic orientations vary both between the examples and over time within each situation." In conclusion, she stated, "On the basis of these four examples, no single political or economic approach can claim greater facility in creating conditions conducive to the improvement of health" (Rosenfield 1985:175). More concerted analysis of political regimes is needed to improve our understanding of government intervention.

Thomas John Bossert has analyzed the impact of regime characteristics on health policy as the dependent variable (rather than on health outcomes as done in the Rockefeller volume). He examined the adoption and implementation of primary health care policies in four Central American countries (Guatemala, Honduras, Costa Rica, and Nicaragua), and considered regime characteristics along four dimensions: strength of the state, stability, ideology, and democracy. Bossert explained the logic of relating these four dimensions to primary health care policy in the following hypotheses (1983:426):

> Strong regimes will have the capacity to adopt and fund innovative health programs because they will be able to extract sufficient resources and distribute those resources to nondominant sectors of society. Stable regimes will be most able to implement these policies because they allow more continuity in the bureaucracy. Progressive regimes will pursue more social welfare policies. Democratic regimes will give more voice to lower class beneficiaries and therefore be more responsive to their demands.

Bossert's study did not find any simple relationships between one dimension of regime characteristics and the adoption of primary health care policies. Both stable (Costa Rica) and unstable (Guatemala and Honduras) regimes adopted the policy, as did reformist (Costa Rica and Sandinista Nicaragua) and status quo (Guatemala and Honduras) regimes. But he did identify several complex "contingent" relationships among the variables (1983:426). Status quo regimes that are threatened with instability have a greater incentive to adopt these policies, as an effort to coopt potential rural support to opposition. "In a status quo regime, instability may be an incentive to adopt minor reforms. The status quo regime that was unstable — Guatemala — was one of the first in the world to adopt the reforms" (1983:436). Without that threat, stable regimes (like pre-1975 Somoza Nicaragua) have little incentive to adopt such reforms.

Bossert reached similarly complex conclusions about implementation, although single dimensions of regime characteristics tended to show greater influence on these processes. Weak and unstable regimes (Honduras and Guatemala) showed a lack of centralization and integration, two important variables for successful implementation, in contrast to the strong and stable regime of Costa Rica. Bossert suggested that weak and unstable regimes may not design policies that can be effectively implemented because of the potential threat that a successful program would pose to political and economic elites. Moreover, when weak states do design primary health care policies they are more likely to depend on foreign funding (such as Guatemala), in contrast to strong states (Costa Rica) that can allocate national resources to rural areas.

Bossert's overall conclusion stressed the importance of regime analysis. "At the very least, this study suggests that advocates of policy changes take into account regime characteristics when they design strategies for the adoption and the implementation of preferred policies" (1983:438). The nature of the political regime will affect the public policies for health, and thereby (presumably) will influence health outcomes. Bossert's analysis also suggests that in addition to the regime, one must also understand the role of political and economic interests in society.

The Role of Interests: Appeals for government intervention in health and for political commitment to equity often approach these as disinterested concepts and normative values, to be accomplished for humanitarian goals. Only rarely do the appeals recognize that politics is not simply a residual variable in public health but a primary determinant of who gets what, and thereby has a major impact on health status. W. Henry Mosley acknowledged the distributional consequences of political and economic interests when he commented, "The real question is not 'What is the cost?' but, rather, 'Who pays and who benefits?'" (1985:244). Improving the health of the majority in a poor country probably involves an income transfer of one sort or another, which affects the distribution of resources in society. The organization of interests in that particular society will influence the adoption and implementation of policies, as well as the ultimate health outcomes.

Compared to the field of health policy, the study of agricultural policy in poor countries has achieved a greater understanding of the role of interests in shaping government intervention. Robert H. Bates argued persuasively that the stated social objectives of governments do not adequately explain the particular forms that agricultural policy takes in the Third World (Bates 1988a). The dominant pattern of agricultural policy, in Africa as in other poor countries, does not favor the majority of producers. Government objectives to increase food supplies, to strengthen incentives for food production, to increase output, and to meet shortages are systematically translated into policies that fail and that tend to impose costs on most agricultural producers. Bates concluded (1988a:345):

> The policy instruments chosen to secure social objectives are...often inconsistent with the attainment of these objectives. And yet the choices of governments are clearly stable; despite undermining their own goals, governments continue to employ these policy instruments. Some kind of explanation is required, but one based on factors other than the social objectives of government.

In short, the notion of governments as "agents of the public interest" cannot explain choices of policy. Bates offered two alternative political explanations.

The first alternative views governments as agents of private interests. Here, public policy results from the pressures of organized interest groups, reflecting an established approach in political analysis. For agricultural policy, governments in poor countries tend to make pricing decisions that benefit urban consumers rather than rural producers, because urban residents often constitute an important political constituency and tend to be better organized and more powerful. Higher food prices can squeeze wages and profits, compelling both workers and employers to pressure governments for price reductions. And small-scale farmers, more often than not, bear the costs of lowered food prices for urban consumers (Bates 1988a:345-351). Small-scale farmers can assert their interests and oppose the urban bias of agricultural policy by influencing national leaders through two methods: organization of pressure groups and participation in competitive elections.[5]

The second alternative proposed by Bates views governments as agencies that seek to retain power. Governments design policies and programs to secure control over the majority of the population and thereby to remain in power. Bates argues that this approach helps explain how African governments can "get away" with policies that adversely affect the interests of most farmers (1988a:351-356). Governments use agricultural policies to organize a rural constituency and to disorganize the rural opposition, through the allocation of investments, jobs and projects as forms of political patronage. In short, "public officials are frequently less concerned with using public resources in a way that is economically efficient than they are with using them in a way that is politically expedient" (Bates 1988a:352). In both organizing a rural constituency and discouraging a rural opposition, governments use regulated markets for political purposes in order to maintain social control and retain governmental power.

The political analysis of agricultural policy in poor countries has direct relevance for health policy. More analysis is needed of the political determinants of health policy in poor countries, especially the influence of private interests on government intervention in health and the government's use of public health resources to protect its access to power.

The analysis of governments as agents of private interests appeared in several chapters of the Rockefeller volume. For example, the historical strength of competitive political processes in Sri Lanka (Gunatilleke 1985:122) and Costa Rica (Rosero-Bixby 1985:126-127) contributed to a redistribution of political power to the rural poor, giving them greater voice in the allocation of health resources. But the volume gave little indication of how these four societies dealt with the most powerful organized interest group in health: physicians. Many analyses of health policy discuss conflicts between the interests of physicians and urban consumers who want high-technology medical care and the interests of rural residents and government officials who favor primary health care (Segall 1983). It would be instructive to know how the four cases of the Rockefeller volume resolved this fundamental conflict in the distribution of medical resources.

But few studies exist on how interest groups, such as physician associations, have influenced specific health policies in the Third World, as has been done, for example, in Britain (Eckstein 1960) and in Japan (Steslicke 1973). One observer of the Indian Medical Association concluded, however, that the group "has not been notably successful in attempting to protect its narrow interests or otherwise to influence policy" (Jeffrey 1988:167). Understanding whether this pattern fits other Third World countries, and the conditions under which physicians exert substantial influence on policy, represents an important area of inquiry. Julio Frenk and Avedis Donabedian have suggested a useful model for thinking about the influence of physician associations on health policy (1987:28-29); their ideas could be developed and applied in several settings to examine the mobilization of interest groups that shape health policy in the Third World countries.

Several studies exist of interventions in health designed to retain power for government organizations. China's emphasis on the mass mobilization of a rural constituency through public health campaigns provided a mechanism that both organized support and disorganized opposition for the government. Similarly, Kerala's emphasis on the rights of the rural poor resulted from a strategic emphasis of government, social movements, and leftist political parties to organize those interests as their key constituents (Nag 1985:58, 70-71; Nag 1989). Additional research is needed to address the political benefits to Third World governments from interventions in health.

Analysis of the political economy of "targeting" health and nutrition programs could improve our understanding of when these efforts succeed at helping relatively powerless groups in society. Advocates of targeting tend to focus on the technocratic aspects of policy design and understate the political difficulties of policy implementation. One recent review concluded, "Targeting social spending to the poor is a bright idea that seems so attractive and sensible that it should take the world by storm. Why would a government *not* want to target its income subsidies to people who need them most?" (Pfeffermann and Griffin 1989:23). The authors answered their own question earlier, by recognizing the political roots of income and consumption subsidies, which "are often distributed so as to secure patronage, votes, or clients rather than assist the poor, who rarely have political clout" (1989:3). They decided, nonetheless, to give only "passing reference" to the political forces that shape the design and implementation of subsidies. More explicit analysis of these forces is needed to explain who benefits and who pays for subsidies.

The use of highly regulated health markets by governments to reward private interests and to retain or gain political power represents another critical area for research. Governments have liberalized pharmaceutical policy, for example, to meet the demands of both domestic and international private companies, as occurred in Sri Lanka following the change in political parties in power in 1977 (Lall and Bibile 1978). And some governments, such as Bangladesh, have been accused of introducing restrictive pharmaceutical policies based on the concept of essential drugs, in order to serve the economic interests of individuals rather than the health needs of the public (Jayasuriya 1985). Overall, much more could be done to analyze the role of interests in shaping and changing government policy on health in poor countries and in producing better (and worse) health outcomes.

Market Forces

Advocates of market forces to improve health conditions in poor countries encounter many of the same problems shown by the proponents of government intervention. Those who call for the market as the solution rarely provide cogent political analysis. They often reduce their recommendations to the familiar neo-classical refrain of using a competitive market to solve the problems of public services. Indeed, they view government intervention and political processes as the sources of social costs that subvert and distort development in Third World countries (Lal 1983). Overall, this school underestimates the problems of the market and overestimates the problems of government, while neglecting the role of politics on both scores. Political analysis of market forces to improve health conditions in poor countries needs to begin with a concept of the role of the state in economic and social development, and then proceed to examine the selection of cases, the trade-offs of markets, and the role of interests.

The Concept of the State: A tendency exists among some market advocates to view the state as equivalent to the government or the public sector, or at least not to distinguish these as separate concepts. General problems of public administration in the Third World are then extrapolated to the state, leading to the conclusion that market forces must be unleashed. These concepts, however, are not one and the same. The term "government" usually refers to the official agencies directly concerned with the tasks of governance at the central and decentralized levels, while the "public sector" includes these plus a broader range of institutions, particularly autonomous state-owned enterprises (Mamalakis 1989:1045).

The concept of the state among contemporary social scientists is strongly influenced by the work of Max Weber, who viewed the state as the institutions that assert control over specific territories and the people within them. Following a Weberian perspective, Alfred Stepan (1978:xii) provided this description:

> The state must be considered as more than the "government." It is the continuous administrative, legal, bureaucratic and coercive systems that attempt not only to structure relationships *between* civil society and public authority in a polity but also to structure many crucial relationships within civil society as well.

A narrow concept of the state, as somehow equivalent to government or the public sector, deprives this approach of its analytic power.

Political economy in the 1970s and 1980s emphasized "bringing the state back in," a major shift away from social science in the previous two decades that stressed pluralist perspectives and structural-functionalism (Evans et al. 1985). Social theorists of the state have sought to explain the state's efforts to pursue goals independent of specific social groups and the state's capacity to achieve those goals despite actual or potential opposition (Skocpol 1985:9). They have employed cross-national and historical analysis to examine why some states are more successful than others in achieving their objectives and why specific states are more capable of intervening in one socioeconomic area compared to another.

The central question for Third World states, in the view of Joel S. Migdal (1988), is explaining their striking duality: "their unmistakable strengths in penetrating societies and their surprising weaknesses in effecting goal-oriented social changes" (1988:9). According to Migdal, conflicts inevitably arise between the state and other social organizations over who has the right and ability to make and enforce binding rules. Simply put, Migdal concluded that weak states and their failures in policy implementation result from strong societies with strong systems of control based in other social organizations that keep the state out. Only after massive social dislocations, often accompanied by war and revolution, have strong states emerged that can challenge previous systems of social control and thereby effectively implement social policies (1988:269). In most Third World countries, however, strong societies compel state leaders to employ the "politics of survival" to assure that state agencies do not become too aligned with social organizations and thereby undermine the leaders' power (1988:209). To protect their power, political leaders undermine the effectiveness of the agencies intended to carry out social policies.

Migdal's analysis suggests that strategies designed to strengthen the market and weaken the state are likely to have counterproductive results. In producing good health, the capacity to intervene effectively in society may be more important than the maintenance of competitive markets. A similar argument has been made about the role of the strong "developmental" state in producing a healthy economy, especially for Japan and the newly industrializing countries of East Asia (Johnson 1981; Johnson 1987). In this view, strong political institutions of the state are necessary to control distributive politics (the efforts by groups to advance their own interests instead of collective welfare) and bureaucratic politics (the organizational rivalry and fragmentation that can obstruct decision making and implementation) (Haggard and Moon 1990). Strong states, however, also have political and economic costs, as noted earlier in the discussion of the trade-offs of government intervention. In considering health improvements associated with the market forces approach, one must also ask whether this strategy is expected to work in all countries, regardless of the state of the state.

Selection of Cases: While the advocates of government intervention have used specific cases to argue their approach to good health, the advocates of "market oriented" policies have not provided a selection of countries in which their proposals would yield better health outcomes. The latter argument implies that market forces should be applied and should succeed in all states, regardless of the particular institutions, values, histories, or power structures. One could ask, however, whether market oriented approaches would have been more effective or appropriate in those countries where government intervention is considered to have played a major role in mortality declines and health improvements. Specifically, for the four governments in the Rockefeller volume: Why were these governments more effective than others in producing good health? Should their methods of government intervention be applied in other countries or subnational entities? Would market oriented approaches have been as effective in producing good health?

Birdsall, in her article on "good health and good government," unfortunately did not directly address these questions and sometimes offered a confusing message. On the one hand, she approvingly cited the Rockefeller volume as demonstrating that government delivery of personal health services "has clearly contributed to the high levels of life expectancy" in the volume's four case studies (1989:95-96). On the other hand, she seemed to question the conclusions of the Rockefeller volume (and her own prior statement) by referring to the "*apparent* success of governments in the developing world in bringing about major declines in mortality" (my emphasis) (1989:96).

The explanation of "apparent success," however, remained ambiguous. In which states was the success of government more apparent than real? Birdsall argued that government intervention worked "in the past" when new health technologies could be introduced without requiring changes in individual behavior. (Importantly, the Rockefeller volume did not reach this technology-based conclusion.) But she did not specify which states are likely to achieve the "future potential" of state involvement. Nor did she indicate which states are likely to deal better with the problems that undermine the effectiveness of government efforts to produce good health: the diminishing returns of health technology, the difficulties of altering individual behavior, the fiscal pressures of growing deficits, and the changing demographic and epidemiologic patterns.

Birdsall divided states into those with "good" governments and those with "bad" governments, and then suggested that the fundamental problem is "the advent of 'bad' government" (1989:106-107). She described bad government as involving "bloated public sectors with substantial internal and external debt," plus problems of increasingly ineffective, inefficient, and inequitable performance. The article, however, provided no persuasive evidence that Third World governments today are substantially worse than those of the 1950s to the 1970s. The murky standard for measuring "good" and "bad" government makes evaluation difficult. In addition, trade-offs exist among the goals of government; for example, in the health sector, pockets of effective performance may result in an inequitable distribution of services. Finally, most of Birdsall's reported problems of "bad" government did not refer to specific countries and seem simply to be politics as usual. What is economically irrational often is perceived as politically essential.

Migdal's categories of strong and weak states, on the other hand, provide some help in discriminating among countries and explaining the problems of implementation. Migdal concluded that strong states, capable of effective implementation, emerge only rarely in the world, when the right confluence of highly disruptive domestic and international political circumstances occurs. He also concluded that weak states rarely can improve policy performance, except under special conditions. Those conditions involve countervailing forces at the regional level to assure that the implementors of policy act responsibly or face sanctions. Migdal held out little hope for the current vogue of solutions: "New policies, management techniques, administrative tinkerings, more committed bureaucrats are all inadequate to change the structural relations between weak states and strong societies" (1988:277). One doubts he would consider a call for good government as likely to be effective in producing good health.

Trade-offs of Markets: In contrast to the advocates of government intervention, who usually ignore the trade-offs of administrative action, the proponents of market forces see mainly the trade-offs of government efforts. Birdsall characterized these two worldviews as the public-interest and the private-interest perspectives of government. Additional consideration of this Manichean split is worthwhile.

The public-interest view sees government intervention as essentially positive, contributing to the improvement of the entire community, and necessary to foster development. In the health sector, government intervention is necessary to assure that the health transitions in poor countries move in positive directions not only for the aggregate but also for specific groups. Government action could have positive outcomes, in terms of access to services or improvements in health, even if specific policies are implemented due to pressure from self-interested groups. According to the public-interest view, government intervention is required because markets fail to produce public goods (preventive health services) or merit goods (freedom from avoidable death or illness) and fail to control bad goods (pollution or traffic hazards).

The public-interest view has both proponents and critics. Proponents consider the concept of public interest as normatively essential. James W. Fesler, reflecting his specialization in public administration, embraced the concept as an ideal (1988:897):

> It is for administrators what objectivity is for scholars — something to be strived for, even if imperfectly achieved, something not to be spurned because performance falls short of the goal. If there is not a public interest then we must denounce the idea of ideals...

Bates, on the other hand, rejected the public-interest perspective as empirically unhelpful: As noted above, he concluded that the public-interest objectives of governments do not explain the specific forms of policy adopted (1988a:343-345). The views of Fesler and Bates may seem mutually exclusive, but are not necessarily so; one could consider the public-interest viewpoint as normatively desirable but empirically unachievable.

The private-interest school of thought on government takes the critique one step further, rejecting the public-interest viewpoint on normative grounds. In the private-interest view, the actions of government are intentionally designed to meet the personal interests of politicians and bureaucrats, not to meet the needs of the population. Government intervention inevitably results in an inefficient allocation of resources due to diversions to meet private interests. In health, for example, the private-interest school would recommend against government provision of health services for the poor at no cost, since "most resources are likely to go to support bureaucratic interests and to reach the poor at higher cost to society than private, voluntary efforts would" (Birdsall 1989:97).

The interpretation of the private-interest view as emphasizing the "personal goals" of bureaucrats is rejected by both Bates and Fesler. Bates supported a broader political interpretation of the private-interest approach, with his interest-group model and power-maintenance models to explain government policy, as described earlier in this chapter. And Fesler argued from personal experience, "No-one who has served in the government, as I was privileged to do, could suppose that the behavior of career civil servants can be summed up as simply self-regarding" (1988:897).

While Birdsall did not advocate a pure private-interest worldview of government, she proposed partial adoption of market forces to correct for the imperfections of government action. Her main recommendations were selective user charges ("particularly charges to the nonpoor for private curative services"), decentralization of government services, and greater government use of the private sector (1989:111). She argued that these "market oriented" policies would lead to more efficient and more effective achievement of health goals than what might be called "government-oriented" policies.

The concept of selective medical user charges (MUC) has direct parallels to the concept of selective primary health care (Walsh and Warren 1979). The latter stressed the point that government could not provide all health services and therefore needed to focus on the high priority, cost-effective items. Selective MUC suggests that government should not charge everyone for all health services, but that those who can pay should pay. Selective PHC argues that equity must be balanced with efficiency in health care, while selective MUC argues that efficiency must be balanced with equity.

The introduction of medical user charges inevitably arouses opposition and imposes political costs. The beneficiaries of free services resist the idea of making even nominal payments. When the beneficiaries have strong political allies, user charges become difficult, if not impossible, to implement. In these cases, the political costs are perceived to exceed the financial benefits, in rich as well as poor countries. In the United States, for example, political opposition in Congress and the Pentagon has blocked efforts by the Office of Management and Budget to introduce user charges for medical services provided to military dependents and retirees. In 1986, when first proposed, reaction to the idea was so strong that Congress passed a law banning such fees for two years (*New York Times* 1988). No one likes to lose existing benefits, and more powerful groups are better positioned to prevent the erosion of their interests.

The debate over medical user charges in poor countries has focused on the impacts on the poor. The market forces school has argued that MUCs are good, because they raise money for the medical care system and improve allocative efficiency (making prices approach marginal costs) (de Ferranti 1985; Jimenez 1986). The government intervention school has responded that free access represents a basic right in many countries and that the poor would suffer most from higher prices and reduced medical utilization (Cornea et al. 1987). Economic modelers have predicted that higher user fees in government clinics would reduce utilization, especially among the poor; and that in urban areas, poor people would probably substitute private care for the previous public care, unless private practitioners raised their prices (Alderman and Gertler 1989). Unfortunately, the modelers did not estimate the probability that such prices would rise in the private sector.

A fundamental problem with advocating greater reliance on market forces to improve health conditions in poor countries is that not enough attention has been given to the political consequences. One review of the "principle and practice" of medical user charges argued that efforts at cost recovery in the rural health sector are regressive and that hospital-based fee systems could redress some inequities in society (Griffin 1988:36). But the author did not analyze the political obstacles to full cost recovery — mentioning political feasibility only once in passing, in parentheses (1988:11) and discussing political costs in one paragraph in the next-to-last Appendix (1988:76). He concluded that "loans or outside assistance" would be needed to compensate for the political costs and to assure "careful timing." In short, political feasibility does not automatically follow economic rationality. These "market oriented" approaches invariably confront significant political barriers; and market oriented economists, ironically, end up recommending administrative intervention (by international agencies) to change the political cost-benefit calculation.

Markets and Interests: Proponents of market forces in the health sector of poor countries tend to assume a separation between markets and interests. These advocates see an idealized vision of the world, in which The Market appears (or is assumed to be) immune to the influence of politics. But in many poor countries, the prevailing reality approaches the opposite: through various mechanisms, the market becomes part of politics.

Bates identified several ways that political actors take over market forces in agricultural policy (1988a:355-356). Price controls below market levels for commodities create opportunities for huge profits and for allocating those benefits as political favors. The power to grant access to regulated markets provides a major method for government leaders to accumulate political influence and secure political allies. Another way that markets become part of politics involves the implementation of rules. Government bureaucrats achieve political influence through their discretion to enforce the rules, for example, of regulated prices for agricultural commodities (1988a:355):

> By allowing exceptions to the rules, the bureaucracy grants favors; by preparing to enforce the rules, it threatens sanctions. Market regulations thus become a source of political control, and this, in a sense, is most true when they are in the process of being breached.

Rationing provides another method for the distribution of benefits to political allies and for depriving one's opponents. Finally, the appointment of allies to positions of power in the regulated market creates ties of political loyalty and a basis for political organization. In their work of coalition building, political actors find the market's invisible glove quite handy in dispensing rewards and punishments.

Similar processes operate for health policy in poor countries. The notion of an "unbridled private market" (Birdsall 1989:97) may represent a theoretical standard against which some economists seek to measure the efficiency of public health programs, but at least some analysts regard this standard as pie-in-the-sky reasoning for rich as well as poor countries (Culyer 1982; Reich 1988a). Price controls on pharmaceuticals provide opportunities to allocate the benefits of profits to political allies, through the distribution of scarce supplies and through the allowance of black market activity. Access to regulated markets for private services, in providing health care and in selling medical products, represents another way of dispensing political favors. Similarly, rationing of scarce resources and appointments to public programs operate as political processes in the health field.

In short, political elites have powerful incentives to use regulated health markets to retain power by rewarding constituents and excluding opponents. Birdsall's notion that a market oriented approach "could encourage a reorientation of government's role toward 'public' goods, especially more public spending on basic care for the poor" (1989:111) ignores these basic political realities. The implementation of selective medical user charges could provide another area for "selectively" dispensing benefits to political allies. Studies on the political economy of introducing medical user charges would improve our understanding of who gains and who loses and how governments adjust the implementation of such policies to fit local interests.

Advocates of market forces have recently begun to promote decentralization of government services, which is supposed to make the public sector more responsive and accountable to local needs. But decentralization can increase rather than decrease the political use of markets, as Birdsall recognized, by creating opportunities for politically tied appointments or by strengthening secessionist tendencies (1989:114). The decentralization of financing for social programs, in order to improve central budgets, can undermine the effectiveness of programs and exacerbate regional inequities (Pfeffermann and Griffin 1989:26). Even calling decentralization a market oriented approach stretches the definition of that concept.

India's long history of decentralized planning illustrates important limits of this proposed remedy. Since its First Five Year Plan, India has sought to decentralize the planning and implementation of development, to achieve more efficient use of resources and more equitable distribution of benefits. The results, according to one review, have been "dismal," despite the establishment of institutional structures, the *panchayati raj,* at the local level (Rao 1989). "Under the prevailing social structure and property relations, the rural elite has often come to dominate these institutions and appropriated a major share of benefits from development so that the improvement in the living conditions of the poor and the underprivileged has been negligible" (1989:412). Without changes in the socioeconomic structure of rural society, through policies oriented toward the poor and through effective social mobilization, decentralization is more likely to perpetuate rather than ameliorate the inefficiencies and inequities of the political use of markets in development. In short, Migdal's notion of a strong state may be more efficient and equitable in promoting development and social welfare for the poor.

The likelihood of implementing decentralized planning increases when political leaders perceive political needs or opportunities to expand their constituencies. In the mid-1970s, decentralization stalled in Kenya, despite the declarations of official policy, the incentives of foreign aid, and the dispatch of technical advisors. Only after a new president took office in 1978 did implementation begin, because the leaders viewed decentralization as a convenient means to expand their political base (Grindle and Thomas 1991:90-91,140). Here, the political cost-benefit analysis produced incentives that made decentralization both feasible and desirable for the political leaders. Whether the circumstances of the rural poor consequently improved is uncertain.

Another popular solution, proposed by international agencies, is to expand the government's use of private sector strategies. One consulting company identified 17 "discrete privatization options" in the health sector, ranging from the transfer of all curative services to the private sector, to the promotion of health maintenance organizations, to the expansion of autonomy for public hospitals and other health facilities (Jeffers 1989). But even this explicitly pro-privatization review concluded with a veiled warning that governments need "careful consideration" whether the supplier industry will remain competitive over the long term, implicitly recognizing, in the article's last sentence, the dangers of becoming a "captive of the private sector" (1989:12). In the absence of perfect competition, privatization can produce a broad arena for political activities, in the assignment of contracts, decisions about fees, and payment for services.

One could argue that the efforts by international agencies to increase the use of markets in Third World countries, in the recent fashion of "conditional" loans, represents a form of administrative intervention in markets. These aid programs seek to reduce the state control of the economy by making loans "conditional" on critical changes in government services and policies, and thereby are supposed to increase overall efficiency and economic growth. The "conditions," however, often impose costs on important political constituencies of the groups in power. In effect, the promise of economic growth and the lure of continued aid represent a "bribe" to powerholders "to embolden them to incur the political cost of taking away rents from those who receive them" and "to buy out some of the restrictive practices by which they currently hold the state together" (P. Mosley 1988:53).

This process of international influence, in Paul Mosley's metaphor, is like "persuading a leopard to change his spots" and requires careful consideration of political feasibility. In Mosley's sample, the two countries that most faithfully implemented World Bank conditional policy-reform packages were Jamaica and Turkey, which had undergone changes in government prior to signing the loan agreements. "The important point is that neither government was significantly obligated to the groups who could be expected to lose from a liberalization of domestic and foreign trade, or could be accused of inconsistency of betrayal of those groups if it went ahead with an economic stabilization program" (1988:78). Indeed, the new governments of these two countries had already committed themselves to liberalization programs prior to completing the World Bank agreements.

Interventions in national markets by international agencies thus are constrained by the structure of political interests. The economic incentives of international persuasion work best when governments have already decided to change their political spots. When pushed to economic brinks, the survival politics of most Third World governments depend more on local constituencies than on world bankers. Government leaders are not easily persuaded by international agencies to implement policies perceived as posing significant political costs to important constituencies, as illustrated by the case of agrarian land reform in the Philippines (Grindle and Thomas 1991:145).

The above analysis suggests that the market has a limited and complicated role to play in health transitions. One should not doubt the ability of user fees, if properly managed, to improve the financial situation of health services in poor countries. But the market (even a market oriented approach) does not provide a panacea for the multiple ills of the health sector or for the problems of development more broadly. Nor does the market necessarily lead to better health for all. Any effort that seeks to impose market solutions, without taking into account the impact of political and economic interests, may end up creating more problems than it solves.

Conclusion

Analysis of political economy constitutes an essential element in understanding health transitions in poor countries — something that Marxian analysts have been saying for a long time. Simple calls for government intervention or for market forces, as the method to improve health conditions in poor countries, are more likely to mystify and confuse than to explain and clarify. Yet most studies of health transitions in the Third World, especially when carried out by economists or health professionals, have underplayed and underanalyzed the pervasive influence of politics.

From a political perspective, the two approaches of government interventions and market forces are imperfect alternatives. Neither strategy is a magic wand to produce health for all in Third World countries. Political processes affect the design and implementation of both government policies and market mechanisms so that actual results often differ dramatically from the stated or intended ones. Indeed, it seems likely that no single path to good health exists. Each country may need to design its own combination of governments and markets to avoid the pitfalls and potholes that plague the implementation of policy and to arrange the political costs and benefits so that stability and positive outcomes result.

The costs of seeking to impose a single solution, in hopes of improving health, need to be explicitly assessed. A strong state may be able to implement public health measures effectively (even ruthlessly). But that implementation may occur at great costs in terms of political liberty and human lives — as in the case of China during the Cultural Revolution. And strong states do not necessarily produce health improvements, as illustrated by the mixed achievements of the command-and-control states of the Soviet Union and Eastern Europe (Eberstadt 1988:207-250). Similarly, a single-minded reliance on market forces may unleash a plethora of health hazards associated with industrialization and urbanization along with positive health consequences for some social groups. The opening of Eastern Europe, for example, could contribute to continued deterioration in health conditions if reliance on the market results in even worse environmental pollution or wider availability of tobacco products.

In order to understand how the politics of governments and markets affect health conditions, both positively and negatively, we need more political inquiries into the patterns of health transitions in different kinds of states. Analysis is also needed of the values that underlie the evaluation of health achievements and the accompanying costs in different states, especially beliefs about how the state should relate to individuals in society and how to assess conflicts between state power and individual freedom.

Attention should also be directed to a third major analytic approach to health transitions in the Third World: that involving competitive political markets. This approach stresses the empowerment of relatively powerless groups in society, the development of mechanisms for state and market accountability, and the emergence of nongovernmental groups that form coalitions and mobilize latent interests. The experiences of Costa Rica and Kerala suggest that these political processes played a major role in shaping both government interventions and market forces in directions that had positive health consequences — and with lower human costs than the strong state approach to good health adopted in China.

This third approach would depend on the role of nongovernmental organizations (NGOs) as agents of political change in promoting good health and development and in addressing the problems raised by government-oriented and market oriented approaches. A growing literature recognizes the potential contributions of NGOs in development (Drabek 1987). NGOs have a number of comparative advantages over states, especially in the quality of relationships with intended beneficiaries and in the autonomy of choice in organizational design and objectives (Fowler 1990a). A political analysis of the role of NGOs in southern Africa pointed out their potential in advancing democratization but also the efforts by national governments and international agencies to contain NGOs (Fowler 1990b). Additional research is needed on the political conditions in which NGOs can promote positive health transitions and how NGOs can manage the obstacles created by both national and international institutions.

NGOs have also demonstrated an ability to affect the health consequences of national and international markets. In the past decade, international networks of NGOs have emerged to exert increasing influence on markets of specific products and on the agendas of international organizations (Reich 1991). The formation of international networks has resulted from two patterns of organizational development: the strengthening of domestic NGOs in poor countries and the internationalization of existing groups in rich countries. On health and environment issues, examples include Pesticide Action Network (PAN), Health Action International (HAI), and the International Network of Victims of Corporate and Government Abuse. The international linkages created and maintained by these networks hold the potential for political action to reduce the negative health consequences of market oriented approaches in both domestic and international markets. To understand when and how these networks succeed, additional research is needed on case studies and political strategies.

A final conclusion of this chapter is the importance of assessing the political feasibility of policies to improve health conditions in poor countries. Policy analysis needs to take into account the vast areas of uncertainty that surround important social issues and the inevitable influence exerted by the values of administrators and experts. Analysis that considers the political implications of policy proposals can help decision makers and the general public "avoid both reckless underestimation and harsh overstatement of the limitations of the possible in public policy" (Majone 1988:165). To do this, analysis must explicitly recognize how governments act as the agents of private interests, how governments act to retain power, and how markets become instruments of political organization. Lastly, greater attention needs to be directed to the international political economy and its impact on national health policy and health conditions.

Acknowledgments

The author appreciates helpful comments on earlier drafts from Barbara Crane, Arthur Kleinman, Lynn M. Morgan, and Diana Cooper Weil, and from participants at several seminars where the paper was presented.

Notes

1 The field of political economy covers a broad range of schools and traditions that involve political and economic analysis in various combinations. Martin Staniland (1985) provides a good map and guidebook to the array of approaches. These include: the new political economy, which applies assumptions of economic rationality to explain political choices in society; "politicist" theories, which argue that power and political institutions take precedence in explaining economic patterns in society; international political economy, which examines political and economic forces in the international arena and includes schools of liberalism, realism, interdependence, and dependency; and Marxian political economy, which includes several traditions with different emphases on internal class structures and external capital influences.

2 Regarding the broad theoretical territory covered by political economy, Staniland (1985:198) wrote, "The term *political economy*, used generically, refers to a continuing intellectual enterprise, a particular agenda, a specific object of theoretical ambition. Because 'political economy' is an agenda rather than a method, there will always be a variety of theories of political economy. And because a variety of assumptions and values underlies such variety of theory, it may be possible (indeed, it is very desirable) to criticize each theory; but it will never be possible to decide between them, to end the debate, and to remove variety by purely logical means."

3 The growing literature on political economy of health in the United States includes the following studies: R. R. Alford, *Health Care Politics: Ideological and Interest Group Barriers to Reform* (1975); T. R. Marmor and J. B. Christianson, *Health Care Policy: A Political Economy Approach* (1982); P. Starr, *The Social Transformation of American Medicine* (1982); L. D. Brown, *Politics and Health Care Organization: HMOs as Federal Policy* (1983); P. J. Feldstein, *The Politics of Health Legislation: An Economic Perspective* (1988); D. M. Fox, *Health Policies, Health Politics: The British and American Experience, 1911–1965* (1986).

4 These two broad approaches, government interventions and market forces, represent a heuristic dichotomy to characterize studies of the political economy of health transitions. Some studies, however, may not fit easily in these two neat categories. For example, I have not included many studies of international political economy of either the dependency or the interdependence type (although the first would probably fit in the government intervention approach, while the second would be compatible with the market forces school). Similarly, Marxian analyses would fit best in the government intervention approach, although such studies also have problems in their political analysis. Finally, the analysis of new non governmental and non market actors does not fit well in either normative school; I discuss some implications of these new actors in the chapter's concluding section.

5 In rare circumstances, when farmers are well organized and connected to national elites, sufficient political pressure can be exerted to shape government policy and resist efforts to push down agricultural prices. In countries where competitive elections occur on a regular and fair basis, agrarian interests can

achieve greater voice and thereby affect national policy, as illustrated by the tendency for politicians to launch major rural development programs just before elections (Bates, 1988a:350). In Africa, as in other parts of the developing world, the weakness of electoral politics means a weakness of rural influence on agricultural policies.

References

Alderman, H., and P. Gertler. 1989. "The substitutability of public and private health care for the treatment of children in Pakistan." Living Standards Measurement Study Working Paper No. 57, Washington, D.C.: World Bank.

Alford, R.R. 1975. *Health Care Politics: Ideological and Interest Group Barriers to Reform.* Chicago: University of Chicago Press.

Bardhan, P. 1988. "Alternative approaches to development economics." In H. Chenery and T.N. Srinivasan, eds. *Handbook of Development Economics,* Volume I. New York: Elsevier Science Publishers.

Barry, M. 1991. "The influence of the U.S. tobacco industry on the health, economy, and environment of developing countries." *New England Journal of Medicine,* 324: 917–920.

Bates, R.H. 1988a. "Governments and agricultural markets in Africa." In R.H. Bates, ed. *Toward a Political Economy of Development.* Berkeley: University of California Press.

Bates, R.H. ed. 1988b. *Toward a Political Economy of Development.* Berkeley: University of California Press.

Berliner, H.S., and C. Regan. 1987. "Multinational operations of U.S. for-profit hospital chains: Trends and implications." *American Journal of Public Health,* 77: 1280–1284.

Birdsall, N. 1989. "Thoughts on good health and good government." *Daedalus,* 118(1): 89–117.

Bossert, T.J. 1983. "Can we return to the regime for comparative policy analysis? or, The state and health policy in Central America." *Comparative Politics,* July: 419–441.

Brown, L.D. 1983. *Politics and Health Care Organization: HMOs as Federal Policy.* Washington, DC: Brookings Institution.

Buchanan, J.M. 1985. *Liberty, Market and the State: Political Economy in the 1980s.* Brighton, England: Wheatsheaf Books.

Caldwell, J.C. 1986. "Routes to low mortality in poor countries." *Population and Development Review,* 12: 171–220.

Caldwell, J.C. 1990. "Introductory thoughts on health transition." In J.C. Caldwell, S. Findley, P. Caldwell, G. Santow, W. Cosford, J. Braid, and D. Broers-Freeman, eds. *What We Know About the Health Transition: The Cultural, Social and Behavioural Determinants of Health, Health Transition Series,* No. 2, Vol. 1. Canberra: Health Transition Centre, Australian National University.

Chen, L.C. 1988. "Health policy: An approach derived from the experiences of China and India." In D.E. Bell and M.R. Reich, eds. *Health, Nutrition and Economic Crises: Approaches to Policy in the Third World.* Dover, MA: Auburn House Publishing Company.

Chilcote, R.H. 1985. "Alternative approaches to comparative politics." In H.J. Wiarda, ed. *New Directions in Comparative Politics.* Boulder, CO: Westview Press.

Cleaves, P. 1980. "Implementation amidst scarcity and apathy: Political power and policy design." In M.S. Grindle, ed. *Politics and Policy Implementation in the Third World.* Princeton, NJ: Princeton University Press.

Cornea, G., R. Jolly, and F. Stewart. 1987. *Adjustment with a Human Face.* Oxford: Clarendon Press.

Culyer, A.J. 1982. "The NHS and the market, images and realities." In G. McLachlan and A. Maynard, eds. *The Public/Private Mix for Health: The Relevance and Effects of Change.* London: The Nuffield Provincial Hospitals Trust.

Davis, C., and M. Feshbach. 1980. *Rising Infant Mortality in the USSR in the 1970s.* Series P–95, No. 74, Washington, DC: U.S. Bureau of the Census, September.

de Ferranti, D. 1985. "Paying for health services in developing countries: An overview." Staff Working Paper 721, Washington, DC: World Bank.

Doyal, L., and I. Pennell. 1979. *The Political Economy of Health.* London: Pluto Press.

Drabek, A.G. 1987. "Development alternatives: The challenge for NGOs — An overview of the issues." *World Development,* 15(suppl): 9–15.

Eberstadt, N. 1988. *The Poverty of Communism.* New Brunswick: Transaction Publishers.

Eckstein, H. 1960. *Pressure Group Politics: The Case of the British Medical Association.* Stanford, CA: Stanford University Press.

Elling, R. 1981. "The capitalist world system and international health." *International Journal of Health Services,* 11: 21–51.

Evans, P., D. Rueschemeyer, and T. Skocpol, eds. 1985. *Bringing the State Back In.* New York: Cambridge University Press.

Feldstein, P.J. 1988. *The Politics of Health Legislation: An Economic Perspective.* Ann Arbor, MI: Health Administration Press.

Feinsilver, J.M. 1989. "Cuba as a 'world medical power': The politics of symbolism." *Latin American Research Review,* 24: 1–34.

Fesler, J.W. 1988. "The state and its study, the whole and the parts." *PS: Political Science and Politics,* Fall: 893–897.

Field, M.G. 1990. "Noble purpose, grand design, flawed execution, mixed results: Soviet socialized medicine after seventy years." *American Journal of Public Health*, 80: 144–145.

Findley, S.E. 1990. "Social reflections of changing morbidity during health transitions." In J.C. Caldwell, S. Findley, P. Caldwell, G. Santow, W. Cosford, J. Braid, and D. Broers-Freeman. *What We Know About the Health Transition: The Cultural, Social and Behavioural Determinants of Health, Health Transition Series*, No. 2, Vol. 1. Canberra: Health Transition Centre, Australian National University.

Fowler, A. 1990a. "Doing it better? Where and how do NGOs have a 'comparative advantage' in facilitating development?" *Agricultural Extension and Rural Development Department Bulletin*, University of Reading. February, pp. 11–20.

Fowler, A. 1990b. "Political dimensions of NGO expansion in Eastern and Southern Africa and the role of international aid." Paper presented at the African Studies Association Annual Meeting, Baltimore, November 1–4.

Fox, D.M. 1986. *Health Policies, Health Politics: The British and American Experience, 1911–1965*. Princeton, NJ: Princeton University Press.

Frenk, J., J.L. Bobadilla, C. Stern, T. Frejka, and R. Lozano. 1991. "Elements for a theory of the health transition." *Health Transition Review*, 1: 21–38. Reprinted in this volume.

Frenk, J., and A. Donabedian. 1987. "State intervention in medical care: Types, trends and variables." *Health Policy and Planning*, 1: 17–31.

Gereffi, G. 1978. "Drug firms and dependency in Mexico: The case of the steroid hormone industry." *International Organization*, 32: 237–268.

Griffin, C.G. 1988. "User charges for health care in principle and practice." EDI Seminar Paper No. 37, Washington, DC: World Bank.

Grindle, M.S., and J.W. Thomas. 1991. *Public Choices and Policy Change: The Political Economy of Reform in Developing Countries*. Baltimore: Johns Hopkins University Press.

Gunatilleke, G. 1985. "Health and development in Sri Lanka — An overview." In S.B. Halstead, J.A. Walsh, and K.S. Warren, eds. *Good Health at Low Cost*. New York: Rockefeller Foundation.

Gwatkin, D.R. 1979. "Political will and family planning: The implications of India's emergency experience." *Population and Development Review*, 5: 29–60.

Haggard, S., and C.I. Moon. 1990. "Institutions and economic policy: Theory and a Korean case study." *World Politics*, 42(2): 210–237.

Halstead, S.B., J.A. Walsh, and K.S. Warren, eds. 1985. *Good Health at Low Cost*. New York: Rockefeller Foundation.

Halstead, S.B., J.A. Walsh, and K.S. Warren. 1985. "Editors' preface." In S.B. Halstead, J.A. Walsh, and K.S. Warren, eds. *Good Health at Low Cost*. New York: Rockefeller Foundation.

Jamison, D.T. 1985. "China's health care system: Policies, organization, inputs and 'finance'." In S.B. Halstead, J.A. Walsh, and K.S. Warren, eds. *Good Health at Low Cost*. New York: Rockefeller Foundation.

Jasanoff, S. 1985. "Remedies against hazardous exports: Compensation, products liability and criminal sanctions." In J. Ives, ed. *The Export of Hazard: Transnational Corporations and Environmental Control Issues*. Boston: Routledge and Kegan Paul.

Jayasuriya, D.C. 1985. *The Public Health and Economic Dimensions of the New Drug Policy of Bangladesh*. Washington, DC: U.S. Pharmaceutical Manufacturers Association.

Jeffers, J.R. 1989. "Conceptual options for public-private partnerships in health care." *The Privatization Review*, Spring: 4–12.

Jeffrey, R. 1988. *The Politics of Health in India*. Berkeley: University of California Press.

Jimenez, E. 1986. "The public subsidization of education and health in developing countries: A review of equity and efficiency." *The Research Observer*, 1: 111–129.

Johnson, C. 1981. *MITI and the Japanese Miracle*. Stanford, CA: Stanford University Press.

Johnson, C. 1987. "Political institutions and economic performance: The government-business relationship in Japan, South Korea, and Taiwan." In F. Deyo, ed. *The Political Economy of the New Asian Industrialism*. Ithaca, NY: Cornell University Press.

Joseph, S.C. 1985. "The case for clinical services." In S.B. Halstead, J.A. Walsh, and K.S. Warren, eds. *Good Health at Low Cost*. New York: Rockefeller Foundation.

Lal, D. 1983. *The Poverty of "Development Economics."* London: Institute of Economic Affairs.

Lall, S., and S. Bibile. 1978. "The political economy of controlling transnationals: The pharmaceutical industry in Sri Lanka, 1972–1976." *International Journal of Health Services*, 8: 299–328.

Lange, P., and H. Meadwell. 1985. "Typologies of democratic systems: From political inputs to political economy." In H.J. Wiarda, ed. *New Directions in Comparative Politics*. Boulder, CO: Westview Press.

Lewis, J.P., et al. 1988. *Strengthening the Poor: What Have We Learned?* Overseas Development Council, U.S. Third World Development Perspectives, No. 10.

Lindblom, C.E. 1977. *Politics and Markets: The World's Political–Economic System.* New York: Basic Books.

Lipton, M. 1977, c1976. *Why Poor People Stay Poor: Urban Bias in World Development.* Cambridge, MA: Harvard University Press.

Mamalakis, M. 1989. "Review of political survival: Politicians and public policy in Latin America." *American Political Science Review,* 83: 1044–1045.

Majone, G. 1975. "On the notion of political feasibility." *European Journal of Political Research,* 3: 259–274.

Majone, G. 1988. "Policy analysis and public deliberation." In R.B. Reich, ed. *The Power of Public Ideas.* Cambridge: Ballinger Publishing Co.

Marmor, T.R., and J.B. Christianson. 1982. *Health Care Policy: A Political Economy Approach.* Beverly Hills,CA: Sage Publications.

May, P.J. 1986. "Politics and policy analysis." *Political Science Quarterly,* 101: 109–125.

Migdal, J.S. 1988. *Strong States and Weak Societies: State-Society Relations and State Capabilities in the Third World.* Princeton,NJ: Princeton University Press.

Morgan, L.M. 1989. "'Political will' and community participation in Costa Rican primary health care." *Medical Anthropology Quarterly,* 3: 232–245.

Mosley, P. 1988. "On persuading a leopard to change his spots: Optimal strategies for donors and recipients of conditional development aid." In R.H. Bates, ed. *Toward A Political Economy of Development.* Berkeley: University of California Press.

Mosley, W.H. 1985. "Remarks." In S.B. Halstead, J.A. Walsh, and K.S. Warren, eds. *Good Health at Low Cost.* New York: Rockefeller Foundation.

Nag, M. 1985. "The impact of social and economic development on mortality." In S.B. Halstead, J.A. Walsh, and K.S. Warren, eds. *Good Health at Low Cost.* New York: Rockefeller Foundation.

Nag, M. 1989. "Political awareness as a factor in accessibility of health services: A case study of rural Kerala and West Bengal." *Economic and Political Weekly,* February 25: 417–426.

Navarro, V. 1984. "A critique of the ideological and political positions of the Willy Brandt report and the WHO Alma Ata declaration." *Social Science and Medicine,* 18: 467–474.

Pfeffermann, G.P., and C.C. Griffin. 1989. *Nutrition and Health Programs in Latin America: Targeting Social Expenditures.* Washington, DC: World Bank.

Przeworski, A., and H. Teune. 1970. *The Logic of Comparative Inquiry.* New York: Wiley.

Rao, C.H.H. 1989. "Decentralised planning, an overview of experience and prospects." *Economic and Political Weekly,* February 25: 411–416.

Reich, M.R. 1987. "Essential drugs: Economics and politics in international health." *Health Policy*, 8: 39–57.

Reich, M.R. 1988a. "International trade and trade-offs for third world consumers." In E.S. Maynes, ed. *The Frontier of Research in the Consumer Interest.* Columbia, MO: American Council on Consumer Interests.

Reich, M.R. 1988b. "Technical fixes and other problems in saving lives in the world's poorest countries." *Journal of Public Health Policy*, 9: 92–103.

Reich, M.R. 1991. "Toxic politics and pollution victims in the Third World." In S. Jasanoff, ed. *Learning from Disaster.* Ithaca, NY: Cornell University Press.

Roemer, M.I. 1987. "Foreign privatization of national health systems." *American Journal of Public Health*, 77: 1271–1272.

Rosenfield, P.L. 1985. "The contribution of social and political factors to good health." In S.B. Halstead, J.A. Walsh, and K.S. Warren, eds. *Good Health at Low Cost.* New York: Rockefeller Foundation.

Rosero-Bixby, L. 1985. "Infant mortality decline in Costa Rica." In S.B. Halstead, J.A. Walsh, and K.S. Warren, eds. *Good Health at Low Cost.* New York: Rockefeller Foundation.

Sagan, L.A. 1987. *The Health of Nations: True Causes of Sickness and Well-Being.* New York: Basic Books.

Segall, M. 1983. "Planning and politics of resource allocation for primary health care: Promotion of meaningful national policy." *Social Science and Medicine*, 17: 1947–1960.

Sethi, S.P., H. Etemad, and K.A.N. Luther. 1986. "New sociopolitical forces: The globalization of conflict." *Journal of Business Strategy*, 6(Spring): 24–31.

Sidel, V.W., and R. Sidel. 1973. *Serve the People: Observations on Medicine in the People's Republic of China.* New York: Josiah H. Macy, Jr. Foundation.

Skocpol, T. 1985. "Bringing the state back in: Strategies of analysis in current research." In P. Evans, D. Rueschemeyer, and T. Skocpol, eds. *Bringing the State Back In.* New York: Cambridge University Press.

Staniland, M. 1985. *What is Political Economy? A Study of Social Theory and Underdevelopment.* New Haven: Yale University Press.

Starr, P. 1982. *The Social Transformation of American Medicine.* New York: Basic Books.

Starrels, J.M. 1985. *The World Health Organization: Resisting Third World Ideological Pressures.* Washington, DC: The Heritage Foundation.

Stepan, A. 1978. *The State and Society: Peru in Comparative Perspective.* Princeton, NJ: Princeton University Press.

Steslicke, W.E. 1973. *Doctors in Politics.* New York: Praeger.

"Summary statement adopted by conferees." 1985. In S.B. Halstead, J.A. Walsh, and K.S. Warren, eds. *Good Health at Low Cost.* New York: Rockefeller Foundation.

Swanstrom, T. 1989. "Homeless: A product of policy." *The New York Times*, March 23: Op-Ed Page.

U.S. Agency for International Development. 1989. *Development and the National Interest: U.S. Economic Assistance into the 21st Century.* Washington, DC: USAID.

Vitta, P.B., n.d.. "Technology policy in Sub-Saharan Africa: Why the dream remains unredeemed." International Development Research Center, Nairobi, Kenya. Mimeo.

Walsh, J.A., and K.S. Warren. 1979. "Selective primary health care: An interim strategy for disease control in developing countries." *New England Journal of Medicine*, 301: 967–974.

Warren, K.S. 1985. "Remarks." In S.B. Halstead, J.A. Walsh, and K.S. Warren, eds. *Good Health at Low Cost.* New York: Rockefeller Foundation.

Wolf, C. 1988. *Markets or Governments: Choosing Between Imperfect Alternatives.* Cambridge, MA: MIT Press.

World Bank. 1988. *World Development Report 1988.* New York: Oxford University Press.

World Health Organization, Advisory Committee on Health Research. 1988. "Health research strategy, priorities in health research and service policies in developing countries, summary." Prepared by T. McKeown, for 29th Session of ACHR, Geneva, October 3–7.

―――. 1988. "Budget office seeks military health care fees." *The New York Times*, December 15.

16

The Political Economy of Health Financing Strategies in Kenya

Göran Dahlgren

Background

This paper analyzes the process of developing a health care financing strategy by the Kenyan government. Like other countries around the world, from 1988–90 the Kenyan government was examining alternative public financing strategies in the context of severe domestic budgetary constraints, exacerbated by pressures from foreign donor agencies. Ultimately, a policy outcome was reached that many considered to be less than ideal. This strategy generated less revenue and produced greater inequities than several other alternatives, but avoided the adverse outcome of public services being transformed into semi-private services primarily focusing on middle and high income groups in the country. Selection of this sub-optimal financing strategy was due neither to insufficient information nor to lack of better alternatives; rather, the government, in the end, adopted a financing strategy which accommodated diverse political and economic influences and interests.

This chapter describes the objectives pursued by the participants in the policy formulation process, and then analyzes the policy choices in terms of the alternatives presented.

Objectives of Strategies

The conceptual framework utilized for this analysis is a health policy assessment matrix, which attempts to match means, or financial resources, with ends, or the objectives to be achieved (Table 16-1). The objectives for health financing strategies may be seen as falling into the following four categories:

Table 16-1   Health policy assessment matrix[1]

Health Policy Objectives/ Financial Sources	Financial objectives	Equity objectives	Efficiency objectives	Health service structure objectives
Taxes				
Direct	++	++		
Indirect	+++	– – –		
Users charges				
Outpatient	++	– –	+–	+–
Inpatient	+	– –	+–	+–
Insurance schemes				
Public	+++	+++		+++
Private	++	– –		– –
External Aid	+ – + –	+ – + –	+ – + –	++
Community contribution	++	+ – + –	++	++

[1] The number of the plus and minus signs indicates the magnitude of positive and negative impact of using alternative financial sources in relation to overall objectives.

- **financial**: to generate sufficient revenue for financing the public health sector;

- **equity**: to increase economic and geographical access to health services, especially in underserved areas and amongst low income populations;

- **efficiency**: to obtain more or better services for the money;

- **structural**: to reduce imbalances among promotive, preventive, and curative services and between primary versus specialized care.

In Kenya, these four objectives were reflected in general policy declarations by the government as well as by donors such as the World Bank and USAID. In principle, a general consensus emerged among all parties regarding the desirability of these objectives and thus the direction of policy reform. In practice, however, the underlying implicit objectives differed significantly from these explicit objectives; the relative weight accorded to various objectives also differed. A critical analysis of this policy-making process reveals that real objectives may only be derived from an examination of specific actions recommended and decisions taken, rather than from a study of more general discussions or rhetoric.

Financing

Kenya's economic growth in the second half of the 1980s averaged 5 percent annually despite rapid population growth, a stagnant economy until the mid-1980s, and heavy borrowing from abroad due to the second oil shock (Odada 1988). Even with these moderately favorable macroeconomic conditions, Kenya had large external debts and was under severe international pressure to reform its economy structurally. Public expenditures in such areas as education and health had placed increasing pressure on government finances. In an effort to clarify priorities, the Kenyan government announced a Budget Rationalization Program in 1986. The development of alternative or complementary ways of financing public expenditures in the social sectors was a high priority for this program.

It was estimated that around 20 percent of the population was effectively covered by comprehensive government health services (Mwabu and Mwangi 1986). Because of limited public financing, it was impossible to make public services available to all Kenyans. Even existing health services were seriously underfinanced. Symptoms of under-financing included inadequate and unreliable drugs and supplies, breakdown of facilities and equipment, lack of transport, and underpaid staff unable to fulfill functions because of lack of ancillary support (Abel-Smith 1989). Therefore, a new strategy for health financing was needed to generate additional revenues, primarily from sources within the health system such as user charges or payments into a National Hospital Insurance Fund (NHIF).

Equity

Income distribution in Kenya is extremely skewed (Odada 1988). The per capita income for 30 percent of the population living at or below the poverty line is fifteen times less than the average of the general population (Van de Moortele and Van der Hoeven 1982). Poverty is particularly concentrated in rural areas, especially among small landholders and pastoralists, and urban poverty has been estimated at over 15 percent. The financing strategy reform, therefore, needed to reduce, rather than increase existing inequities in the country.

Efficiency

A great potential existed to improve efficiency within the Kenyan public health care system. This was partly a matter of better management and partly an issue related to the financial system. Under-utilization of resources was also a major problem. While an increasing proportion of the recurrent budget was used for salaries, many staff lacked the means to perform their duties. The financing strategy, therefore, needed to serve as a management tool for improved efficiency.

Structural

"The inverse law of care" — that the greater the need the fewer resources available — is evident in this Kenyan case. The lack of balance in health between rich and poor, and between urban and rural areas, was reflected in the high health care consumption of affluent urban groups in comparison to rural poor groups. In 1990-91, the funds allocated to disease prevention and health promotion were only 3.4 percent, compared to more than 70 percent for curative care. Reduction of the resource gaps between urban and rural areas, between health centers and hospitals, and between preventive and curative services was, therefore, another objective of policy development.

Sources of Financing

Five basic sources of financing were available to the Kenyan Government — taxes, user charges, insurance, external aid, and community contributions. Direct and indirect taxes in Kenya are the main sources of financing for public services, including health. Direct taxes, around 25 percent of public funds, have a slightly progressive distributional impact, while indirect taxes, about 45 percent of total public funds, are usually regressive. The net effect of all general taxes at the time in Kenya was probably regressive. The political reality was that additional health funds could not be generated by increasing either direct or indirect taxes on products such as alcohol, tobacco, or luxury goods.

The two main sources for generating additional public funds were "user charges" and "public insurance schemes." Financially, the public insurance scheme had great potential, while the potential of user charges was more limited. User charges could cover 10 percent of the recurrent budget if economic access to health care was to remain secure (Abel-Smith 1989), while the corresponding figure for an insurance scheme was around 25 percent. These two sources of revenue differed significantly in terms of equity: the flat rate of user charges constituted another regressive tax, while a pooled insurance fund, depending upon its ultimate allocation, could be more equitable.

Neither external aid nor community contributions promised to help solve the bulk of Kenya's financing dilemmas. External aid was reserved almost exclusively for the development budget, not the recurring health budget. Although local communities in Kenya often contributed both in cash and kind to various development activities, including health, these were usually intended for investment rather than recurring costs. Many experimental efforts were made, but the prospect of developing a voluntary system generating a steady, ongoing flow of resources for public health was considered limited.

The Policy Process

Given the objectives and means of policy development, a new financing strategy focused on two primary sources of additional revenue — user charges and pooled insurance funds. Within this decision-making context, several more specific policy questions emerged. What type and level of user charges should be introduced? How much could be paid, by whom, and for what, within the health insurance system? How would the alternatives fulfill the basic objectives of the policy reform?

Very different answers to these questions were offered by the diverse actors engaged in the policy process: the World Bank, USAID, the Ministry of Health, an independent advisor, the Kenyan Cabinet, and even the country's President.

The Starting Point

The very process of formulating a new strategy for financing health care was quite dramatic as there was considerable pressure from external donors to institute reform. Traditionally, a negative attitude towards fees prevailed, while the idea of tax-financed social services was deeply rooted in Kenyan society. Direct-user charges for public health, like other social services, were few and at a very low level. Thus, an unexpected high user charge for services could be perceived as an introduction of the criterion of ability to pay rather than of need.

Increasing financial problems during the 1980s and pressure from the World Bank and USAID had already created consensus that some additional fees should be introduced, provided economic access was not compromised and the quality of services could be improved, particularly the availability of drugs. The question, therefore, was not whether user charges should be increased, but what fee levels and the rules for waiving fees should be.

At the same time, the situation of the National Hospital Insurance Fund (NHIF) was quite unique. With this fund, established before independence, a flat rate of 20 Kenyan shilling (kshs) was the compulsory contribution from all employees earning 1,000 kshs or more per month. Although the contributions were very modest, the NHIF had accumulated a considerable surplus over the years, because few of the insured could actually afford to use it. The low reimbursement rate meant that private funds were needed to cover the remaining payments for private care. Unable to match the reimbursement with private funds, the less well-to-do resorted to using the free public health services, in the same way as the non-insured. The net effect of this asymmetry was that contributions from the less wealthy subsidized those able to use the NHIF. To rectify this problem, the government considered a new fee structure based on 2 percent contribution of income earned from both employees and employers.

The dynamics regarding the shaping of these user fees and the insurance fund went through five phases, summarized graphically in Figure 16-1. In each phase, the actors emphasized different aspects of these two sources of financing, reflecting their priorities and generating differing impacts on the objectives of the reform.

Figure 16-1   The Policy Process (January 1988 – February 1990)

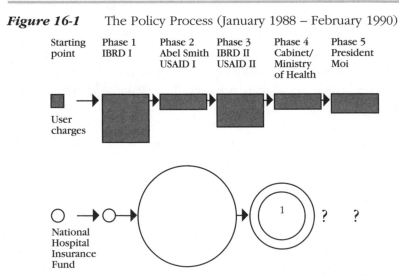

The size of squares and circles indicate the magnitude of revenue generated for public health services via user charges and NHIF, respectively.
[1] The smaller inner circle represents the policy in IBRD II, the outer the policy indicated in USAID.

Phase I (IBRD-I)

In the first five months of 1988, the initial proposal for a new financial strategy was presented to the Ministry of Health by a World Bank team. This strategy (IBRD-I) was based on high user charges. The Bank mission assumed that 90 percent of users would pay fees. Since only 10 percent of users would be unable to pay, a cost recovery of between 20-30 percent of the recurrent budget would be generated.

Considering the prevalence of poverty in Kenya, others felt it was more realistic to assume that some 40 percent, not 10 percent, of the population would be unable to pay the lowest fees suggested by the Bank, and 55 percent of the population the higher fee level (Abel-Smith 1989). Further analysis and discussion between the Government and the Bank led to the conclusion that the Bank's suggestion of very high fee levels was entirely unrealistic. After some months, the Bank accepted this conclusion and the proposal was discarded.

Phase II (AS-USAID I)

The main actors between January and April of 1989 were Professor Brian Abel-Smith, USAID and the Kenyan Ministry of Health. Abel-Smith served as a consultant to the World Bank, but was paid by the Swedish International Development Authority (SIDA). He was supposed to join a Bank team that was subsequently cancelled. Thus, he independently presented a proposal to the Bank suggesting a fairly modest level of user charges and a complete restructuring of the NHIF. Financially, he envisaged the NHIF as generating an annual revenue corresponding to 30 to 50 percent of the total recurrent health budget. This could be achieved by introducing compulsory contributions from employers and employees of 2 percent of income earned. Part of the NHIF revenues would cover medical services for the insured, most of whom would use private health services. Consequently, most of the funds following the insured would go to private providers, both commercial and non-profit. Abel-Smith also proposed that efforts be made to increase the proportion of insured using public facilities; he argued that part of the NHIF funds should be reallocated to the public health system, thereby advancing both equity and structural objectives.

The Abel-Smith proposal was not welcomed by the Bank. Even the Ministry of Health had to make several requests to the Bank to obtain a copy of the report, despite the fact that Ministry staff had collaborated in its preparation. Nevertheless, at this stage, the Ministry shared the views expressed in Abel-Smith's report. The "2 + 2 percent" financing for the NHIF was in fact very similar to proposals previously developed within the Ministry itself.

USAID also demonstrated interest in the report. It focused more on the potential of the NHIF, both as a revenue source and as a tool for reducing inequities. A USAID proposal presented later in this phase elaborated some key elements of Abel-Smith's proposals, such as the explicit mechanisms for reallocating funds generated via user charges and the NHIF to underserved areas. A constructive dialogue emerged between USAID and the Ministry, resulting an apparent consensus as to how a more equitable strategy for health financing could be developed.

Phase III (IBRD-II)

A two-week World Bank mission between May and July of 1989 resulted in a new Bank proposal (IBRD-II). IRBD-II proposed a reduction in user charges compared to IBRD-I; however, charges remained far above the levels envisaged by Abel-Smith and USAID (Mwabu and Mwangi 1986). The Bank did not accept the idea of reallocating funds generated via user charges from wealthier to poorer districts. More importantly, the Bank accepted only a partial restructuring of the NHIF. The 2 percent compulsory contribution from employees was agreed upon, but the Bank did not accept another 2 percent contribution by employers; they suggested instead a symbolic 0.2 percent. Furthermore, the Bank resisted the idea of reallocating funds from the NHIF to underserved areas. Insurance funds should, according to the Bank, follow the insured. The Bank also linked the outcome of the negotiations with the Kenyan government to prospects of future Bank loans, e.g., to the Kenyatta National Hospital, which was in need of infrastructural investment. Finally, the Bank imposed a deadline for finalization of the negotiations and implementation of recommendations of the end of August, 1989.

Dialogue between the Bank and USAID seemed to be quite intense before and during phase III. One outcome was that USAID changed its policy and presented a second proposal — "USAID II" — more in line with the Bank's IBRD-II. In USAID-II, the critical NHIF restructuring was postponed for further study (Dahlgren 1989a).

Phase IV (Cabinet)

The Kenyan Cabinet approved the Bank's proposal in August 1989. Changes were made, however, including major reductions in the in-patient fees and elimination of out-patient fees at the dispensary level (van der Moortele and van der Hoeven 1982). The new fee structure would begin in December, 1989. In the meantime, the Ministry of Health would work out the necessary administrative procedures, including criteria for waiving fees (Dahlgren 1989b).

Phase V (President Moi)

The final phase in the policy process was intervention by President Moi in early 1990, only one month after the introduction of the new fee structure. Responding to the reduced economic access to health services being experienced by the poor, the President made two major reductions in fee levels. In a Presidential directive on cost-sharing charges for women delivering babies, it was stated that "all mothers delivering babies in health centers and hospitals should only pay 20 kshs per day after delivery until they leave the hospital instead of the earlier charges of 50 and 100 kshs respectively" (Ollech 1990). A few weeks later, the President announced that the daily fee of 100 kshs for in-patient care at Kenyatta National Hospital should be reduced to 20 kshs. In so doing, the President established a fee level quite close to that considered realistic in Phase II.

In August 1990 President Moi, facing increasing public dissatisfaction, decided to abolish all new user charges at all public hospitals for inpatient as well as outpatient services.

Assessment of Alternative Strategies

An ex-ante assessment of the alternatives presented during these five phases is necessary in order to understand the impact of these alternatives in terms of the objectives of developing a new health financing strategy for Kenya.

Financing Objectives

Revenues anticipated from user charges in the different alternatives could not be estimated precisely because of difficulties in: (1) assessing people's ability to pay, (2) identifying the proportion of the population for which the user charges would be waived, and (3) estimating the administrative costs of managing user fees. Some evidence, however, suggested that increasing fees could significantly dampen the demand for health services. In one rural experiment in Kenya, for example, an increase in dispensary outpatient fees from 2 to 4 kshs reduced the demand for services by 50 percent (Abel-Smith 1989). Moreover, operational terms were needed to implement the waiving of fees. These computations were not included in any of the proposals. Information on the additional expenses for employment, training and supervision of the administrative staff needed to implement the user charge system was also unavailable.

The revenue implications of the NHIF restructuring were much easier to estimate, as Kenya's income structure is known and can serve as a basis for computing compulsory contributions to the NHIF. Abel-Smith (1989) noted that "about 3.85 million persons could be covered by such a scheme and the revenue (part of which would go to private hospitals) would be around half the recurrent expenditure of government health services." The challenging questions involved estimating how much of the insurance funds would be paid to private versus public health institutions, and to what extent, if any, funds could be reallocated to public health services.

Despite such uncertainties, it is possible to rank these options. Even if exact levels cannot be calculated, it is possible to estimate whether one alternative, *ceteris paribus*, would generate more financing than another. Table 16-2 presents the ranking of the five proposals in terms of their capacity to address diverse objectives. On strictly financial grounds, the most attractive alternative is the AS-USAID I proposal combining lower user charges with an expansion of the NHIF. The unrealistically high user charges of the IBRD-I option places second. The IBRD-II proposal is third, because the Bank did not accept the 2 percent employer contribution to the NHIF.

Table 16-2   Ranking of Recommendations of Phases I-V on the Basis of Criteria of Financing, Equality, Efficiency and Structural Improvements

Phases	Financing	Equity	Efficiency	Structural
I IBRD–I	2	5	5	5
II AS-USAID I	1	1	1	1
III IBRD–II	3	4	4	4
IV Cabinet	4	3	3	3
V* President Moi	5	2	2	2

* Ultimately selected

The Bank never stated explicitly why it had rejected these urgently needed NHIF resources from employers. The only written argument, one sentence in the final document, was that charging employers would create unemployment. This assumption was challenged by Abel-Smith, who observed, "The weight of evidence is that contributions levied on employers are rapidly passed on to employees particularly when there is inflation. Thus employers very quickly prevent them from increasing their costs. Making employees pay employers' contributions as well as their own in this way is likely to lead to less pressure for wage increases than making them pay for their health services as they use them. Thus, there is little force in the argument that employers' contributions lead to inflation or to a fall in employment" (1990). Moreover, several Kenyan economists supported employers contributions to the NHIF as real wages would soon be increased, the contribution would not spur inflation, and it was more equitable.

Informally, some Bank economists also argued that NHIF contributions from the government as an employer would raise taxes, which is against the government's tax policy. This argument was questionable, since the government itself had initially considered a 2 percent contribution to the NHIF from employers. One plausible explanation is that the Bank's tax policy, not the government's, was of crucial importance in its policy recommendations to the government.

Equity Objectives

Two different sets of questions are related to the equity objectives. The first set is: Who is paying for whom? To what extent, if any, are the wealthier groups paying for the poor or vice versa? User charges, as noted earlier, are regressive, while the NHIF approach could be progressive.

The second set of questions relates to access to health services. A distinction should be made between those who have no access and those with access to free or almost free services. The first group resides in underserved areas of the country. Introduction of user charges for non-existing services would be of marginal interest to them. The AS-USAID I proposal explicitly stated that funds from both user charges and the NHIF should be transferred from well-served to underserved areas. "IBRD-II" as well as Cabinet decision favored a model where 75 percent of the funds generated via user charges would remain at the institution collecting the money; only the remaining funds would be used for primary/preventive health care, and then only within the same district

(Dahlgren 1989b). Under these two schemes, the wealthier districts with more health facilities would retain their resources, while the poorer districts with few health institutions and a higher proportion of impoverished people would receive no public transfers.

These negative distributional effects could be counter-balanced at least partly by a reallocation of existing government funds from richer to poorer areas. Experience indicates, however, that given the political power of those with greater resources, this is generally not feasible. Furthermore, user fee funds were seen as additional to, not a replacement for, the normal government budget allocations. The possibility of reallocating funds among districts in the existing budget was limited.

Differences in abilities to pay fees among socioeconomic groups in diverse geographical locations is a major equity issue. Kenya's poor have a per-capita cash income of 100-200 kshs per month. They spend an average of 1-2 kshs per capita per month on modern health services, including drugs. Between 1981 and 1983, lower income groups in urban areas spent an average of 4 to 5 kshs per capita monthly on health services, compared to 19 kshs in middle income groups (Abel-Smith 1989). One can appreciate the additional burden of asking patients to pay 100 kshs for in-patient treatment at a district hospital. It is also in this context that the cumulative effects of inflation, reduced real wages, new and higher school fees, water tariffs and user charges for health services may be assessed. A family may have to sell land or animals to pay a hospital bill that it was forced to accept in its attempt to save the life of a child.

Together with UNICEF and USAID, the Ministry of Health tried to assess the ability to pay of different socio-economic groups. These findings were presented to the Bank at an early stage of phase IBRD-II. The final IBRD-II proposal did not even cite these findings. The Bank seemed to favor a wait-and-see approach, in which the reduction of access to health care would be monitored before any mitigating action would be considered. In terms of everyday life this meant that many would have to suffer, perhaps even die, before evidence sufficient to start a discussion was collected. Acting first and then, perhaps, mitigating the negative consequences of the actions taken is contrary both to common sense and to development theory. This includes the theories officially supported by the Bank, which stress the importance of integrating rather than separating economic and social objectives.

The Kenyan Cabinet/Ministry of Health managed to reduce, but remained far from eliminating, these risks of reduced access by lowering some of the fees proposed by the Bank. The fee for out-patient casualties, for example, was reduced from 100 to 20 kshs per visit at a provincial hospital (Mbiti 1989). However, the approved fee structure still included some very high rates. One was the in-patient fee at the only public hospital for highly specialized care: Kenyatta National Hospital (KNH). A fee of 100 kshs per day without maximum limits was approved, as proposed by the Bank. The average stay at KNH is 11 days, generating an average total cost of 1,100 kshs per stay. In a country where the majority of people earn less than half of this amount per month, the introduction of this fee level had to imply one of the following two consequences: either the fee would be waived for at least 70-80 percent of the patients, or only those able to pay the fee would be admitted for care at KNH.

Against this background, it may seem strange that the Cabinet/Ministry of Health did not reduce these unrealistically high in-patient fees. One probable reason was the likelihood of pressures from the Bank, which directly linked acceptance of these high fee levels to a subsequent loan for rehabilitation of the KNH. Regardless of the reasons for this decision, subsequent events showed that after the fees were introduced, President Moi was obligated to act to reduce the in-patient fee from 100 to 20 kshs per day.

Looking back, we see that the introduction of user fees had a profound effect on access and utilization. Even an in-patient fee of 20 kshs was too high for the poor. A leading Kenyan daily paper, *The Nation,* described the situation 6 weeks after the introduction of the new user charges: "General hospitals across the country, once notorious for over-crowding, now find themselves in the unfamiliar position of being deserted. It is not the illnesses which have mysteriously disappeared, it is the assumption that every sick person can afford 20 kshs which was way off the mark. The introduction of cost sharing therefore except in terminal cases, made the common illnesses a luxury. People simply choose not to seek treatment" (January 12, 1990). A few months later, the magazine *New African* reported that "patients are being locked up at hospitals after treatment for being unable to pay full fees." The official Kenyan policy, as expressed by the director of medical services, is "to treat the patients first and seek money later." As a result, the director has "found himself in the difficult position of having to ask hospital authorities to free patients who are being held for non-payment" (April 1990, p. 39).

Against this background, the ranking of the various alternatives in terms of equity objectives would clearly favor the AS-USAID-II plans (Table 16-2). President Moi's final decisions place second, with the others following. The IBRD proposals were last in terms of equity objectives.

Efficiency Objectives

The introduction of user charges may be used as a management tool. Improved efficiency was stressed in particular by the Bank, which argued that differentiated fees would reduce over-utilization of tertiary services and increase the utilization of primary care facilities.

One starting point for considering the effect of different strategies upon wasteful demand is to identify which groups are likely to overutilize health services. Focusing upon actual utilization in relation to need in various socio-economic groups, it can be postulated that the risk of demanding unnecessary services is greatest among affluent groups. In Kenya, the most affluent 4 percent of the population consume 25 percent of the recurrent cost of health care. The need for health care within this group, however, may be perhaps 5 to 10 times less than the need among the 30-35 percent of the population living at or below the poverty line.

The Bank's assumption that patients would be guided to the appropriate level of care by a differentiated fee structure may have been built upon questionable assumptions. Decisions regarding appropriate levels are made not only by individual consumers, but by professional care providers as well. The decision-making function of clinicians was not built into the Bank's assumptions. The introduction of higher fees for tertiary specialized in-patient care would have only a marginal effect on efficiency as it does not directly affect decisions concerning referrals made by doctors. From the patient's viewpoint, referral may be perceived as a kind of punishment for having a particular type of health problem. The Bank's proposals never distinguished between primary and secondary demands for health services. The health system was viewed as a producer of services to consumers. Consequently, the recommendation of differentiated fees to stimulate patients to select appropriate levels of care is like using a hammer to drive a screw. It is simply the wrong tool, as the instrument fails to focus upon those who make the decisions about referrals.

The Bank's proposals not only neglected the need to reduce over-utilization by affluent groups, they may have stimulated these groups to increase their demand for scarce health resources. Increasing the demands of the affluent was built into the proposal to increase the NHIF reimbursement to private hospitals. In spite of its general "wait and study" attitude toward changes in the public insurance system, the Bank had no hesitation in shifting additional funds to the private sector.

Against this background, the Kenyan Government in the second half of 1989 decided to use the NHIF surplus to double reimbursements to private health care providers, including expensive private commercial hospitals. Unlike reallocating these funds to primary health care in underserved areas, this action increased unnecessary demand, thus reducing cost-effectiveness. Moreover, the efficiency of private hospitals is not directly influenced by these reimbursement shifts. Directing additional funds to rural health programs is, on the other hand, very likely to increase efficiency. Such a move both frees under-utilized manpower by providing funds for various field activities and reduces capital wastage by providing funds for the maintenance of cars, equipment and buildings.

The policy of the Bank can best be described as a missed opportunity for increasing efficiency. Ranking the alternatives assessed in terms of efficiency is very difficult, but the Abel-Smith/USAID-I probably would have generated the greatest efficiency, followed by President Moi's decisions (Table 16-2).

Health Service Structure

Kenya's official policy, as expressed in development plans, is to strengthen rural primary care by reallocating funds from hospitals to rural health centers. The reality has been, as in so many other countries with the same policy, a growing gap between well-served and under-served areas and between specialized hospitals and primary health care services. The professional and political power structure simply does not reflect plans or rhetoric when general policies are transformed into actual budgets and services.

A new financial system, based partly on user charges and funds from the NHIF, offers fresh opportunities for achieving the stated objectives, as it is easier to allocate new funds than to reallocate existing funds. Both USAID and Abel-Smith proposed a system for directly reallocating funds to under-served rural health services. In spite of this, the Bank favored a system where all funds generated in a district would remain in that district. No mechanisms for reallocating funds from better-off to poorer districts was considered. This was the Bank's position despite the fact that almost half of the Kenyan population had no, or very limited, geographical access to any form of modern health care. The Kenyan Cabinet and Ministry of Health followed the Bank's recommendation.

The ranking of alternatives in terms of reducing gaps between urban-rural, rich-poor, curative-preventive, and primary-tertiary can thus be summarized as follows. Again, the Phase II proposals of Abel-Smith and USAID receive top rank, followed by President Moi's decisions. The Bank schemes fare the worse in terms of efficiency (Table 16-2).

Conclusion

The AS-USAID I proposals receive the highest ranking on all four objectives. Trade-offs between the diverse objectives did not seem to be necessary. On the basis of this analysis, the two Bank proposals receive the lowest ranking. Considering the fact that all parties were in consensus regarding the explicit objectives, other explanations must be sought to explain the positions adopted and the actual policy process.

One way to understand the Bank's approach is to attempt to derive its implicit objectives by considering the likely consequences of proposed policies. Those policies primarily benefited the middle and high income groups rather than the poor majority of Kenyans. For example, if combined with quality improvements, the introduction of high user charges at the Kenyatta National Hospital offered an opportunity for better-off groups to obtain high quality subsidized specialized care at a lower price than presently offered by private commercial hospitals. For the poor it meant that tax-based subsidies to public health services enjoyed by the rich would be increased, at the same time that they experienced a dramatic decline in access to needed specialized care.

The Bank policy of blocking the transfer of user charge funds from richer to poorer provinces favored the rich. Blocking the transfer of NHIF funds to public health services would "safeguard" the better-off from providing subsidies to less fortunate groups. Moreover, increasing NHIF reimbursements to private for-profit hospitals would reduce direct costs for hospital care for those who can afford to use the services offered. This reduction of direct fees for the wealthiest groups would be partly financed by low and middle-income groups who cannot afford to use these services. The introduction of a differentiated fee structure at various levels of care meant that the wealthiest Kenyans could obtain desired care without having to compete, on the basis of medical or economic need, with poorer patients unable to pay the fees.

The Bank policy of improving public health services primarily for those who can afford to pay the new charges could also be combined with the objective of "freezing" the recurrent budget for the health sector. Consequently, the Bank policy seems to be logical and efficient in terms of improving the quality and reducing the costs of health services for fairly privileged groups. The weakness of the Bank proposal was that it did not advance these measures for the less well-off. The policies developed by Abel-Smith and by USAID were more equitable, and satisfactory in terms of the other objectives as well.

The policy finally adopted by the Kenyan Government may be described as a second-best solution. The reason for choosing the second-best alternative, not the best, was presumably the power of the Bank. This power is largely derived from the fact that negotiations about health financing are integral parts of an overall structural adjustment program designed by the Bank and the International Monetary Fund. Considering these external factors, it is a remarkable sign of strength from a Kenyan perspective that the financial strategy ultimately adopted was a second-best alternative, scoring much higher than the Bank's proposals on equity, efficiency and structural objectives.

The price to be paid by the Kenyan Government for attaining a second-best outcome is the low revenue it will generate. This is because the government had to accept that the NHIF funds could neither be increased by a "2% contribution" from employers nor be partly reallocated to the public health sector. The Cabinet and Ministry of Health, then President Moi, recognized the necessity of securing the equity objectives. Thus their only real option, without a way of increasing the revenue base through NHIF, was to reduce proposed user charges.

Acknowledgement

An earlier version of this chapter was published in the *Scandinavian Journal of Social Medicine,* 46 (Suppl):67-81, 1990.

References

Abel-Smith, B. 1989. "Issues and options in health financing." Discussion paper. Nairobi, January.

Abel-Smith, B. 1990. Comments to G. Dahlgren via fax April 20.

Dahlgren, G. 1989a. World Bank Aide Memoir on Health Financing (draft 11.5.89): Some comments and recommendations. Nairobi, Ministry of Health, Internal Working Paper.

Dahlgren, G. 1989b. United States Agency for International Development Kenya Health Care Financing (KHFC) Programme: Some brief comments. Nairobi, Ministry of Health, Internal Working Paper.

Godfrey, M. 1986. "Kenya to 1990: Prospects for growth." Economic Intelligence Unit, London.

Mbiti, D.M. 1980. Permanent secretary, Ministry of Health "Re: Cost sharing policy." (Ref No B/13/1) 18A. 30 October.

Mwabu, G.H., and W.M. Mwangi. 1986. "Health care financing in Kenya: A simulation of welfare effects of user fees." *Social Science and Medicine,* 22(7): 763–767.

Odada, J.E.O., and A.B. Ayako. 1988. "The impact of structural adjustments policies on the well being of the vulnerable groups in Kenya, Nairobi." UNICEF Kenya Country Office and Kenyan Economic Association.

Ollech, J.S. 1990. Presidential directive on cost sharing charges for delivering mothers, 24th January. Office of the Director of Medical Services.

Van de Moortele, J., and R. van der Hoeven. 1982. "Income distribution and consumption patterns in urban and rural Kenya by socio-economic groups." World Employment Programme Research Working Paper WEP I: 32/WP 46. Geneva: International Labour Organization.

———.1990. "Medical fees pays for the drugs also". *Daily Nation,* January 12.

17

Promoting Health: Implications for Modern and Developing Nations

David Mechanic

Promoting Health

Health promotion has become very fashionable. At a major conference in Berlin on this topic, Dr. Halfdon Mahler, Director-General Emeritus of the World Health Organization, was only one of a number of speakers at the first evening's plenary session who reiterated the need for more attention to improved lifestyles, particularly in such areas as smoking, drinking, nutrition, and exercise. The session then adjourned to dinner festivities that featured liquor and beer, salted snacks, and a variety of bratwursts. This instance would be unworthy of comment except that it typifies the enormous gap between our rhetoric and our behavior, and helps to highlight the challenge that serious health promotion efforts must face.

The main point of this paper is simple but crucial: most behavior, whether conducive or detrimental to health, is influenced as much or more by the routine organization of everyday settings and activities as by the personal decisions of individuals. Health education efforts that ignore this principle are destined to fail.

The Status of Health Promotion

American society places a high value on health. We see this in public attitudes, in the more than half-trillion dollars per year expended for health services, and in the immense interest reflected in the media. Health consciousness has been growing in this country since the 1970s. Efforts to induce an increased sense of personal responsibility for physical fitness and improved behaviors in health-related areas have also been increasing. These developments are in part motivated by the uncontrollable escalation of medical care costs (Lalonde 1974; Knowles 1977; United States Assistant Secretary for Health 1979).

Whether we consider education campaigns directed toward cigarette smoking, alcohol and drug use, or those devoted to exercise, nutrition, and safety, it is clear that health promotion has become a growth industry. The threat of the AIDS epidemic and its close link to personal sexual and drug use behavior reinforce the shared view that individuals play a major role in their own destinies and can, through personal action or restraint, shape their vitality, their health, and their longevity.

The elimination of noxious habits and other known risk factors must have some impact on those involved. But health education campaigns are commonly ineffective. When they do succeed in changing behavior, the change usually lasts only for a limited time. Yet both the faith and the potential persist, and there have been some notable successes. A good example is the impressive drop in cigarette smoking among men — from 52% to 32% from 1965-87 (Centers for Disease Control 1989, p. 96). The comparable decrease for women, from 34% to 27%, is more disappointing, given the enormous effort and attention devoted to the smoking issue.

In other areas, such as alcohol consumption, drug use, excess weight, high risk cholesterol levels, and even blood pressure control, the progress achieved is even less impressive. In still other areas, such as homicide, adolescent pregnancy, and suicide, we have made no progress, or worse, lost ground over the past 40 years. The age-adjusted death rate for homicides, for example, increased from 5.4 to 9 deaths per 100,000 residents between 1950 and 1986 (Centers for Disease Control 1989, p. 62).

It would be foolish to place too much faith in the capacity of health education as we know it to contain high risk behaviors, morbidity, and mortality. The determinants of health risks are far too complex and powerful to succumb simply to ordinary efforts to change the practices of the public through information. Effective health promotion will require deeper scrutiny of the structure of communities and the routine activities of everyday life. Stronger interventions than current efforts, whose effects are marginal, will also be needed.

The Importance of Group Structure

Almost one hundred years ago, Emile Durkheim published his classic study of suicide, in which he examined the links between suicide rates and the social constraints characteristic of varying situations and groups (Durkheim 1951 [translation]). He identified two processes that were associated with suicide, but in somewhat different ways. First, a loosening of social constraints, whether characteristic of egoistic suicide or anomie, was linked to elevated rates. Alternatively, a high level of social integration associated with a tradition of ritualistic suicide in response to duty could also lead to high rates.

Durkheim's insights into how group structures constrain individual behavior are important for developing appropriate strategies for change. The strength of the individual's ties to the immediate social context determines the scope of influence exercised by that context over behavior. As the level of social integration diminishes, the group — whether family, neighborhood, or larger social entity — is less successful in enforcing its expectations. When group commitment and social integration is strong, the specific norms characteristic of the group and its normal settings shape the boundaries of permissible behavior and define the limits of deviance.

Most of the behaviors we view as health relevant are in daily structures and routines. The regularity of daily functions, such as eating and sleeping habits, routine exercise and levels of exertion, and many more, are substantially programmed for us. The norms of our social contexts also define the appropriateness of a wide range of risk behaviors and the circumstances under which such behaviors are permitted. Expectations, and the shame of nonconformity, set the standards for our efforts and motivate our achievements. These very basic group structures and processes account for much of the behavior we observe.

Explaining Health Indicator Trends

The relevance of social relationships for explaining patterns of morbidity and mortality is well documented. Personal attachments consistently predict mortality in both sexes, even after adjusting for other risk factors known to affect death. The magnitudes of these relationships are comparable to those cited by the Surgeon General in his 1964 report linking cigarette smoking with disease and death (House, Landis, and Umberson 1988). The specific mechanisms, and how they function, are not well understood. But an appreciation of the ways in which individuals are tied to social structures, and an understanding of how groups exercise influence, help to explain a variety of seemingly unrelated findings in the health care literature.

Disease causation is multifaceted and complex. There is a compelling need to separate selection from true causal factors, and to disentangle many interrelated influences. Yet, it is intriguing that such measures as socioeconomic status, marital status, and religiosity and church attendance are consistently associated with health outcome measures (Mechanic 1978; Zuckerman, Kasl and Ostfeld 1984; Levin and Vanderpool 1987). A particularly important challenge is to clarify the association between indices of low socioeconomic status and poor health (Henry J. Kaiser Family Foundation 1989). The fact that many subgroups in the population have favorable health experiences despite low socioeconomic status suggests that poverty is not a sufficient explanation.

While the relationships noted above involve a variety of interpretative issues, they have an underlying factor in common. In each case, those with the poorest health experiences come from disrupted social settings. They are less constrained, or protected, by family and community expectations. Such indicators as marriage, religiosity, church attendance, community participation, and higher socioeconomic status may have varying meanings and impacts, but they all imply a certain conventionality and regularity in style of living. In contrast, high rates of morbidity and mortality among the divorced, the socially alienated, the lowest socioeconomic strata, and among disadvantaged minority groups in part reflect the loss of authority of the family and the neighborhood over behavior. Family disruption removes many of the constraints on living that give daily life a predictable rhythm.

Women have benefited greatly from increased education and growing equality. But the relaxing of cultural constraints on women brought about by gender equality has also meant that they have equal opportunity for good and bad. As a consequence, women drink and smoke more than in previous decades and more commonly confront such problems as lung disease and alcoholism. Age-adjusted death rates among white women in the United States for cancer of the respiratory system rose from 4.6 per 100,000 in 1950 to 23.1 per 100,000 in 1986, surpassing the rate for breast cancer. Rates of death from chronic obstructive pulmonary disease (COPD) increased from 2.8 to 13.3 per 100,000 during this same period.

For black women, the data are similar. The death rate from respiratory cancer among black females rose from 4.1 per 100,000 in 1950 to 23.3 per 100,000 in 1986. Black female deaths from COPD are also rising, although the information available is less complete.

Ironically, these increases come during a period when the overall death rate for women has declined substantially. The age-adjusted overall death rate for white women decreased from 645 to 388 between 1950 and 1986, while the comparable rates for black women decreased from 1107 to 588. Only two major causes of death besides respiratory cancer and COPD have not substantially decreased; these are suicide and homicide. In fact, rates of death from homicide among white women doubled between 1950 and 1986 (Centers for Disease Control 1989, pp. 62-63).

The Constraints of Culture

In his classic book, *Who Shall Live?*, Victor Fuchs (1974) explains the huge difference in death rates between the contiguous states of Utah and Nevada. He points out:

> Utah is inhabited primarily by Mormons, whose influence is strong throughout the state. Devout Mormons do not use tobacco or alcohol and in general lead stable, quiet lives. Nevada, on the other hand, is a state with high rates of cigarette and alcohol consumption and very high indices of marital and geographic instability (p. 53).

Fuchs goes on to show that the two states are comparable on many of the indices associated with mortality, such as income and schooling. They are also similar in terms of climate, urbanization, and concentration of health care resources.

Fuchs is surely correct in a general sense. However, Mormonism and its influence encompass a variety of features that not only affect health indices but are also related to other factors, e.g., low rates of delinquency, crime, and violence; high educational achievement; and a purposeful orientation. In these respects, Mormons are not unlike other cultural groups, such as Jews, Chinese, and Japanese, who also perform well on many health and welfare indices.

Like other groups with good health indices, Mormons have a strong kinship structure. This structure serves as a solid base for childhood socialization, and fosters a positive attitude toward education. It also creates an ethic that gives work a meaningful place in the group's value structure.

The Mormon church teaches the importance of family, parenthood, and family relationships, while also encouraging a strong orientation toward mastery of the environment. Active effort and accomplishment, together with the acquisition of skills and education, are emphasized.

The following excerpt, from T.F. O'Dea's *The Mormons* (1957), illustrates:

> Life is more than a vocation, more than a calling; it is an opportunity for deification through conquest, which is to be won through rational mastery of the environment and obedience to the ordinances of the church. This doctrine, permeating individual and community life, is expressed today in a configuration of attitudes clustering around activity and development. This configuration represents an important aspect of the individual's integration into the life of the Mormon group, or it relates the striving of individuals to collectively prescribed ends. Moreover, since it is taught by exhortation and example from early childhood, this set of attitudes becomes second nature to those brought up in the Mormon home and community environment (O'Dea: 143-44).

Mormons have good health not simply because they value health and refrain from smoking and drinking. Their health also derives in part from daily routines evolving out of accepted patterns of everyday living — family, work, and play.

The presence of a well-knit group structure that demands a person's loyalty and commitment is, however, only an enabling factor. More important are the particular values, goals, and preferences that are taught and rewarded. For example, early studies of medical care utilization among ethnic groups in New York City found that ethnic exclusivity and cohesiveness resulted in greater skepticism of medical care (Suchman 1964, 1965). In contrast, a similar study focusing on Mormons suggests that a cohesive group structure may encourage high acceptance and use of medical services (Geertsen, Klauber, Rindflesh et al. 1975). Group structures provide a basis for influence, but it is the content of values that shapes behaviors.

Socioeconomic Status, Race, and Health

Socioeconomic status (SES) and race are associated with almost every health index, and these relations have received much attention (Henry J. Kaiser, Family Foundation 1989). While aggregate associations are important, it is essential to identify those specific factors linked to SES and race that account for observed relationships. Many disadvantaged subgroups perform well on important measures of health and well-being despite low incomes and limited education. For example, immigrants to the United States early in this century generally had high rates of infant mortality relative to native born whites. But as Anderson (1958) noted:

> Even though the Jewish group was foreign-born, lived in as crowded conditions as other foreign-born, bore just as many children...and enjoyed an income which was much lower than that of native born whites, this group experienced the lowest infant mortality of all groups (p.21).

Some of this effect may have been due to breastfeeding, which was more prevalent among Jewish mothers. But concern for the health of children and a resulting solicitude within traditional Jewish culture also have been commonly noted (Mechanic 1963; Zborowski and Herzog 1952). As in the case of Mormons, a strong family structure and an emphasis on children and their development have contributed not only to health awareness, but also to educational and occupational achievement.

Thus health outcomes are substantially dependent on patterns of family life and social participation and on the structuring of everyday activities. The aggregate associations between SES and health summarize the product of many different processes pertinent to both. Effective action therefore requires a better understanding of the underlying patterns of relationships that result in these correlations.

Cross-national Considerations

The United States and other developed countries have reached relatively high levels of health and longevity compared to most underdeveloped and developing nations. Thus, the factors essential to enhancing health and longevity may not be as apparent in developed societies as in other regions of the world. The fact that large variations in health and mortality exist among poor nations allows us to better understand broad influences. Developing countries that have achieved levels of life expectancy at birth approaching those of developed nations are those that have been generally successful in reducing fertility and infant mortality and in improving child health.

Caldwell (1986) has identified several areas with low per capita GNP but exceptional success in reducing infant mortality. In his analysis, he focuses on four states and countries that have low infant mortality relative to income — Kerala (India), Sri Lanka, Costa Rica, and Jamaica. Caldwell also discusses countries, like China and Cuba, that have used aggressive political organization to reduce infant mortality through the establishment of an institutional infrastructure for maternal and infant health. For our immediate analytic purposes, the former examples are more important than the latter, although the existence of alternative pathways to achieving varying health targets is worth noting.

As health is multidimensional, an active, motivated population is especially important for achieving favorable health status. In this respect, Caldwell finds female schooling to be a particularly crucial element in the health equation. Those countries with a high proportion of females in primary school in 1960 had the lowest infant mortality rates and the highest expectation of life at birth in 1982. In contrast, those countries with the poorest mortality outcomes were Islamic nations, where contact between the sexes has traditionally been discouraged and where strong constraints have typically been placed on the social participation of women outside the household. Compared to the poor nations that achieved good health, some of these countries (Saudi Arabia, Libya, Iraq, Iran, Oman) are relatively affluent, indicating that wealth is no more than a potential enabling factor.

Female education is a complex indicator. Part of the reason for this is that in many of the countries studied, levels of schooling are modest by Western standards. Caldwell places great emphasis on the position of women, their levels of autonomy, and their political participation, each of which is associated with female education. He also notes that education and accessibility of health facilities are a powerful combination in reducing infant mortality.

The fact that education has also been an important predictor of health outcomes in Western countries is another indication that this variable should be examined more closely. The relationship of education to various health behaviors and outcomes appears to be linear, even at relatively high educational levels.

Why is Education Important?

Education is the single most important determinant of "psychological modernity." Persons who have developed attitudes of "psychological modernity," in Alex Inkeles' terms, take on "new transformative roles within their societies and in their more immediate social networks." Such persons:

> ...adopt different social roles than do their less modern country-
> men. They are more active in voluntary organizations and

participate more in politics; they practice birth control more regularly and have fewer children as a result; they are quicker to adopt innovative practices in agriculture and are more productive as workers in industry; they keep their children longer in school and encourage them to take up more technical occupations; and in general, they press more actively for social change (Inkeles 1983:26-27).

Inkeles argues that schooling imparts the attitudes, values and psychological dispositions essential to psychological modernity. In his view, however, much of this learning occurs not as a result of the formal curriculum, but rather through ordered sequences of activities, role modeling, and other psychosocial processes that are inherent in the structure of the classroom situation (Inkeles and Smith 1974:140-42). Inkeles' concerns are directed toward modernization in the developing countries, but it should be clear that the concept of psychological modernity applies to problems in modern nations as well.

Schooling is particularly important because of its association with a wide range of psychosocial and interactional capacities, including cognitive complexity, self-concept, active coping, self-efficacy, openness to information, and the conceptual skills required for managing information (Mechanic 1989). Persons with more schooling not only have greater knowledge, but are inclined to acquire more. Also, when presented with information, they show higher levels of acquisition than the less educated (Feldman 1966). Spaeth (1976) has argued that socioeconomic levels are indicators of cognitive complexity, and that children exposed to better educated models, whether parents or teachers, learn to cope actively with complex stimuli.

Although the schooling variable points to options for possible interventions, it also has limitations. As an enabling factor, schooling facilitates a variety of outcomes. Its consequences, however, are dependent on values that may be exogenous. In developing countries, schooling is associated with increased female autonomy, control of fertility, and a higher quality of prenatal and infant care. But in modern societies, female autonomy may be associated with a variety of increased health risks, such as smoking or use of alcohol and drugs. This suggests the complexity of causal pathways.

Furthermore, experience in modern nations amply demonstrates that getting children to school doesn't necessarily mean they will find there a culture that promotes values of academic achievement, skill acquisition, or positive health behavior. Schooling is a measure of exposure, but in some contexts it remains a "black box."

Finally, the process of school entry, progression and attrition is a complex social selection process that may result in our mistakenly attributing more influence to the content of schooling than to the capacities, personal characteristics, and values of families that persist in keeping children in school despite economic and other costs.

The foregoing suggests, at very least, a two-stage process of enablement and action. Schooling establishes the conditions for positive health by encouraging an active and informed orientation to the environment. Education fosters the ability to use information and plan for the effective implementation of values and intentions. But the active inclinations that schooling induces should be separated from the values or instruction that push these inclinations in one direction or another. Encouraging psychological modernity through schooling and other means, shaping values and preferences in health relevant directions, and providing the accessible services necessary for effective prevention and care are distinct objectives that require separate initiatives. In combination, they offer a powerful mechanism for promoting positive health outcomes.

Practical Implications

A difficulty with the type of analysis presented here is that its focus on deeper dimensions of culture and social structure leaves the practitioner initially frustrated. Practitioners are quite comfortable launching an anti-smoking or good nutrition campaign, but have no idea how to initiate culture change or modify social structure. Admittedly, these are difficult challenges, requiring a relatively long time perspective. But thinking at this broader level allows us to build more effective strategies that integrate our efforts in a synergistic way. The alternative is to accept fragmented, and largely unsuccessful, individual efforts.

Culture change requires collective action. It depends on the principles by which social movements become established and innovations diffuse among populations. The process itself involves several interrelated requirements. First, there must be an agenda — a set of ideas and practices seen as conducive to some valued goal. The presence of credible innovators who model the desired practices is a second requirement. Third, there has to be some motivating force, shared by the larger target population, that can encourage adoption of the new practices. Reinforcers, who sustain a new practice until it becomes part of the natural flow of everyday activities, represent the final step in the process.

In many instances, there may be strong forces working against behavior change. Many behaviors detrimental to health offer immediate short-term rewards. Or they may be so integrated into current cultural practices that they are inadvertently reinforced in normal, day-to-day life. Under these circumstances they will be strongly resistant to change.

Often, harmful behaviors are also sustained by powerful economic interests that promote their perpetuation. In the case of smoking, for example, even the sustained and well-publicized efforts at reduction pale in comparison to the well-financed and strategically targeted advertising campaigns encouraging this behavior (Warner 1985).

In fact, as noted earlier, the recent campaign to reduce smoking may be considered reasonably successful in light of the intense advertising efforts of the industry. It is impossible to untangle the influences that have resulted in lower tobacco consumption, but it is clear that changes at the cultural level, as well as the level of individual behavior, are involved. Smoking has been prohibited in many public places and restricted in public transportation, restaurants, and workplaces. Moreover, social norms have been modified sufficiently to put smokers on the defensive. It is no longer embarrassing to ask people not to smoke in social settings, and smokers increasingly are made to feel apologetic about their behavior. Such normative changes may not induce many people to give up cigarettes, but they will probably change the frequency and context of smoking, making it easier for those who do want to quit.

Perhaps most important is the fact that young people are growing up in contexts where they sense increasing disapproval of smoking. This may serve as a deterrent to initiating the behavior.

Other types of behavior, such as the use of alcohol, are so much a part of social gatherings that participants feel strong inducements to partici-pate even if they prefer not to. Drink is associated with occasions of conviviality and recreation, serving as a lubricant for sociability. More-over, the tendency to consume alcohol at parties, taverns, athletic events, and the like virtually ensures that drinking will be associated with driving. While such devices as collecting car keys at teenage parties or using designated drivers for partying groups may be marginally beneficial, the organization of social life does much to induce and sustain drinking and to link drinking with driving.

Nutrition is a third area where forces working to counteract health-promoting behaviors may be observed. Both the fast food industry and increasing preferences for eating outside the home encourage less than optimal practices. Some changes in restaurant fare are evident, such as low-calorie and low-salt meals, more salads, and a greater variety of fish. The fact remains, however, that it takes considerable awareness and conscious effort to practice good nutritional behavior in these contexts. Any set of practices that requires vigilance and effort is not likely to be consistently sustained.

What has been briefly noted about smoking, drinking, or nutrition can also be said about almost any common behavior that is immediately rewarding but detrimental to health. These behaviors flourish in contexts that routinely sustain them. Usually efforts at resistance require vigilance and conscious choice. The challenge is therefore to alter the balance of influences by defining points of leverage that can redirect the flow of everyday activities in more positive directions. This requires coordinated programs with interventions that are regulatory, technological, and educational.

Our culture generally resists the regulation of personal choice. It is clear, however, that the consumption of harmful substances is facilitated by ease of access. Cigarettes available through self-serve machines are more accessible to youngsters than those purchased over the counter (Altman et al. 1989). The age at which drivers' licenses may be obtained is linked to injury and death (Robertson 1983). Taxes on alcohol and cigarettes affect levels of consumption (Cook 1981; Lewit and Coate 1982; Harris 1982). Thus, a reluctance to prohibit access notwithstanding, regulations restricting accessibility remain viable options. These regulations are likely to have the greatest effect on youth, who are, after all, the proper targets of such efforts.

Good health practices can be promoted independently of conscious positive health behavior by incorporating them into technology. We are all familiar with inflatable air bags and involuntary seat belts, safe cigarettes, low-salt food products, and fireproof clothing. The success of such technical approaches to reducing risk depends on their cost and their acceptability to consumers. Much more could be done to develop health-promoting technologies and potential markets for such products. Industry is extraordinarily adaptive in responding to consumer demands. Encouraging the development and expansion of health-enhancing products and activities should therefore be part of any long-range strategy for change.

Health educators seek interventions that will motivate individuals to take responsibility for their health. This task is complicated by the fact that health-related behaviors are a product of many different motives and processes.

Health-related behaviors typically are only loosely associated and may, in some instances, be negatively correlated (Mechanic 1979; Mechanic and Cleary 1980:808). For example, exercise has been shown to be linked to behaviors that put an individual at risk for ill health — both possibly influenced by an underlying activity factor.

Despite this, there is consistent evidence that well-integrated group settings that encourage positive health behaviors have far-reaching impact. Also, affective factors are powerful reinforcers of cognitive processes. In our studies of adolescents, we find that young people's perceptions of how much their parents care about them are better predictors of positive health behavior than specific admonitions or even parents' health behavior. Most parents care deeply about their children, and most parents, regardless of their own habits, want their children to avoid behavior that is obviously dangerous. Most people, at least on a cognitive level, understand the risks of smoking, drinking, and drug use, and most youngsters share this awareness. Feelings of acceptance and love in a context that defines these behaviors as damaging seem to help insulate young people from many unacceptable behaviors.

We live in a culture where health is an important shared value and where there is much readily available health information. Those with more conceptual skills assimilate information and use it more wisely than those with fewer skills. Conceptual skills not only make complex information more understandable, they also give individuals the resources to plan and use information aggressively. The acquisition of conceptual skills, like other behaviors, is facilitated by group expectations and influences (Bock and Moore 1986).

We have no assurance that the improvement of conceptual skills will in itself enhance health. However, such improvement has benefits that transcend health concerns. As an indirect influence, improved general education may do more to promote the subcultures and health goals that we seek than many of the public information campaigns designed to shape specific behaviors in a particular way.

Psychological Modernity and Health Behavior in Developing Countries

Inkeles (1983) has defined the essence of "psychological modernity" as follows:

> Central to this syndrome are: (1) openness to new experience, both with people and with new ways of doing things such as attempting to control births; (2) the assertion of increasing independence from the authority of traditional figures, such as parents and priests, and a shift of allegiance to leaders of government, public affairs, trade unions, cooperatives, and the like; (3) belief in the efficacy of science and medicine, and a general abandonment of passivity and fatalism in the face of life's difficulties; and (4) ambition for oneself and one's children to achieve high occupational and educational goals. Men who manifest these characteristics (5) like people to be on time and show an interest in carefully planning their affairs in advance. It is also part of this syndrome (6) to show strong interest and take an active part in civic and community affars and local politics; and (7) to strive energetically to keep up with the news, and within this effort to prefer news of national and international import over items dealing with sports, religion, or purely local affairs (p. 101).

Both the concept of psychological modernity and the pragmatic indicators used to operationalize it in research have been subjects of debate. Despite disagreement about particulars, however, the concept appears to tap an orientation of significance. Health behavior can be thought of as having four underlying components: motivation, cognition, an activity pattern, and affect.

The cognitive component reflects the individual's meaning system and beliefs. In the case of psychological modernity, cognitive components include an orientation toward planning for the future and a belief in the efficacy of science, technology, and medicine.

At the motivational level, psychologically modern persons tend to be open to new experiences and innovative practices. They have ambitions for themselves and their children, and they seek to maintain a reasonable independence from traditional society. They think for themselves.

At the activity level, persons with a modern orientation engage issues, organize their lives around time and schedules, participate in civic and community affairs and local politics, keep up with the news, and press for social changes. They also activate their orientation toward planning in significant ways, as evidenced in the practice of birth control and planned family growth.

The role of affect in modernity is less clear. However, there is considerable evidence to support the motivating role of affect. Affect also triggers the enactment of important health behavior sequences.

There is considerable convergence in the research literature among concepts seeking to measure the extent to which individuals control, or believe themselves to control, their environments: mastery, self-efficacy, locus of control, and helplessness (in this instance, its obverse). Control over the environment is typically manifested through a thought-plan-action sequence. The lack of a plan often inhibits the expression of intention. When a plan exists, its enactment tends to be facilitated by arousal, or affect, which contributes to motivation. For example, Leventhal (1970) has noted that fear is a motivating factor when individuals know how to cope (i.e., have a plan). Without a plan, high fear often leads to denial and inaction. Thus, the plan is the map for coping, but a motivational impetus is necessary to activate it. This helps to explain why publicity about a well-known person's illness often leads to help-seeking on the part of those who fear they may have a similar condition.

It is useful to think of health care improvement in developing countries as a process that takes place in various stages. In the initial stage, educational and public health measures are directed at infectious and communicable diseases that can be reduced through appropriate interventions. These include insuring a safe source of water, appropriate management of waste products, adequate sanitation, and the application of preventive health care (prenatal care, safe childbirth practices, immunization, and appropriate infant nutrition). Since these interventions are relatively focused and effective, impressive advances can occur relatively quickly. These are indexed by sharp reductions in infant, child, and maternal mortality. The implementation of the first stage usually requires some degree of community mobilization and a primary health care system that is accessible and oriented to public health practice. Some degree of "psychological modernity" is also necessary if the population is to be motivated to use primary health care facilities, cooperate in care, and adhere to advice and instruction. However, the necessary level of modernity and the educational experience needed to produce it are relatively modest if the system of primary care is economically, physically, and culturally accessible and if it maintains a preventive orientation with aggressive community outreach. A strong psychological modernity orientation can overcome an inefficiently organized primary care system, but a well-organized system of care can have impressive results, even in highly traditional contexts.

The second stage of the health transition encompasses a broader range of the life cycle, a multiplicity of diseases with varying causes, and less proven social and technological interventions. Accordingly, it poses more difficult challenges. Here the goal is to add increments of health and increased longevity at various points in the life cycle, including old age. The instruments to be employed are both more varied and less well understood. Moreover, interventions directed toward later life stages, such as those related to diet, work and environmental dangers, accidents, and high risk behaviors, have much broader economic implications and often involve competing priorities. At any given level of economic development, progress in the second stage is likely to depend in a much deeper sense on the degree of "psychological modernity".

In many areas of the world, efforts to promote even the initial stage of health improvement remain underdeveloped. This situation is a reflection of extreme poverty, poor access to basic public health and preventive health care services, and highly traditional cultures that pose major barriers to health innovations. Cultural patterns that inhibit female education and social participation, and discriminate against females with respect to nutrition, medical care and schooling, are formidable problems. These patterns are typically quite resistant to change techniques outside the context of significant economic development and modernization.

Not much is known about how to effectively introduce modern medical and fertility planning in these contexts or about which approaches are most persuasive when fertility control challenges important principles of traditional culture. This is probably one reason education is such a powerful proxy for modernization. Schooling offers an alternative to the traditional culture while also teaching some of the habits and skills essential for participation in a more modern social system.

We might conceive of the fulfillment of a particular health objective as the endpoint on a continuum that involves a variety of barriers. These barriers may entail tangible costs, such as embarrassment, stigma, or social distance. They might be modified either by reconceptualizing the organization of service delivery (e.g., through improved physical access, outreach, and increased sensitivity to cultural concerns), or by teaching individuals the confidence and skills they need to overcome roadblocks to appropriate care. While the latter approach might seem preferable, the former is probably more readily achieved in the short run.

But even with the organizational approach, there is a need for a clear understanding of how notions of health and illness are constructed in varying cultural circumstances, how attributions are made about cause and threat, and how meanings are assigned. This requires some local anthropology to assess how misunderstanding can best be avoided, how behavioral modifications might best be achieved, and what types of indigenous networks might be mobilized to accomplish health objectives.

In sum, an examination of some of the evidence concerning health promoting processes points to the importance of understanding how to bolster group influences in the direction of health-enhancing values. An appreciation of how our lives are patterned by the structure of everyday expectations and activities is particularly crucial. It is undoubtedly true that individual motivation to improve health is important. However, many influences on behavior are less conscious and, perhaps, less obvious, by virtue of being routine. Health actions that must depend on persistent conscious motivation are unlikely to succeed in the long course. But once imprinted on our habits and routines, they are likely to be effective regardless of where we direct our attention.

Acknowledgements

Sections of this chapter are adapted from the author's "Promoting Health," *Society,* January/February 1990, and are republished with permission of Transaction Press.

References

Altman, D., V. Foster, L. Rousenick-Douss, and J. Tye. 1989. "Reducing the illegal sale of cigarettes to minors." *Journal of the American Medical Association,* 261: 80–83.

Anderson, O.W. 1958. "Infant mortality and social and cultural factors: Historical trends and current patterns." In E.G. Jaco, ed. *Patients, Physicians and Illness: A Sourcebook in Behavioral Science and Health.* New York: Free Press.

Bock, D.R., and E.G.J. Moore. 1986. *Advantage and Disadvantage: A Profile of American Youth.* Hillsdale, NJ: Lawrence Erlbaum Associates.

Caldwell, J.C. 1986. "Routes to low mortality in poor countries." *Population and Development Review*, 12: 171–220.

Centers for Disease Control. 1989. *Health, United States, 1988.* Hyattsville, MD.: DHHS Pub. No. (PHS) 89–1232.

Cook, P.J. 1981. "The effect of liquor taxes on drinking, cirrhosis, and auto accidents." In M.H. Moore and D.R. Gerstein, eds. *Alcohol and Public Policy: Beyond the Shadow of Prohibition.* Washington, DC: National Academy Press.

Durkheim, E. 1951. *Suicide: A Study in Sociology.* New York: Free Press.

Feldman, J. 1966. *The Dissemination of Health Information.* Chicago: Aldine.

Fuchs, V.R. 1974. *Who Shall Live: Health, Economics, and Social Choice.* New York: Basic Books.

Geertsen, R., M.R. Klauber, M. Rindflesh, et al. 1975. "A re-examination of Suchman's view on social factors in health care utilization." *Journal of Health and Social Behavior*, 16: 226–237.

Harris, J. 1982. "Increasing the federal excise tax on cigarettes." *Journal of Health Economics*, 1: 117-120.

Henry J. Kaiser Family Foundation. 1989. *Socioeconomic Status and Health.* Menlo Park, CA.

House, J., K.R. Landis, and D. Umberson, 1988. "Social relationships and health." *Science*, 241: 540–545.

Inkeles, A. 1983. *Exploring Individual Modernity.* New York: Columbia University Press.

Inkeles, A., and D.H. Smith. 1974. *Becoming Modern: Individual Change in Six Developing Countries.* Cambridge, MA: Harvard University Press.

Knowles, J.H. 1977. "The responsibility of the individual." *Daedalus*, 106: 57–80.

Lalonde, M. 1974. *A New Perspective on the Health of Canadians: A Working Document.* Government of Canada, Ottawa.

Leventhal, H. 1970. "Findings and theory in the study of fear communications." In L. Berkowitz, ed. *Advances in Experimental Psychology*, 5: 119–186. New York: Academic Press.

Levin, J.S., and H.Y. Vanderpool. 1987. "Is frequent religious attendance really conducive to better health?: Toward an epidemiology of religion." *Social Science and Medicine*, 24: 589–600.

Lewit, E.M., and D. Coate. 1982. "The potential for using excise taxes to reduce smoking." *Journal of Health Economics*, 1: 121–145.

Mechanic, D. 1963. "Religion, religiosity, and illness behavior: The special case of the Jews." *Human Organization*, 22: 444–453.

Mechanic, D. 1978. *Medical Sociology.* Second edition. New York: The Free Press.

Mechanic, D. 1979. "The stability of health and illness behavior: Results from a 16-year follow-up." *American Journal of Public Health,* 69: 1142–1145.

Mechanic, D. 1989. "Socio-economic status and health: An examination of underlying processes." In J.P. Bunker, D.S. Gomby and B.H. Kehrer, eds. *Pathways to Health: The Role of Social Factors.* Menlo Park, CA: Kaiser Family Foundation.

Mechanic, D., and P. Cleary. 1980. "Factors associated with the maintenance of positive health behavior." *Preventive Medicine,* 9: 805–814.

O'Dea, T.F. 1957. *The Mormons.* Chicago: University of Chicago Press.

Robertson, L.S. 1983. "Injury epidemiology and the reduction of harm." In D. Mechanic, ed. *Handbook of Health, Health Care, and the Health Professions.* New York: Free Press.

Spaeth, J.L. 1976. "Cognitive complexity: A dimension underlying the socioeconomic achievement process." In W.H. Sewell et al., eds. *Schooling and Achievement in American Society.* New York: Academic Press.

Suchman, E.A. 1964. "Sociomedical variations among ethnic groups." *American Journal of Sociology,* 70: 319–31.

Suchman, E.A. 1965. "Social patterns of illness and medical care." *Journal of Health and Social Behavior,* 6: 2–16.

United States Assistant Secretary for Health. 1979. *Healthy People: The Surgeon General's Report on Health Promotion and Disease Prevention.* Washington, DC: Government Printing Office.

Warner, K.E. 1985. "Cigarette advertising and media coverage of smoking and health." *New England Journal of Medicine,* 312: 384–388.

Zborowski, M., and E. Herzog. 1952. *Life is with People.* New York: International Universities Press.

Zuckerman, D., S.V. Kasl, and A.M. Ostfeld. 1984. "Psychosocial predictors of mortality among the elderly poor." *American Journal of Epidemiology,* 119:410–423.

18

Responding to Health Transitions:
From Research to Action

David E. Bell
Lincoln C. Chen

Introduction

In this chapter, we will argue that recent research on health transitions, some reported in this volume, can make a major contribution to practical policy decisions in the health field. Although still in the stage of intellectual development, the concept of health transitions, we believe, can inform health policy choices and can guide health actions in developing as well as industrialized countries. In this chapter, we will discuss the linkages between health transition research and action in three arenas of decision making: (1) improving health resource allocation and planning; (2) recognizing heretofore under-appreciated health problems; and (3) promoting non-medical interventions for health and development.

In many ways, the role of knowledge in achieving health improvements seems obvious. After all, much of this century's remarkable health progress worldwide can be attributed to the advancement of modern health knowledge. Yet, the connections between the production of knowledge, the mechanisms through which knowledge flows to action, and the impact of specific research endeavors remain poorly understood. One purpose of this chapter is to explore these questions with regard to recent social research on health transitions.

One framework for analyzing how research advances the health status of populations was proposed by the Commission on Health Research for Development (Commission 1990). Research may be hypothesized to advance health through four pathways: (1) improving the assessment of health problems, (2) facilitating health actions, (3) developing new technologies, and (4) advancing basic knowledge. Biomedical and clinical research based upon the natural sciences are primarily directed at the third and fourth pathways — developing new tools for the control of disease and advancing basic knowledge related to health. Social science research on health transitions ultimately may be hypothesized to contribute principally to the first two pathways — improving the recognition, assessment, and measurement of dynamic changes in health conditions, and strengthening the efficiency and effectiveness of health policies and actions. Like the natural sciences, however, the social sciences also contribute to the advancement of basic knowledge and to the development of new health technologies.

Concepts and Attributes

Before analyzing these linkages between health transition research and health action, several attributes of the health transition concept are worth underscoring because of their practical relevance. Concepts of health transitions, while as yet neither comprehensive nor definitive, build upon earlier transitional theories in demography and epidemiology. The "demographic transition" describes the transition of societies from high to low fertility and mortality regimes, with consequent changes in population growth, age distribution, and other demographic characteristics. The "epidemiologic transition" describes shifts in the patterns of causes of death that accompany the process of mortality decline and socio-economic development. Health transition research combines the two to describe and anticipate patterns of change in population numbers, age structure, and causes of death. In addition, the parameters of concern are extended to include morbidity and disability as key health outcomes, social and behavioral health problems in populations, and most importantly the changing demands upon and responses of health policy and the health care system — all as they accompany the process of socio-economic change.

As Frenk and colleagues make clear in their chapter in this volume, the patterns of health transitions are far from uniform within and between populations, and there are no guarantees of progression or even ultimate outcome. Moreover, there are important differences in the nature and timing of change in different countries and communities. Nevertheless, it is clear that there is sufficient regularity to permit a sensible structuring and use of empirical data across time and space, to understand what is happening to the health status of a population, to help to analyze the determinants and consequences of these health changes, and to address the changing issues of health policy and health action. Because of their concern for health policy and action, concepts of health transitions appear to be particularly valuable for informed policy analysis and decision making. Useful attributes in particular are:

Dynamism: Transition research *a priori* assumes rapid and continuing changes in the level, causes, structure, determinants, and consequences of health. Research on health transitions explicitly seeks to understand these changes, and through adopting assumptions, projects their trajectories into the future. Unlike most research that attempts to describe the present or understand the past, health transition research assumes dynamic changes over time, thereby enabling anticipatory actions to respond to evolving health challenges.

Equity: Transition research also explicitly considers the distribution of health across groups within and among national populations. Thus, not only aggregated averages are considered, but the distributive impact of the changing burdens of ill health within and across societies. Most importantly, the impact of alternative health care responses may be considered with regard to their differential impact across population subgroups.

Multidisciplinary: As illustrated in many chapters of this volume, health transition research is fundamentally multidisciplinary. The concept of health transitions thus provides a unifying analytical framework for bringing together the contribution of diverse disciplines — economics, anthropology, political sciences, and the health sciences. Indeed, some of the health transition hypotheses can only be examined with the participation of several disciplines. Transition research also relates health changes to other dimensions of socioeconomic development, considering health within the context of social, political, economic, and behavioral factors, in addition to health care.

For illustrative purposes, this chapter examines the contribution of transition research to three major areas of health policy and decision making. Before considering these areas, it would be useful to review our assumptions regarding the multiple levels of society at which knowledge translates into health action.

Individual and Community Levels: In recent years, there has been growing recognition of the importance of health action at individual and community levels. Health promotion and disease prevention, as well as health seeking behavior, are primarily individual and household actions. Community-level organizations, formal and informal, are means of organizing resources for advancing the health of communities. The chapters in this volume by Condran and Preston on health behavior, LeVine et al. on maternal education and competence, and Kunitz on cultural dimensions of health, illustrate how decisions at individual and community levels can improve the health status of populations.

National Level: Health action may also be improved by national policies that meet the health needs of a country efficiently, effectively, and equitably. Health transition research can describe the dynamic changes in a nation's health and the match between health needs and national health expenditures. Also, use of the health transition framework means that national health plans may be more readily related to and considered within overall national development plans.

International Level: Some health problems, both new and old, are transnational in scope and require regional or global action if an appropriate response is to be mounted. An example is the worldwide eradication of smallpox, which required global action. Health threats are increasingly assuming global dimensions; examples include AIDS, environmental assaults, and the upsurge of behavioral pathologies.

Illustrations

We have selected three arenas of health decision making within which to illustrate the potential applicability of health transition research for improving and informing the quality of health policy and action. These are: (1) improved resource allocation and health planning; (2) emerging challenges of behavioral health pathologies; and (3) implications of health for overall development policies.

Improving Resource Allocation: Health planning anticipates health needs and attempts to organize human action to maximize health advances within limited human and financial resources. Since resources are limited, especially so in developing countries, resource allocation in health requires tough implicit or explicit choices regarding the efficiency, effectiveness, and equity impact of health expenditures. Health transition research can clearly inform tough choices on expenditure options.

A common challenge, for example, in developing countries is to decide what share of health resources should be allocated to controlling the poverty-linked diseases of infection, malnutrition, and reproduction affecting mostly children and women, and what share should be concentrated on the growing proportion of chronic and degenerative diseases that mostly affect adults and the elderly. Health transition research can provide estimates of the numbers of persons who are and will be affected by these two types of conditions, and can show how the resources of a society are in fact being allocated (Evans, Hall, and Warford 1981). Such research can clarify central issues. Are resources being directed at the health problems that are most significant for today and the near future? Should health care investments be targeted at sophisticated urban-based hospitals or paraprofessional field workers serving rural populations?

Thus health transition research can provide a base of knowledge and analysis for rational decision making about resource allocations (National Academy of Sciences 1991). Moreover, such research can provide a common, easily-understood basis for communication among officials in health ministries and officials in ministries of finance and planning.

But we note immediately three major cautions. First, little is known about the costs and benefits of alternative health interventions. For example, Bobadilla et al. (1993) have noted that the Mexican government policy of requiring that all births take place in medical institutions is not feasible; it is not realistically possible for Mexico to provide enough hospital and clinic beds to carry out that policy. This is a useful negative conclusion stemming directly from health transition research. But to lead to improved resource allocations, this negative judgment needs to be followed by a substantial program of follow-up research to answer the question, in the circumstances of Mexico, what would be appropriate alternative arrangements for achieving safer births at feasible costs?

We believe it is fair to make the general claim that health transition research, by illuminating mismatches and disjunctions between the nature of a country's health problems and the allocation of its health resources, will open up a large and productive agenda of investigations into how to achieve more health gains by re-allocating and using more efficiently the limited health resources that are available.

A second caution is that knowledge and analysis are, by themselves, not enough as a basis for improved decisions. For example, health transition research may show trends in diseases, and identify the gains that may be made for each disease by applying the best available interventions efficiently. But arriving at policy choices will require another step. The fact that not all needs can be met requires value judgements about which needs are most important. As in other areas of social decision, rational analysis can clarify the issues and alternatives, but cannot eliminate the necessity of making value judgments.

Finally, our third caution is that policy decisions in the practical realm of action, whether on the grand scale of nations or the small scale of families and communities, reflect not only knowledge and values but also coalitions of interests and the distribution of power. No country's health situation illustrates this point more sharply than that of the United States, where the infant mortality rate for children of African-American descent stubbornly remains twice as high as the rate for children of European descent, even though the technical means of achieving greater equality are well-known. It is not knowledge and analysis that are lacking, but political and economic power exercised on behalf of the disadvantaged.

In his chapter in this volume, Reich describes how the interplay of political and economic interests, working through both governments and markets, affect health outcomes in the developing world, typically to the disadvantage of the poorer and less powerful groups in the population. He suggests that in addition to analyzing government interventions and market forces, "a third major analytic approach to health transitions in the Third World revolves around competitive political markets: the empowerment of relatively powerless groups in society, the assurance of fair and free elections, and the ability of groups to form coalitions and mobilize latent interests."

We believe Reich's prescription is correct, but incomplete. To his emphasis on the importance of broadening the political process, we would add another major element: the importance of deepening the base of knowledge and understanding. The policy process is not, in our experience, simply about politics. It is about blending politics with substance. To improve the health of poor and less powerful people does indeed require astute and energetic pursuit of political influence. But it also requires penetrating and accurate analysis of what their health problems are, how those problems are changing over time, and what the most effective means are of responding to them. This is the role of health transitions research.

In contrast, most health policy analysis and research concerned with developing countries over the past two decades have focussed on primary health care and the "child survival revolution." While this focus has produced many useful results, it has been concerned principally with health technology and health care delivery systems. It has not linked health centrally to other aspects of social policy, nor has it addressed the rapid pace of health change. A review of recent research experience concluded: "The economic crisis of the 1980s, the rapid changes in the age structure of the population, the rise in the prevalence of risk factors for communicable diseases, and the escalation of health care costs are demanding a comprehensive review of priorities and criteria to allocate resources in the health sector." (Jamison and Mosley 1991).

Emerging Social and Behavioral Pathologies: A second means through which health transition research can contribute to better health policy and action is in improving recognition of under-appreciated health problems. Several of the chapters in this volume, including those by Sugar et al., Kleinman, and Christakis et al., have spotlighted growing or emerging health problems that are of major importance but have been heretofore under-recognized. Examples are socio-behavioral pathologies, including addictive (drug and tobacco) substance abuse, sexual health (teenage pregnancy and sexually transmitted diseases, including HIV/AIDS), environmental health threats (air, water, and chemical pollution), and the epidemic of violence (intentional and unintentional) around the world.

Why have these health problems been under-recognized? One clear reason is that these behavioral problems are primarily linked to illness, sickness, and suffering; they are not well reflected by mortality statistics. Until recently, health policy analysis has been heavily focused on causes of death; little attention was given to morbidity. A second reason for neglect is that many of these health problems are socially stigmatized, and thus passed over in silence by both lay and professional communities. A third reason is that many of these behavioral problems may not have been thought of primarily as health issues. Drug addiction has been considered by many as resulting from moral weakness, and therefore beyond the province of the health professions. Automobile accidents have been thought of as the business of licensing authorities and traffic engineers, not of health policy analysts.

Health transition research focuses attention on health problems of these types, because it asks the questions: what is the array of illnesses and injuries from which people are actually suffering, how are the numbers of such problems changing over time, and how do these health outcomes relate to the socioeconomic transformations through which societies are progressing? To answer these questions, transition research must dig out data that have been comparatively neglected, and explore new research fields, such as the measurement of morbidity and the epidemiology of substance abuse. Moreover, health transition researchers must link up with other professional colleagues beyond their usual community of health specialists — such as traffic planners and community organizers.

Such linkages are important not only for measuring health problems more accurately and completely. Health transition research does not stop with measurement, but also includes questions about what is being done to respond to the problems identified, and what better possibilities might exist? Consequently, health analysts must team up with a wide variety of experts and researchers from other disciplines to develop policy responses in these neglected areas. Information dissemination through the mass media, for example, a tool typically not well understood by health researchers, may be crucial for dealing with behavioral pathologies. Structural change in the physical or social environment, for example, physical and regulatory management of automobile accidents or control of advertising and trade in addictive substances, may need to be included in a broad social response to health problems.

In summary, we argue that by throwing the spotlight on the actual nature of health problems in a society and the policies (or lack of policies) intended to deal with those problems, health transition research forces a recognition of major issues that have been widely neglected (Bobadilla and Possas 1992). The results are very valuable for persons in the health field seeking to deal with the reality of health circumstances and how they can be improved. We would hypothesize, moreover, that such research can provide a basis for easy communication and collaboration with persons in other disciplines who come to such problems from non-health backgrounds.

Advancing Health and Development: Health transition research, through its emphasis on the linkage between changes in health and changes in the broader socioeconomic sphere, has underscored the importance of many development factors beyond medical care that profoundly influence the health of populations. Examples in this volume are found in the chapters by Condran and Preston on the effects of personal hygiene and individual behavior on child mortality improvements in the United States; by LeVine et al. on the impact of maternal education on child health; and by Potter on the social mediation of mortality and fertility declines. Other obvious health and development linkages are the bi-directional relationships between economic poverty and health and between environmental pollution and health.

Recognizing the importance of such linkages can lead to significant practical consequences. One is the potential value of integrating health impact assessments into the consideration of broader development policies. Experience with impact assessments in other sectors has been mixed. Environmental impact assessments, for example, have sometimes achieved the desired effect of bringing to light potential environmental gains or losses from policies or projects in other fields. Sometimes, however, such assessments have turned out to be lengthy bureaucratic processes with no real effect. It may well be that project-by-project assessment would not be the most useful procedure for analyzing the potential health effects of investments in other fields. Perhaps more useful would be the development of specific sector-by-sector analyses of proposed activities and their potential health impact. It is recognized that the primary goal of these non-health sector investments is not health but rather education, economic growth, environmental preservation, employment, or other concerns. But nevertheless it seems reasonable to hypothesize that explicit data and analysis of health linkages should improve health consequences while retaining these other primary goals.

Important follow-up research related to recognition of the close linkages between changes in health and broader changes in socio-economic development also remains to be done. An example of such research in the developing world stems from the experience of the 1980s, during which most developing countries suffered crushing debt burdens and economic stagnation. Contrary to what might have been expected, however, while the health status of specific high risk groups may have been compromised, the remarkable secular decline of overall mortality seems to have continued (see Chapter 1). What explains this? Is there a threshold of household knowledge and practice above which people maintain their progress toward better health even though their economic circumstances have taken a turn for the worse?

Another example of needed research is from the industrialized world. There is a surprising degree of similarity in the outcomes of the health transitions thus far in countries as culturally different as Japan and Sweden. Presumably this reflects a set of common factors, such as high incomes by world standards, ample nutrition, good health care, and extensive education. But more than material factors must be involved. Even allowing for the pervasiveness of favorable material supports, it is astonishing to find so much similarity in health outcomes. In every industrialized country without exception, for example, fertility has declined to below replacement levels, a social and behavioral phenomenon of truly remarkable uniformity in a disparate world. Comparative analysis of such outcomes has hardly begun.

Conclusion

The concept of health transitions is a new and evolving construct, which has raised many questions not yet answered. One clear component of health progress, however, is health knowledge, which has contributed greatly to health advancement around the world. No other factor explains health progress, and continuing health disparities, better than the unequal distribution and application of health knowledge in diverse countries and communities. "More than natural resources, more than cheap labor, more than financial capital, knowledge is rapidly becoming the key factor of production...[To reduce the knowledge gap], developing countries need...to plug into the growing global knowledge base; to develop a complementary local knowledge base; to promote the rapid dissemination and effective use of knowledge; to invest in technical human capital and in institutional capital." (World Bank 1992).

As health transition research is in its early stages, many major questions remain unanswered. Among the most puzzling and important is: what happens to morbidity as mortality declines in health transitions? The usual assumption has been that morbidity and mortality shift in parallel ways, but recent research suggests uncertainty. A recent study using data from four industrialized countries (Japan, the United Kingdom, the United States and Hungary) suggests that "the epidemiologic transition...is a shift in the leading causes of death from acute to chronic diseases, and it is a shift from brief to protracted maladies" (Riley 1990). Whether this description will turn out to apply to developing countries remains to be seen.

Another unanswered question is: how are health changes related to developments in other sectors? Patterns of socioeconomic development presumably influence the determinants of disease in different ways, and no single health pattern can be expected to accompany diverse patterns of socioeconomic development. Until these questions are better explored, the concept of health transitions will be only partially useful.

There are some major health issues on which health transition research has thus far shed little light. One example is the question of the mix of public and private care. Publicly supported and operated health care systems have been the most usual government policy in developing countries. Recently, however, there has been very rapid growth of private, commercial medical systems. Questions about the relative efficiency and effectiveness of public and private systems need answers (Frenk et al. 1989).

Finally, it is important to underscore the fact that health transition research can lead to highly valuable knowledge and analysis, but cannot provide automatic decisions. Intellectual enlightenment can provide a basis for sound decision making, but decisions also involve values, interests, and power. Most of all, knowledge is only one component of what is called wisdom.

References

Bobadilla, J.L., J. Frenk, T. Frejka, R. Lozano, and C. Stern. 1993. "The epidemiologic transition and health priorities." In D.T. Jamison, W.H. Mosley, A.R. Measham, and J. Bobadilla, eds. *Disease Control Priorities in Developing Countries*. New York: Oxford University Press.

Bobadilla, J.L., and C.A. de Possas. 1992. "How the epidemiological transition affects health policy issues in three Latin American countries." World Bank Working Paper WPS 987, October.

Commission on Health Research for Development. 1990. *Health Research: Essential Link for Equity in Development*. New York: Oxford University Press.

Evans, J.R., K.L. Hall, and J. Warford. 1981. "Shattuck Lecture: Health care in the developing world: Problems of scarcity and choice." *New England Journal of Medicine*, 305:1117–1127.

Frenk J., J.L. Bobadilla, J. Sepúlveda, and M. Lopez-Cervantes. 1989. "Health transition in middle-income countries: New challenges for the organization of services." *Health Policy and Planning*, 4:29–39.

Jamison D., and W.H. Mosley. 1991. "Disease control priorities in developing countries: Health policy responses to epidemiological change." *American Journal of Public Health*, 81(1):15–22.

National Academy of Science Committee on Population. 1991. Workshop on Policy and Planning Implications of the Epidemiological Transition in Developing Countries. Washington, D.C. November 20–22.

Riley, J.C. 1990. "The risk of being sick: Mortality trends in four countries." *Population and Development Review*, 16:403–432.

World Bank. 1992. "Marshalling knowledge for development." *World Bank Policy Research Bulletin*, 3:2, March–April.

Index